RENAL AND UROLOGIC DISORDERS

URINARY INCONTINENCE

CAUSES, EPIDEMIOLOGY AND TREATMENT

RENAL AND UROLOGIC DISORDERS

Additional books in this series can be found on Nova's website under the Series tab.

Additional e-books in this series can be found on Nova's website under the e-book tab.

RENAL AND UROLOGIC DISORDERS

URINARY INCONTINENCE

CAUSES, EPIDEMIOLOGY AND TREATMENT

ERIC CHUNG
EDITOR

NOVA BIOMEDICAL

New York

For permission to use material from this book please contact us:
Telephone 631-231-7269; Fax 631-231-8175
Web Site: http://www.novapublishers.com

Library of Congress Cataloging-in-Publication Data

Library of Congress Control Number: 2013935078

ISBN: 978-1-62618-482-4

Published by Nova Science Publishers, Inc. † New York

Contents

Preface

Urinary incontinence can affect men and women of all age-groups with varying degrees of severity and bother. It is becoming an increasingly dominant health care issue with enormous economic burden and places considerable impact on the overall quality of life, impairing several areas with physical, social, emotional and sexual limitations. It is obvious that continuing efforts must be made to better understand the different types and management strategies of urinary incontinence.

An exact diagnosis is the first step necessary for adequate and optimal therapy. However, an in-depth understanding of the patho-physiology of voiding dysfunction is critical and paramount for the clinician to manage patients with urinary incontinence. In the last few years, there has been an explosion in literature regarding various patho-physiologies and treatments armamentarium for the different types of urinary incontinence. Therefore, we cannot guarantee that every bit of information is absolutely accurate and/or complete. The book chapters were written based on the current available literature and represented a state-of-review by the experts in this field. However reader should affirm that cited recommendations are reasonable still, by reading the original articles, checking other sources and recent literature before applying them.

In the process of preparing this book, the question arises as to whether another publication in the field of urinary incontinence is necessary or mandatory. The abundance of medical books and overwhelming amount of literature in this field rather predicates the contrary. However on reviewing the book chapters, I feel justified and believed that this book provides an important overview and emphasis was placed on detailing new concepts and emerging diagnostic techniques and therapies. I hope that medical students, residents and fellow physicians/surgeons as well as the general public will find this book useful and educational. I am extremely grateful to our contributing authors for their superb effort in completing this work. I would also like to take this opportunity to thank everyone associated with Nova Science Publishers for their support and patience.

Eric Chung, FRACS

In: Urinary Incontinence
Editor: Eric Chung
ISBN: 978-1-62618-482-4

Chapter 1

Pathophysiology of Urinary Incontinence and Pelvic Floor Dysfunctions in Females

Bernhard Liedl,* Martina Riegel and Oliver Markovsky
Pelvic Floor Centre Munich, Department of Urogenital Surgery,
Munich, Germany

Women can develop stress urinary incontinence, urgency, frequency and nocturia, voiding dysfunction, fecal incontinence, obstructed defecation in pelvic pain with increasing age. All these symptoms can often be present without any signs of urological, metabolic or cardiac disease.

More and more evidence evolve that pelvic floor defects, which present as vaginal descensus or prolapse at difference sites, are responsible for development of pelvic floor dysfunctions and symptoms. So, in this chapter, pathophysiology of symptoms and dysfunctions should be presented which can be derived from the pelvic floor itself.

1. Which Tissue Changes of the Pelvic Floor Are Responsible for Vaginal Descensus and Prolapse?

The pelvic floor consists of muscles and connective tissue. The muscles are the active components which contract and relax and are responsible for different functions. The connective tissue acts as structural support of the pelvic organs, which care for the special architecture within the pelvic floor. The muscles, which insert at the pelvic ligaments and fascias, have optimal insertion areas and the muscle lengths enable the muscles to work optimally. With afferent and efferent nerve fibers the pelvic floor is connected with the spine and brain. All functions are controlled by the nervous system.

* Tel: +49-89-92794-1522, Fax: +49-89-92794-1523, E-mail: liedl@bbzmuenchen.de.

Is Partial Denervation an Important Cause of Pelvic Floor Deterioration?

Smith et al. (1989) and Snooks et al. (1984) showed that partial denervation of the pelvic floor can occur after childbirth. Lin et al. (2009) performed vaginal distentions in female mice and observed reduced leak point pressure which was reversible within 20 days. They could observe repair of the sphincter muscle and reinnervation of the urethra. Pierce et al. (2008) performed bilateral levator ani neurectomy in monkeys. The monkeys developed atrophy of levator muscles, but no prolapse, suggesting that connective tissue components compensate for weakened pelvic floor muscles. Thus it seems that denervation is not an important factor for the development of vaginal prolapse.

Are Muscle Changes Responsible for Vaginal Prolapse?

Perucchini et al. (2002) observed a decrease in the number and density of urethral striated muscle fibers with age. Jundt et al. (2004) showed that with age and after vaginal childbirth, histomorphologic muscle cell changes can be observed but there was no significant difference between nullíparas, male and female incontinence or prolapse.

Muscle avulsions have been reported at the pelvic floor (Dietz and Lanzarone 2005, Dietz et al. 2007), but dislocation of insertion areas of muscle is more likely than muscle tears (Petros 2008).

Connective Tissue Changes as Important Cause of Prolapse and Pelvic Floor Dysfunctions

The connective tissue with elastic and collagen fibers and the extracellular matrix cares for structural support of the vagina and organs like the uterus, urethra, bladder and rectum (Abramovich 2009). It has been shown that connective tissue changes occur during pregnancy (Rechberger et al. 1988, Harkness 1959) and in patients with pelvic organ prolapse (Budatha et al. 2011, Connell et al. 2011).

Weakening of collagen cross bonding (Rechberger et al. 1988), added to dilatation of the vaginal canal at childbirth, can lead to over distension or rupture of connective tissue. The first vaginal birth is particularly associated with development of prolapse, whereas additional vaginal birth was not associated with a significant increase in the odds of prolapse (Quiroz et al. 2011).

Increasing age is characterized with loss of collagen, degeneration of the elastic fiber network and loss of hydration as a result of an imbalance between biosciences and degradation (Uitto and Bernstein 1988, Campisi et al. 1998).

Furthermore, there is a huge variability of tissue due to inborn variations (Dietz et al. 2004) and collagen associated disorders (Lammers et al. 2011, Campeau et al. 2011). Surgical procedures can reduce the structural support of the organs, especially those which cut or displace the uterosacral and cardinal ligaments during hysterectomy or which partially resect vaginal tissue or perineal body during colporrhaphy. Reay-Jones et al. (2003) could show that utero-sacral ligament resilience was significantly reduced in symptomatic utero-vaginal prolapse. There was a significant decrease in utero-sacral resilience with vaginal delivery, menopause and older age.

Kefer et al. (2009) performed a dissection of the pubo-urethral ligament in female rats and could observe that it caused long lasting urinary stress incontinence, which was comparable to those animals after dissection of the pudendal nerve. All these findings give high evidence that connective tissue changes are important for the development of vaginal prolapse and pelvic floor dysfunctions.

In 1993 Petros and Ulmsten stated: “Symptoms of stress, urge and abnormal emptying mainly derive, for different reasons, from laxity in the vagina or its supporting ligaments, a result of altered connective tissue”.

The connective tissue alterations, mainly looseness, can result in pelvic organ or vaginal prolapse. This alters the insertion points of the muscles which can be overstretched. At this point it is very important to understand that muscle action depends on muscle length.

After Gordon (figure 1) each muscle has a distinctive length in which the muscle force is optimal. If the muscle is shortened or over-lengthened the muscle force goes dramatically down towards zero.

This means that looseness of connective tissue can cause reduced muscle force. Reduced muscle force leads to reduced function. Thus the hypothetical statement of Petros and Ulmsten (1993) now has a pathophysiological basis.

2. Pelvic Floor Muscles and Important Connective Tissue Structures at the Pelvic Floor

Pelvic floor muscles and ligaments have immense importance for stress incontinence, micturition and anorectal functions. It was P. Petros who explained the directional muscle forces (Petros and Ulmsten 1993, Petros and Ulmsten 1997, Petros and Swash 2008).

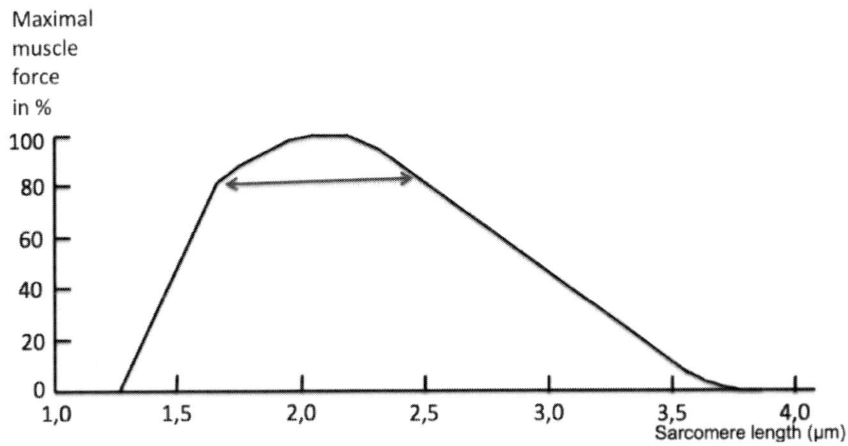

Figure 1. Maximal muscle force in relationship to muscle (sarcomere) length (modified after Gordon 1966). High muscle strength (>80% of maximal force) is exerted over a very short length (red line between arrows). Contractile strength falls rapidly with muscle lengthening and shortening, for example, due to lax connective tissue attachments.

Important Pelvic Floor Muscles

From a functional aspect, 4 major muscle groups of the pelvic floor have to be considered, which are able to move the vaginal wall and pelvic floor organs (Petros 2010):

a. The anterior and medial portions of the pubococcygeus muscle (PCM), arise on either side from the inner surface of the pubic bone and attach to the lateral walls of the distal vagina (Zacharin 1963, Petros und Ulmsten 1997, Corton 2009) This muscle portion, called pubococcygeus muscle (PCM) by Petros and Ulmsten (1993) and the pubovaginal muscle by Corton (2009) can pull the distal vagina forward to close the distal urethra during effort (coughing or straining). This muscle needs intact pubo-urethral ligaments for optimal action.
b. The levator plate in the upper layer runs horizontally into the posterior wall of the rectum, and thus plays a major role in any backward movement of this organ. This muscle needs intact pubourethral and uterosacral ligaments and an intact perineal body to optimize its various actions.
c. The conjoint longitudinal muscle of the anus (LMA) is a striated muscle which constitutes the middle layer. It is vertically oriented, creates the downward force for bladder neck closure during effort and stretches open the outflow tract during micturition. It takes fibers superiorly from the levator plate (LP), lateral part of the pubococcygeus muscle and puborectalis. It is well anchored by extra-anal sphincter (Courtney 1950). This muscle needs intact uterosacral ligaments for optimal action.
d. The puborectalis muscle (PRM) originates just medially to PCM and traverses all three muscle layers. It is orientated vertically and runs forward medially below PCM. It is closely applied to the lateral walls of the rectum and surrounds them (Courtney 1950).

The lower layer of pelvic floor muscles is an important anchoring layer. It consists of perineal membranes and component muscles - bulbocavernosus, ischiocavernosus and the deep and superficial transverse perinei muscles. The deep transverse perinei muscle anchors the upper part of the perineal body to the descending ramus. It is a strong muscle and it stabilizes the perineal body laterally. The external anal sphincter acts as a tensor of the perineal body and represents the principal insertion point of the LMA.

The bulbocavernosus muscle stretches and anchors the distal part of the urethra. The ischiocavernosus muscle helps stabilize the perineal membrane and may act to stretch the external urethral meatus laterally via its effect of the bulbocavernosus. Between the extra-anal sphincter and the coccyx lies the postanal plate, a tendinous structure which also contains striated muscles inserting into the extra-anal sphincter (Petros 2010). The striated rhabdosphincter of the urethra surrounds the urethra in the middle third of its length for approximately 1,5 cm (Oelrich 1983).

Important Connective Tissue Structures at the Pelvic Floor (Figure 2)

After Petros (2010) 9 sites of connective tissue can be defined. With regard to its function they can be divided into three zones: anterior, middle and posterior zone.

a. The anterior zone, which reaches from the external meatus of the urethra to the bladder neck, embraces three important structures: The extra urethral ligament runs from the pubis anteriorly to the meatus urethrae anterior to the perineal membrane. The pubourethral ligament, a ligament with key relevance for stress urinary continence, originates from the lower end of the posterior surface of the pubic symphysis and descends like a fan to insert into the pubococcygeus muscle and lateral part of the mid urethra (Zacharin 1963, Petros 1998). The suburethral vagina acts as a hammock for the urethra. The antero-medial portion of the pubococcygeus muscles is attached laterally on each side of the hammock.
b. In the middle zone, which reaches from the bladder neck to the cervix, three further structures are important: The arcus tendineus fascia pelvis (ATFP) are horizontal ligaments which arise just superior to the pubourethral ligaments at the pubic symphysis and insert into the ischial spine. The vagina is suspended from the ATFP by its fascia, much like a sheet slung across two washing lines (Nichols 1989) The cardinal ligaments are attached to the cervical ring and pubocervical fascia and extend laterally towards and above the ischial spine. The cervical ring surrounds the cervix and acts as an attachment point for the cardinal and uterosacral ligaments as well as the pubocervical and rectovaginal fascia. It consists mainly of collagen. The "pubocervical fascia" – a term still used by surgeons - stretches from the lateral sulci of the vagina to the anterior part of the cervical ring, it is a vaginal muscularis and fibromuscular wall (Corton 2009).
c. In the posterior zone, which reaches from the cervix to the anal canal, the following 3 structures are relevant. The uterosacral ligaments arise from the sacral vertebrate S2,3,4 and attach to the cervical ring posteriorly. It is an effective insertion point of the downward muscle force, the longitudinal muscle of the anus (LMA). The rectovaginal fascia extends as a sheet between the lateral rectal pillars, from the perineal body below to the levator plate above. It is attached to the uterosacral ligaments (USL) and the fascia surrounding the cervix. The perineal body lies between the distal third of the posterior vaginal wall and the anus below the pelvic floor. It is 3-4 cm long. According to DeLancey (1999), it is formed primarily by the midline connection between the halves of the perineal membrane. It is the insertion point of bulbocavernosus muscle and the deep and superficial transverse perinei muscles.

3. Pathophysiology of Pelvic Floor Dysfunctions in the Female

a. Stress Urinary Continence and Incontinence

During stress (coughing or straining) the intraurethral pressure rises in normal patients. The rise in pressure within the urethra precedes the rise in pressure in the bladder by 160-240 milliseconds (Enhorning 1961, Constantinou and Govan 1982, van der Kooi et al. 1984, Pieber et al. 1998). This means that the increased pressure within the urethra during stress must be due to an active muscle contraction and cannot be a passive transmission of the abdominal pressure.

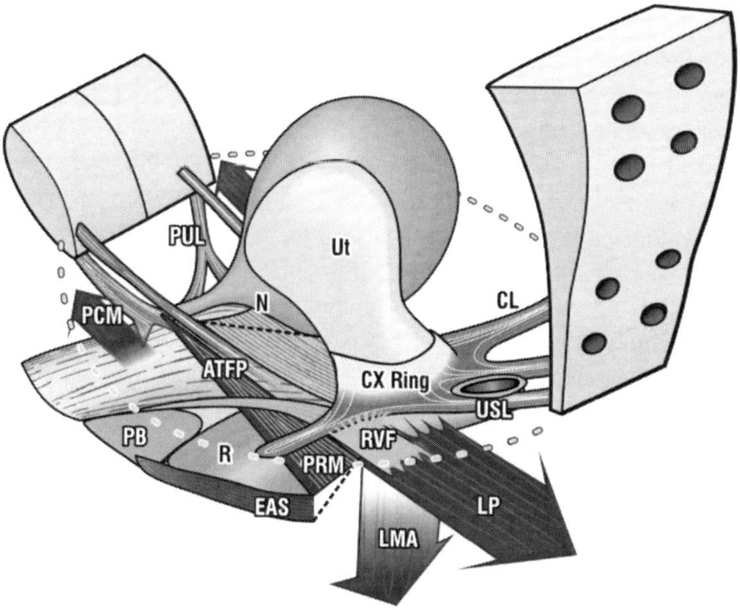

PCM: pubococcygeus muscle, LP: levator plate, LMA: longitudinal muscle of the anus
PRM: puborectalis muscle, EAS: extra anal sphincter
PUL: pubourethral ligament, ATFP: Arcus tendineus fasciae pelvis, CL: cardinal ligament
CX-Ring: cervical ring, USL: uterosacral ligament, RVF: rectovaginal fascia
PB: perineal body, B: bladder, Ut: uterus, R: rectum
N: stretch receptor at bladder base

Figure 2. Important muscles and connective tissue structures at the pelvic floor (from P. Petros 2010, by permission).

In addition to the contraction of the rhabdosphincter at midurethra, the PCM pulls the distal vagina forward to close the distal urethra. Furthermore, the bladder and posterior vaginal wall is pulled backwards (by levator plate) and downwards (by LMA). With intact pubourethral ligaments the urethra is stretched and angulated to "kink" the proximal urethra (Petros and Ulmsten 1995). This action is an important closing mechanism, which, as known, helps many patients maintain continence after excision of the distal urethra.

The Integral Theory (1990, 1993) states that "stress urinary incontinence...derives mainly from laxity in the vagina or its supporting ligaments, a result of altered collagen/elastin". A hypermobile urethra results from loose connective tissue. In stress situations, abdominal forces stretch loose tissues in the anterior zone (pubourethral ligament, extraurethral ligament, hammock), leading to overlengthening of the rhabdosphincter.

According to Gordon`s relation between muscle length and muscle force (figure 1), muscle overlengthening causes reduced muscle force and reduced intraurethral pressure, the patient is stress incontinent. Overstretched connective tissue also leads to an increased radius within the rhabdosphincter and the urethra. According to Laplace's law, the pressure within the urethra correlates inversely to the radius within the rhabdosphincter. In loose connective tissue, the pressure within the urethra thus diminishes in line with the increasing radius.

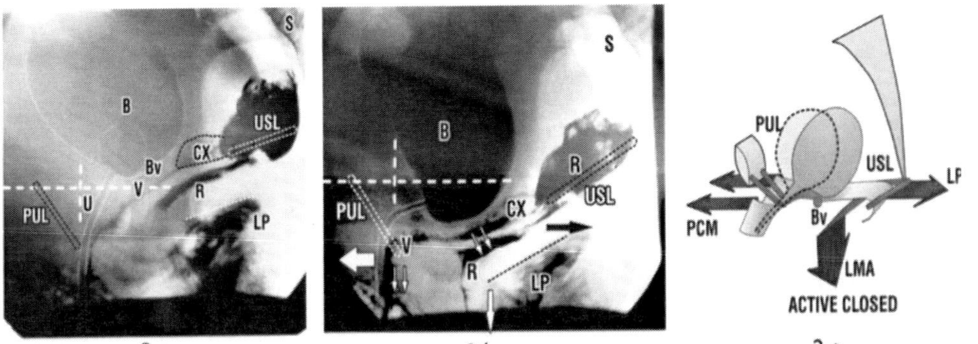

3 a 3 b 3 c

(B = bladder; U = urethra; V = vagina; CX = cervix; R = rectum; PUL = pubourethral ligament; Bv = attachment of bladder base to vagina; LMA = conjoint longitudinal muscle of the anus; LP = levator plate; USL = uterosacral ligament (from P Petros 2010, by permission).

3a) lateral X-ray in resting position, sitting

3b) lateral X-ray during straining, same patient, shows forward movement of distal vagina and urethra and backward/downward rotation of proximal vagina and urethra around the pubourethral ligament (PUL) at the midurethral point

3c) Muscle actions during effort – schematic view. PCM pulls the distal vagina forwards to close the distal urethra! LP/LMA stretch the proximal vagina and urethra backwards/downwards to close off the proximal urethra.

Figure 3. Movements of bladder and urethra during effort.

The Hagen-Poiseuille`s law is also helpful in describing continence. The resistance to flow within the urethra in stress situations correlates directly to the length of the urethra and indirectly to the radius within the urethra in the 4th power (Bush et al. 1997). Stress in patients with loose connective tissue will open the urethra. The stress flow then correlates to the radius of the urethra in 4th power.

In other words, loose connective tissue can lead to reduced muscle force by overstretching the muscle, reduced urethral pressure by increasing the radius within the rhabdosphincter, and reduced resistance to flow by widening the urethral radius.

These correlations have a major impact on interpretation of urodynamic results and should be considered in the future. The missing predictive value of urodynamics on outcome after midurethral sling surgery (Houwert RM 2009, Palma and Hermann 2007) can be explained by the concept of loose connective tissue in stress urinary incontinence in women.

Petros has been developing the midurethral sling since 1986 based on research on the laxities of the vagina and supporting ligaments and loose connective tissue. (Petros and Ulmsten 1990, 1993, Petros 2010)

b. Normal Micturition and Abnormal Emptying of the Bladder

Micturition is another complex mechanism, which is influenced by the pelvic floor. Not only sphincter relaxation and detrusor contraction have to be taken into consideration; EMG-measurements in the posterior fornix have demonstrated commencement of muscle contraction prior to commencement of voiding (Petros 2010).

Radiologically, it was shown that the anterior vaginal wall is stretched and moved backward and downward during micturition (Figures 4a and 4b). The bladder also moves backward and downward in the proximal urethra funnels. This can only be explained by active muscle contractions of the levator plate (LP) and longitudinal muscle of the anus (LMA).

Relaxation of the forward force (PCM) and relaxation of urethral sphincter allows the backward and downward forces to open up the outflow tract (figure 4.c).

The posterior muscles (LP and LMA) only contribute in opening the bladder neck and urethra when the connective tissue architecture and its insertion points are intact in a way that they can pull normally (see figure 1). If the uterosacral ligaments are loose (insertion points of the LMA) or a cystocele is present the posterior forces cannot pull normally, the muscles are shortened or overstretched and have reduced force.

Even a minor degree of prolapse can be the cause of defective micturition. Kinking of the urethra by prolapse can also be a cause of abnormal emptying of the bladder.

A location of the tape too high up the bladder neck, a proximal urethra as well as anterior fixation of the bladder neck after colposuspension can disturb funnelling of the urethra.

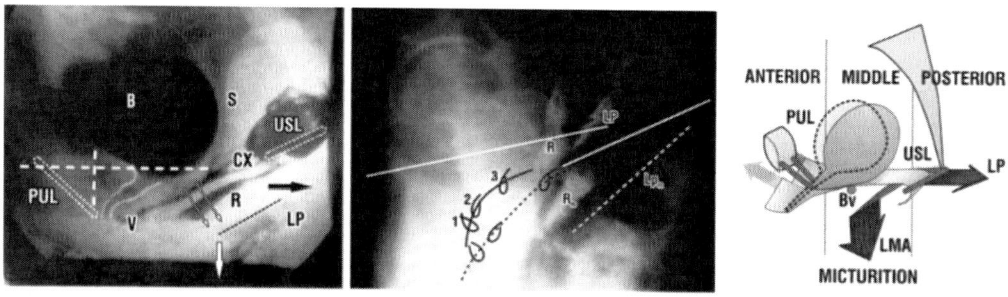

4a 4b 4c

a) Lateral x-ray, same patient as fig. 3. During micturition, the bladder and vagina move backwards and downward, opening out the posterior urethral wall.
b) Superimposed lateral x-rays. At rest (unbroken lines) and micturition (broken lines) vascular clips placed at midurethra “1”, bladder neck “2” and bladder base “3”.
c) Muscle actions during micturition. PCM relaxes. This allows the posterior muscle forces LP/LMA (red arrows) to stretch the vagina and posterior urethral wall backwards/downwards to open out the outflow tract. Same labelling as fig. 3. (From P. Petros 2010, by permission)

Figure 4. Normal micturition.

c. Stability at the Bladder Base by a Tensioned Vaginal Wall, Urgency and Frequency

In their first publication of the “Integral theory” Petros and Ulmsten (1990) stated that “symptoms of stress and urge derive mainly from laxity in the vagina or its supporting ligaments, a result of altered collagen/elastin”. Following their publication, evidence was increasingly found that supported their claim that a correlation between the prolapse and an overactive bladder exists (de Boer et al. 2010).

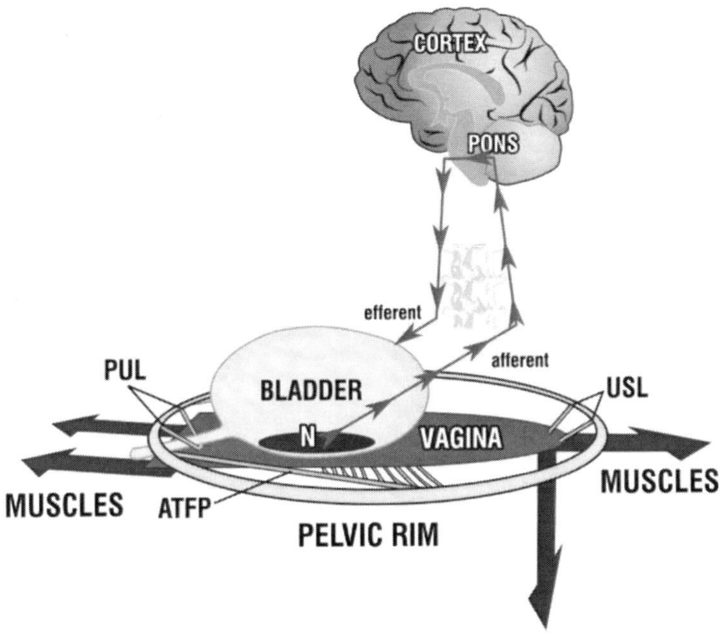

Figure 5. Stability at the bladder base by a tensioned vaginal wall. "Trampoline analogy" (from P. Petros 2010, by permission).

Figure 2.a, 2.b and Figure 5. show that the bladder lies anterocranial (at rest) or cranial (during effort) on the vaginal wall. With effort the posterior vaginal wall is orientated horizontally and the bladder lies on this part of tensioned vaginal wall (Figure 2b), which acts as a "trampoline". The vagina is attached to the pelvic rim by the uterosacral ligaments posteriorly, the arcus tendineus and the cardinal ligaments laterally as well as the pubourethral ligament anteriorly.

Anterior and posterior muscle forces (red arrows in Figure 5) add to tension in the vaginal wall. While the slow twitch fibers are active when at rest, the fast twitch fibers are active during effort. At the bladder base stretch receptors are present which are connected by afferent nerves to the cortex (Wyndaele et al. 2008, Everaerts et al. 2008, Petros and Ulmsten 1990). Efferent nerves can activate the pelvic floor musculature (Figure 5).

Petros and Ulmsten (1993) postulated that urgency could lead to a premature activation of the micturition reflex. A lax vagina at the anterior, middle or posterior zone reduces the tension of the vagina below the bladder base. The stretch receptors can be activated by afferent nerves. The cortex gets the information of full bladder and this creates the sensation urge. Prematurely the micturition reflex can be activated and even urge incontinence can occur.

d. Nocturia

Some patients with vaginal vault or uterine prolapse – even if of a minor degree – complain about nocturia. Figure 6. explains the mechanism that leads to nocturia. When the patient is asleep, the force of gravity pulls down the bladder base.

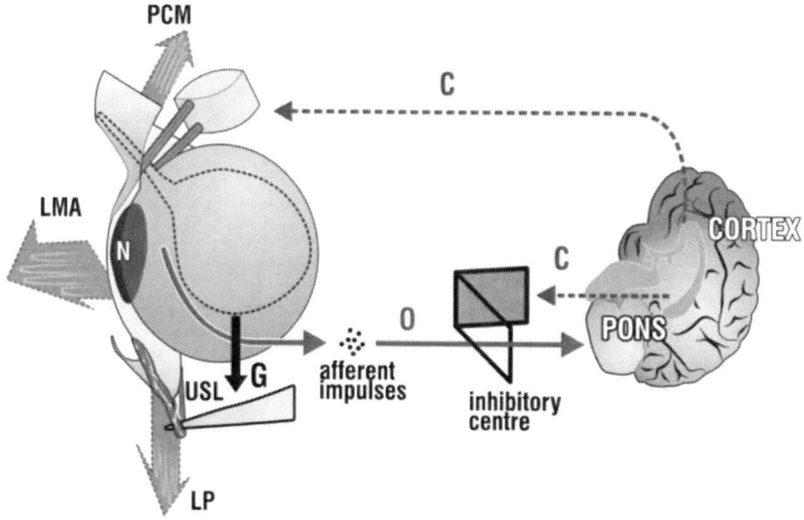

Figure 6. Mechanism of nocturia - schematic view- patient asleep.

Normally, with firm uterosacral ligaments, the bladder is held high (dotted line in Figure 6). When the patient is asleep and the uterosacral ligaments are loose, the pelvic floor muscles are relaxed, the bladder descends posteriorly, the bladder base is stretched and the stretch receptors "N" are stimulated. The pelvic muscles (arrows) are relaxed. As the bladder fills, it is pulled downwards by the force of gravity 'G'. In the normal patient, bladder descent is limited by the uterosacral ligaments "USL". If "USLs" are loose, the bladder descends more, the stretch receptors "N" are stimulated, and the micturition reflex is activated at a low bladder volume, "nocturia". (from P. Petros 2010, by permission)

e. Anorectal Function, Fecal Incontinence and Obstructive Defecation

The anecdotal observation that midurethral slings and repair of loose uterosacral ligaments can cure fecal incontinence has led Petros and Swash (2008) to establish a new theory of anorectal function. A new complex musculo-elastic sphincter mechanism was detected. Its mechanism is similar to that of bladder neck closure. Directional muscle forces stretch the rectum backwards and downwards around an anus firmly anchored by the puborectalis muscle. Anorectal closure occurs when the backward muscle forces of LP and LMA stretch the rectum around the anus, which is anchored by PRM-contraction. Upon comparing Figure 3b with Figure 3a, the rectum above the anal canal has been markedly angulated (and closed) by muscle actions during effort. Upon relaxation of PRM, LP/LMA vectors open out the anal canal for evacuation (broken lines, Figure 2). Fecal incontinence can occur when connective tissue at the anterior zone is loose. Then the insertion points of the puborectalis muscle are dislocated and the muscle is weak. Furthermore, the anterior insertion points of the levator plate are loose and the muscle is weak and the anorectal closure is also weak. When connective tissue at the posterior zone is loose, the muscles also cannot act optimally and fecal incontinence can occur. Lax uterosacral ligaments can explain rectal intussusception and obstructive defecation. The levator plate cannot tension the rectovaginal fascia. The perineal body is an important anchoring point and, if loose, it can contribute to fecal incontinence and obstructive defecation (Petros 2010, Abendstein and Petros 2008).

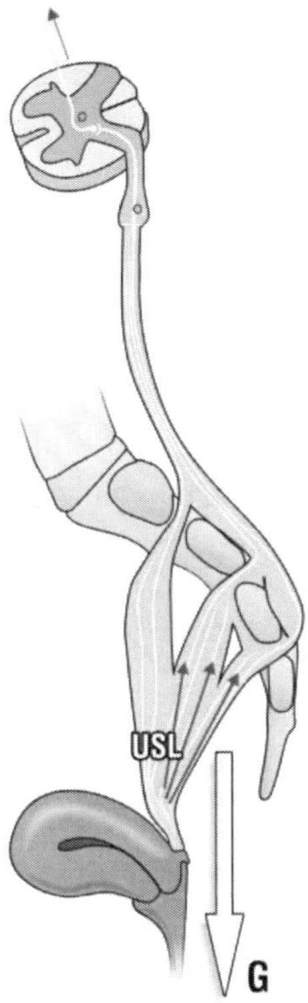

Figure 7. Pelvic pain caused by loose uterosacral ligaments (USL). Especially in the standing position, the uterus or vaginal vault prolapses under the influence of gravity 'G'. The unmyelinated nerves which run along the USLs are stretched by 'G', causing pain (from P Petros 2010, by permission).

f. Pelvic Pain

Some patients with vaginal vault prolapse or uterus prolapse report pelvic pain, a low abdominal dragging pain which occurs mainly in an upright position and is generally relieved in a lying position. This pain may be associated with vulvodynia. Both types of pain have been temporarily relieved by injection of local anaesthetic into the uterosacral ligaments (Bornstein et al. 2005, Petros et al. 2004), supporting the hypothesis that this pain is a referred pain arising from the inability of lax uterosacral ligaments to support the nerves running along the ligament. These nerves are stretched by gravity or during intercourse to cause pain. This pain is almost invariably associated with other symptoms deriving from posterior zone laxity, Figure 8. In a recent study, restoration of uterosacral ligament tension using a posterior tensioned sling showed improvement in posterior zone symptoms as follows: nocturia >2/night 83%; urge-incontinence >2/day 78%; abnormal emptying, 73% ; pelvic pain, 86% fecal incontinence, 87% (Petros PEP, Richardson PA, (2010).

g. The Association of Pelvic Floor Dysfunctions and Different Zones of Connective Tissue Looseness at the Pelvic Floor (Figure 8)

The three zones of connective tissue looseness (see above) are associated with different symptoms. Petros (2010) developed the diagnostic algorithm (Figure 8) by considering the pathophysiology of dysfunctions and through practical experiences with the patients that had different forms and degrees of descensus/prolapse of the vaginal wall. Many symptoms are associated with these different forms of descensus/prolapse: stress urinary incontinence, abnormal emptying of the bladder, urgency and frequency, nocturia, fecal incontinence, obstructed defecation and pelvic pain.

It summarizes the relationship between structural damage (prolapse) in the three zones and the respective functions (symptoms). The size of the bar gives an approximate indication of the prevalence (probability) of the symptoms. Stress urinary incontinence is mainly caused by anterior defects. Defects in the posterior zone cause different dysfunctions like abnormal emptying of the bladder, frequency and urgency, nocturia, fecal incontinence, obstructed defecation, pelvic pain known as the "posterior fornix syndrome" (Petros and Ulmsten 1993).

Anterior zone (meatus urethrae to bladder neck)	**Middle zone** (Bladder neck to cervix)	**Posterior zone** (cervix to anal canal)
Extraurethral ligament (EUL) Pubourethral ligament (PUL) Hammock	Pubocervical fascia (PCF) Arcus tendineus fasciae pelvis (ATFP) Cervical ring (CXring)	Uterosacral ligament (USL) Rectovaginal Fascia (RVF) Perineal body (PB)
Hypermobile urethra	Cystocele	Enterocele Uterine prolapse Vaginal vault prolapse rectocele

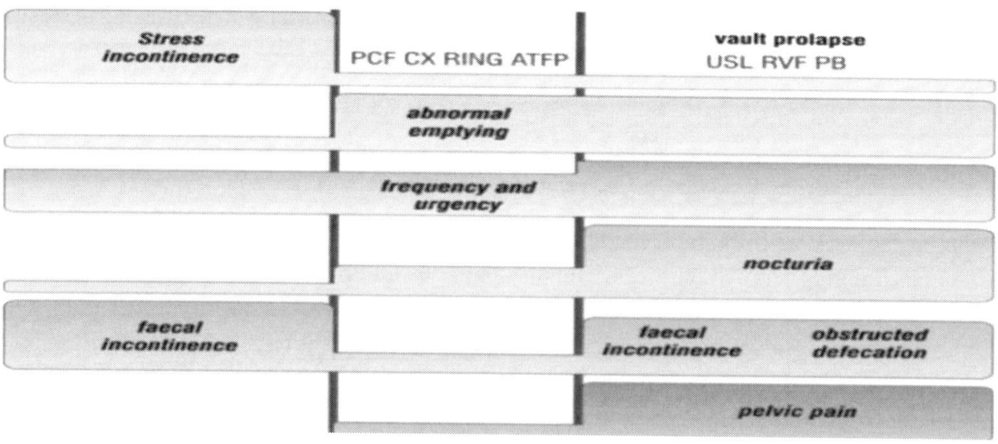

Figure 8. Diagnostic algorithm. Pictorially elaborates the association between connective tissue looseness at different zones, their relationship with specific prolapses and symptoms, and how repair of the ligaments/fascia in each zone may cure or improve both the prolapse and the symptom(s). The size of the bars gives an approximate indication of the prevalence (probability) of the symptom (modified after Petros 2010, by permission).

Nocturia and pelvic pain are specific for posterior zone. Cystoceles are mainly associated with symptoms of abnormal emptying of the bladder and frequency and urgency. The significance of the association between zones and the respective symptoms has been shown by Hunt et al. (2000) using Bayesian networks and decision trees.

h. Tethered Vagina Syndrome

All defects in the three zones in figure 8 represent looseness of connective tissues. After previous surgery at the bladder neck of the anterior vaginal wall the opposite situation can occur. Normally the vaginal tissue below the bladder neck can be stretched by the backward and forward muscle actions (figure 3c, 5). This area is called the "zone of critical elasticity" (Petros 2010).

Scars in this area (after colporhaphy) contracts and can tether the more powerful backward forces to the weaker forward forces. Especially when the patient gets out of bed in the morning, uncontrolled urine leakage occurs as soon as the patient`s foot touches the floor.

The more powerful backward force opens the bladder neck. When urine enters the proximal urethra the mictiurition reflex is activated and the patient loses a lot of urine.

4. Consequences for Surgical Treatments

The detection that connective tissue alterations are important factors in the development of pelvic organ prolapse and pelvic floor dysfunctions led to important surgical developments. "Restoration of form (structure) leads to restoration of function" (Petros 2010). This principle directly applies Gordon`s law: exact restoration of the insertion areas of the pelvic floor muscles allows the muscles to act optimally. The function – even if complex – should thus have the optimal chance to recover.

When repair of weak tissues by conventional techniques such as suturing is not possible (for example, repair of a loose pubourethral ligament for cure of stress urinary incontinence), or the recurrence rate is too high, the use of alloplastic materials is an option. Because normal function requires a neurologically complex co-ordination of smooth and striated muscle, any surgery must mimic the natural anatomy as closely as possible if it is to restore function.

The axis of the posterior vagina is nearly horizontal because the uterosacral ligaments insert dorsally between S2-4. Elevation of the vagina to the promontorium is too high, while fixation of the vagina to the sacrospinous ligament is too caudal.

It is a surgical compromise to use these areas for easy and safe fixation but the site of the uterosacral ligament remains the optimal site for its reconstruction. The uterus needs to be conserved whenever possible. It is the central anchoring point for the posterior ligaments, the rectovaginal fascia and the pubocervical fascia. The descending branch of the uterine artery is a major blood supply for these structures, and should be conserved where possible even if subtotal hysterectomy is performed.

It is important to understand that tissue structure is often displaced laterally (e. g. cardinal ligaments, uterosacral ligaments, rectovaginal fascia, pubocervical fascia, hammock, perineal body). Surgical techniques, which bring the tissues together in the midline or bridge it with alloplastic tapes at the anatomically correct place, should be applied and further developed. Simply applying a large mesh provides a barrier to the prolapse and seem not to restore the damaged anatomy or function efficiently.

Instead, such meshes have the tendency to shrink and reduce elasticity of tissues. Furthermore, they obliterate the organ spaces. This may cause pain, dyspareunia, and erosions and may negatively affect the dissection required in cases where the patient develops rectal or bladder carcinoma.

The use of alloplastic materials has to be reduced to the necessary amount and their application sites carefully considered. The conventional techniques have to be evaluated following these fundamental principles.

In order to minimize pain, surgery to the perineal skin and tension when suturing the vagina should be avoided. Vaginal excision should be avoided even in patients with large bulging prolapse. After repair of underlying ligamentous fascial defects, the vaginal wall contracts and will be more elastic than after excision. Tightness or elevation of the bladder neck area of the vagina as well as indentation of the urethra with a midurethral sling should be avoided in order to avoid urinary retention. .

Looking at the bladder neck closure mechanism the midurethral tape should be positioned along the pubourethral ligament, which inserts retropubically. This seems especially important in patients with severe stress urinary incontinence or recurrence.

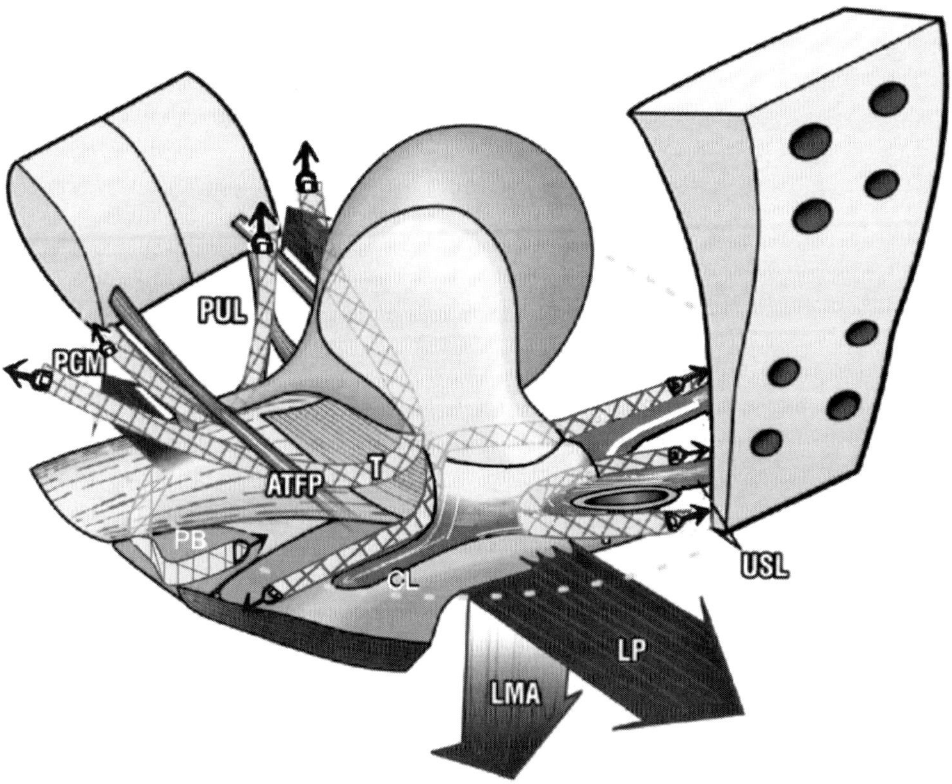

Figure 9. The use of tensioned tapes to strengthen the principal connective tissue structures which support the vagina, bladder, uterus and rectum: pubourethral ligament (PUL), arcus tendineus fascia pelvis (ATFP), cardinal ligament (CL), uterosacral ligaments (USL), perineal body (PB). These 5 structures are the effective insertion points of the directional muscle forces (arrows) which support the organs, and which open and close the urethra and anorectum, anteromedial part of the pubococcygeus muscle (PCM), levator plate (LP) and longitudinal muscle of the anus (LMA) (from P. Petros 2010, by permission).

In order to fix such loose ligaments Petros et al. (1990) have introduced alloplastic material for planned formation of an artificial ligament. From this basic research, new surgical techniques have been developed, such as tapes for midurethral slings (TFT, TOT) and for repair of other pelvic floor ligaments (Petros 2010). The new developments and the recent focus on connective tissues are important, not least because looseness of tissues can be repaired surgically. New techniques using mini tissue anchors have been developed to fix connective tissue at the main sites of structural support: pubourethral ligament (PUL), arcus tendineus fasciae pelvis (ATFP), cardinal ligament (CL), uterosacral ligament (USL), perineal body (PB) (figure 9).

Petros and Ulmsten (1993) stated early that looseness or laxity of the vagina and its supporting ligaments could cause stress incontinence as well as urge. Since then the theory has been expanded to include other symptoms such as pelvic pain, voiding dysfunction and more recently, fecal incontinence and constipation (Petros and Swash 2008).

We now recognise that symptoms of different degrees and combinations can be present in different forms and degrees of prolapse, as seen in figure 8. Because of the peripheral neurological origin of some symptoms such as urgency and pain, major symptoms may occur with only minimal prolapse. Therefore the new anatomical and functional findings, as summarized in figure 8, have to be considered in modern pelvic floor surgery.

References

Abramowitch SD (2009) Tissue mechanics, animal models, and pelvic organ prolapse: A review. Eur J Obstet Gynecol Reprod Biol 144S: S146-S156

Abendstein B, Petros PE, Richardson PA, Goeschen K, Dodero D (2008) The surgical anatomy of rectocele and anterior rectal wall intussusception. Int. *Urogynecol. J. Pelvic. Floor Dysfunct.* 19: 705-710.

Budatha M, Roshanrava S, Zheng Q, Weislander c, Chapman SL, Davis EC, Starcher B, Word A, Yanagisawa H (2011) Extracellular matrix proteases contribute to progression of pelvic organ prolapse in mice and humans. *J. Clin. Invest.* 121:2048-2059.

Bush MB, Petros P, Barrett-Lennard BR (1997) On the flow through the human urethra. *Biomechanics* 30: 967-969.

Campisi J (1998) The Role of Cellular Senescence in Skin Aging. *Journal of Investigative Dermatology Symposium Proceedings* 3:1-5.

Campeau L, Gorbachinsky I, Badlani GH, Andersson KE (2011) Pelvic floor disorders: linking genetic risk factors to biochemical changes. *BJU Int.* Aug 26 (Epub ahead of print).

Connell KA (2011) Elastogenesis in the Vaginal Wall and Pelvic-Organ Prolapse. *N. Engl. J. Med.* 364 (24):2356-2358.

Constantinou CE, Govan DE (1982) Spatial distribution and timing of transmitted and reflex generated urethral pressures in healthy women. *J. Urol.* 127:964-969.

Corton MM (2009) Anatomy of Pelvic Floor Dysfunction. *Obstet. Gynecol. Clin. N. Am.* 36:401-319.

Courtney H (1950) Anatomy of the pelvic diaphragm and ano-rectal musculature related to sphincter preservation in ano-rectal surgery. *American Journal Surgery* 79:155-173.

De Boer TA, Salvatore S, Cardozo L, Chapple C et al. (2010) Pelvic Organ Prolapse and Overactive Bladder. *Neurourol. Urodynam.* 29: 30-39.

DeLancey JOL (1999) Structural anatomy of the posterior pelvic compartment as it relates to rectocele. *Am. J. Obstet. Gynecol.* 180:815-823.

Dietz HP, Eldridge A, Grace M, Clarke B (2004) Pelvic organ descent in young null gravid women. *Am. J. Obstet. Gynecol.* 191:95-99.

Dietz HP, Lanzarone V (2005) Levator trauma after vaginal delivery. *Obstet. Gynecol.* 106:707-712

Dietz HP, Gillespie AV, Phadke P (2007) Avulsion of the pubovisceral muscle associated with large vaginal tear after normal delivery at term. *Aus. N. Z. J. Obstet. Gynaecol.* 47: 341-344.

Enhorning G. Simultaneous recording of intravesical and intraurethral pressure. *Acta Chir. Scandinavica*, (1961), (Supplement) Vol. 27:61-68.

Everaerts W, Gevaert T, Nilius B, De Ridder D (2008) On the origin of bladder sensing: Tr(i)ps in urology. *Neururol. Urodyn.* 27:264-273.

Gordon AM, Huxley AF, Julian FJ (1966) The variation in isometric tension with sarcomere length in vertebrate muscle fibers. *J. Physiol.* 184: 170-192.

Harkness MLR, Harkness RD (1959) Changes in the Physical Properties of the Uterine Cervix of the Rat during Pregnancy. *J. Physiol.* 148:524-547.

Houwert RM, Venema PL, Aquarius AE, Bruinse HW, Kil PJ, Vervest HA (2009) Predictive value of urodynamics on outcome after midurethral sling surgery for female stress urinary incontinence. *Am. J. Obstet. Gynecol.* 200: 649.e1-649.e12.

Hunt M, von Konsky B, Venkatesh S, Petros P (2000) Bayesian Networks and Decision Trees in the Diagnosis of Female Urinary Incontinence. Engineering in Medicine and Biology Society 2000. *Proceedings of the 22nd Annual International Conference of the IEEE.* Volume 1 Issue: 551-554.

Huisman AB. Aspects on the anatomy of the female urethra with special relation to urinary continence. *Contr. Gynecol. and Obstets.* (1983), Karger Basel, Vol.10:1-31.

Hvid LG, Ortenblad N, Aagaard P, Kjaer M, Suetta C (2011) Effects of aging on single muscle fibre contractile function following short-term immobilisation. *J. Physiol.* 2011 Aug 8 (Epub ahead of print).

Lammers K, Lince SL, Spath MA, van Kempen LC, Hendriks JC, Vierhout ME, Kluivers KB (2011) Pelvic organ prolapse and collagen-associated disorders. *Int. Urogynecol. J.* Aug 3 (Epub ahead of print).

Lexell J, Taylor C., Sjostrom M (1988) What is the cause of the ageing atrophy? Total number, size and proportion of different fiber types studied in whole vastus lateralis muscle from 15- to 83-year-old men. *J. Neurol. Sci.* 84:275-294.

Lin YH, Liu M, Xiao N, Daneshgari F (2010) Recovery of continence function following simulated birth trauma involves repair of muscle and nerves in the urethra in the female mouse. *Eur. Urol.* 57:506-512.

Nichols DH and Randall CL (1989) Vaginal Surgery, 3rd Ed, Williams Wilkins, Baltimore. 1-46.

Oelrich TM (1983) The striated urogenital sphincter muscle in the female. *The Anatomical Record* 205:223-232.

Palma P, Herrmann V (2007) Urodynamics and stress urinary incontinence: the dark side of a gold standard. *Int. Urogynecol. J. Pelvic. Floor Dysfunct.* 18:1385-6.

Perucchini D, DeLancey JO, Asthon-Miller JA, Peschers U, Kataria T (2002) Age effects on urethral striated muscle. I. Changes in number and diameter of striated muscle fibers in the ventral urethra. *Am. J. Obstet. Gynecol.* 186:351-355.

Petros PE and Bornstein J Vulvar vestibulitis may be a referred pain arising from laxity in the uterosacral ligaments - a hypothesis based on 3 prospective case reports, *ANZJOandG* (2004) 44: 483–486.

Petros PEP, Richardson PA, TFS posterior sling improves overactive bladder, pelvic pain and abnormal emptying, even with minor prolapse – a prospective urodynamic study, (2010) *Pelviperineology 29*: 52-55.

Petros PE, Ulmsten U (1990) An Integral Theory of female incontinence. Acta Obstetrica et Gynecologica Scandinavia, *Supplement* 153, Vol 69: 1-79.

Petros PE, Ulmsten U (1993) An Integral Theory and its Method for the Diagnosis and Management of Female Urinary Incontinence. Part II. The biomechanics of vaginal tissue, and supporting ligaments with special relevance to the pathogenesis of female urinary incontinence. *Scand. J. Urol. Nephrol. Supp.* 153: 29-40.

Petros PE, Ulmsten U, Papadimitriou J (1990) The Autogenic Neoligament procedure: A technique for planned formation of an artificial neo-ligament. *Acta Obstetrica et Gynecologica Scandinavia*, 69 (Suppl. 153) 43-51.

Petros PE, Ulmsten U (1993) An Integral Theory and its Method for the Diagnosis and Management of Female Urinary Incontinence. Part I. Theory, morphology, radiographic correlations and clinical perspective. *Scand. J. Urol. Nephrol. Supp.* 153: 5-28.

Petros P, Ulmsten U (1993) Bladder instability in women: A premature activation of the micturition reflex. *Neurourol. Urodynam.* 12:235-239.

Petros PE, Ulmsten U (1995) Urethral and bladder neck closure mechanisms. *Am. J. Obstet. Gynecol.* 173: 346-347.

Petros PE, Ulmsten U (1997) Role of the Pelvic Floor in Bladder Neck Opening and Closure I: Muscle Forces. *Int. Urogynecol. J.* 8:74-80.

Petros PE (1998) The pubourethral ligament - an anatomical and histological study in the live patient. *Int. J. Urogynecology* 9:154-157.

Petros PE (2010) The Female Pelvic Floor. Function, Dysfunction and Management According to the Integral Theory. Springerverlag, Berlin-Heidelberg.

Petros PE (2008) Pubovisceral muscle avulsion. *Aust. N. Z. J. Gynaecol.* 48:124.

Petros PE, Swash M (2008) The Musculoelastic Theory of anorectal function and dysfunction. *J. Pelviperineology* 27:89-93.

Petros P, Swash M, Kakulas B The Musculo-Elastic Theory of anorectal function and dysfunction, Experimental Study No. 8: Stress urinary incontinence results from muscle weakness and ligamentous laxity in the pelvic floor. Pelviperineology 2008; *27*: 106 - 109.

Pierce LM, Coates KW, Kramer LA, Bradford JC, Thor KB, Kuehl TJ (2008) Effects of bilateral levator ani nerve injury on pelvic support in the female squirrel monkey. *Am. J. Obstet. Gynecol.* 198: 585.e1-585.e8.

Pieber D, Zivkovic F, Tamussino K (1998) Timing of urethral pressure pulses before and after continence surgery. *Neururol. Urodyn.* 17:9-23.

Quiroz LH, Munoz A, Shippey SH, Gutman RE, Handa VL (2010) Vaginal parity and pelvic organ prolapse. *J. Reprod. Med.* 55:93-98.

Rechberger T, Uldbjerg N, Oxlund H. (1988) Connective tissue Changes in the Cervix Curing Normal Pregnancy and Pregnancy Complicated by Cervical Incompetence. *Obstet. Gynecol.* 71:563-567.

Smith ARB, Hoskel GL, Warrel DW (1989) The role of partial denervation of the pelvic floor in the etiology of genitourinary prolapse and stress incontinence of urine: a neurophysiologic study. *Br. J. Obstet. Gynaecol.* 96:24-28.

South MM, Stinnett SS, Sanders DB, Weidner AC (2009) Levator ani denervation and reinnervation 6 months after childbirth. *Am. J. Obstet. Gynecol.* 200:519.e1-7.

Snooks S J, Swash M, Setchell M and Henry M M. Injury to innervation of pelvic floor sphincter musculature in childbirth. *LANCET* 1984 2 546-550.

Swash M, Henry MM, Snooks SJ Unifying concept of pelvic floor disorders and incontinence. *Journal of the Royal Society of Medicine*, (1985),78: 906-911.

Ulmsten U, Henriksson L, Johnson P, and Varhos G, An ambulatory surgical procedure under local anesthesia for treatment of female urinary incontinence, *Int. Urogynecol. J.* (1996); 7: 81-86.

Uitto J, Bernstein EF (1998) Molecular Mechanisms of Cutaneous Aging: Connective Tissue Alterations in the Dermis. *Journal of Investigative Dermatology Symposium Proceedings* 3:41-44.

Van der Kooi JB, van Wanroy PJ, De Jonge MC, Kornelis JA (1984) Time separation between cough pulses in bladder, rectum and urethra in women. *J. Urol.* 132: 1275-1278.

Wyndaele JJ, De Wachter S (2008). The sensory bladder (1): an update on the different sensations described in the lower urinary tract and the physiological mechanisms behind them. *Neurourol. Urodyn.* 27: 274-278.

Zacharin RF (1963) A suspensory mechanism of the female urethra. *Journal of Anatomy* 97:423-427.

In: Urinary Incontinence
Editor: Eric Chung

ISBN: 978-1-62618-482-4

Chapter 2

Urodynamics Assessment in Urinary Incontinence

William Bowes[1], Eric Chung[2] and Peter McTaggart[1]
[1] Department of Urology, Queens Elizabeth II Hospital, Brisbane QLD, Australia
[2] Department of Urology, Princess Alexandra Hospital, Brisbane QLD, Australia

Introduction

Urodynamics study (UDS) involves the use of specialised tools for objective measurement of the various parameters related to the lower urinary tract. It allows the clinician the ability to diagnose both functional and anatomical abnormalities that lead to lower urinary symptoms.

It is particularly useful in cases of complex urinary incontinence, to confirm the diagnosis and exclude confounding pathology prior to incontinence surgery, and also the evaluation of recurrent or new symptoms following surgical intervention [1].

In general, the aims of urodynamic assessment are:

- To reproduce the patient's symptoms and correlate these with urodynamic findings
- The assessment of bladder capacity and sensation
- The assessment of detrusor activity and function
- The assessment of urethral function during the filling/storage phase
- The assessment of outlet function during voiding
- The measurement of residual volume [1]

History

There has been significant evolution in the field of UDS since the genesis of the concept in the late 19th century [2]. The work of several pioneering clinicians, combined with the technological revolution of the latter half of the 20th century, resulted in modern UDS with reproducible and clinically relevant investigational modality.

In 1927, Rose [3] introduced the cystometer, the first UDS instrument to reliably measure detrusor pressure during filling and voiding. The next innovation was the invention of the uroflow-meter in 1946 by Drake [4]. This has arguably become the most widely-used urodynamic instrument in modern practice.

The advent of electronics led to further improvements, with von Garrelts developing an electronic uroflowmeter. This device calculated flow based on increasing weight (and therefore volume) of urine over time [5]. It was found to be accurate and consistent [6], and the basic principle is still employed in contemporary devices.

As far as electromyography is concerned, Du Bois-Reynard published his discovery that muscle contractions produce an electrical current that can be measured in 1848 [7]. In 1852, von Helmholtz devised a method of measuring nerve conduction velocity [8]. This work laid the foundation for subsequent developments in EMG. The first documented application in UDS was in 1955, when Franksson and Peterson used EMG to measure the activity of the external urethral sphincter in various types of incontinence and voiding dysfunction [9].

Video-fluoroscopy was first used to visualise the lower urinary tract during voiding by Miller in 1954 [10]. In 1967, he took this innovation a step further by developing a technique for simultaneously displaying video-fluoroscopy and plots from pressure-flow studies [11]. This method was further refined in the 70's by prominent researchers such as Whiteside and Bates [12-14].

In the same way that these conceptual breakthroughs have been a cornerstone of UDS, so too are those in the technological realm. Advances in the fields of electronics, computers, software, materials engineering, mass production methods and information dissemination have all contributed to making UDS a valid and accessible tool [15].

Consensus by the ICS

The aforementioned early pioneers were a small part of a multitude of workers worldwide, who were engaged in the practice and research of UDS. It soon became clear that many of these groups were unable to reliably compare and share their results, due to the heterogeneity of terminology and protocols.

The International Continence Society (ICS) was established in 1971 in Exeter, when it became clear that this deficiency ought to be addressed. Its goal was to provide (often in collaboration with various other organisations) a standardised framework of terminology and protocols, allowing better communication between researchers and clinicians.

Examples of topics covered by ICS publications include:

- Standards for digital exchange of UDS study data [16]
- Terminology and classification of:
    - Symptoms and signs
    - Pathology [17, 18]
    - Complications of surgery [19]
- Recommendations for the conduct of clinical trials/research studies

- Management guidelines [20]
- Protocols and recommendations for the conduct of UDS studies [21]

Access to these documents is provided via the ICS website, located at www.icsoffice.org. It is important that urodynamic studies are conducted to these standards.

What Is Being Measured?

UDS is the measurement of several specific physical parameters for evaluation, in association with the physical examination and possibly imaging, to deduce the likely cause of an effect.

It is important to note that urodynamics measurement devices are currently not in themselves able to make a definitive analysis. There are not enough inputs. The instruments cannot be put into action to produce a diagnosis; they are simply measurement tools.

The clinician is in control, not the recording system, and his/her actions during measurement determine the outcome.

Parameters

- Fill volume (V_{fill}) and voided volume (V_{void}) in ml
- Voiding flow rate (Q_{void})in ml/s
- Primary pressures of intravesical pressure (P_{ves}), abdominal pressure (P_{abd}) and urethral pressure (P_{ura}) in cmH_2O (**measured pressures**)
- Subtracted pressures: detrusor pressure ($P_{det} = P_{ves} - P_{abd}$) and urethral closure pressure ($P_{uc} = P_{ves} - P_{ura}$) in cm$H_2O$ (**calculated pressures**)
- Muscle bioelectric activity for EMG in mV

At this juncture, it is useful to consider the scale of pressures being measured. Atmospheric pressure at sea level is usually 1034 cmH_2O, whereas the maximum pressures generated during UDS are 100 to 200 cm H_2O. It is also important to understand that what is being measured is not absolute pressure, but pressure change relative to atmospheric pressure.

Components of UDS

1. Uroflowmetry:
   - Description: Uroflowmetry is, simply, the measurement of urine volume passed per unit time.
   - Equipment required:
     i. Uroflowmeter
2. Residual volume:

- Description: Determination of the residual urine volume in the bladder after voiding. Some authors perform this by means of catheterisation [15].
- Equipment required
  i. Portable ultrasound bladder-scanner OR
  ii. Catheter

3. Pressure studies
   - Description:
     i. Urethral pressure measurement: Urethral pressure (p_{ura}) is defined as the pressure required to open a closed urethra. It is possible to measure the pressure at specific *points* in the urethra, or to obtain a *urethral pressure profile(UPP)* by withdrawing the tip of the pressure probe catheter through the urethra at a constant rate while a pressure measurement is being taken continuously. Urethral pressure is usually measured supine, but some investigators also take measurements erect, ambulatory or during straining/Valsalva. Simultaneous recording of intravesical pressure (P_{ves}), allows for the calculation of urethral closure pressure ($P_{uc} = P_{ves} - P_{ura}$) [22]. Other more sophisticated measures, such as stress urethral pressure profile and micturitional pressure profile, can be performed. However, much controversy surrounds the use of UPP, and many critics have shown it to both unreliable and replaceable by other measures (such as leak-point pressures) [23].
     ii. Cystometry (multichannel UDS): This is the most accurate tool available for assessing the passive filling component of bladder function [15]. It is performed by filling the bladder, whilst measuring the intravesical pressure (P_{ves}) and abdominal pressure (P_{abd}). Depending on circumstances and equipment, the urethral pressure (P_{ura}) during this phase may also be measured. Apart from pressures, other parameters that are assessed include bladder capacity and sensation, the presence/absence of detrusor overactivity, and the presence/absence of incontinence. Various manoeuvres, such as cough, strain, or Valsalva, may be employed during this phase of the study to elicit stress incontinence. During Valsalva, it is possible, with fair precision, to establish the abdominal pressure at the moment that incontinence occurs, thus yielding the Valsalva leak-point pressure (VLPP). Generally, a VLPP lower than 60 cmH_2O is associated with intrinsic sphincter deficiency, whilst higher pressures usually indicate urethral hypermobility. In some cases, such as patients with neurological disease who have reduced bladder compliance and incontinence, it is important to measure the detrusor leak-point pressure (DLPP). This is the P_{det} at which incontinence occurs in the absence of a detrusor contraction. Pressures of greater than 40 cmH_2O are marker for possible upper tract deterioration [24].
     iii. Video-cystometry: Video-UDS allows for simultaneous evaluation of the physiology and anatomy of the lower urinary tract. This is usually accomplished by means of fluoroscopy (with a mixture of contrast medium and water/saline instilled during filling), but some investigators assert that real-time ultrasonography is equivalent [25-27]. Useful information, such as

bladder contour, VUR, bladder neck/base and urethral mobility during Valsalva, bladder calculi, fistulae, urethral diverticula and bladder neck anatomy during voiding, can be obtained with this modality.

- Equipment required:

i. Catheters (for filling bladder)

ii. Pressure probes and transducers

1. Urethral and Vesical: these are available in many configurations. These include single-lumen (requiring separate catheters for fill, Pves and Pura), dual-lumen (fill and P_{ves}), and triple-lumen (fill, P_{ves} and P_{ura}). The relationship between catheter and pressure transducer (device that converts kinetic energy/pressure into electrical energy/signal) also varies.
   a. Extracorporeal strain-gauge with fluid-filled probe catheters
      i. Disposable dome: these are relatively robust, with a lower disposable cost, but are affected by hydrostatic pressure heads
      ii. Fully disposable: more costly, but perform better due to a lower displacement volume, and are also affected by hydrostatic pressure heads
   a. MTC: these catheters have a miniature pressure-transducer at the tip of the catheter (intracorporeal strain-gauge). They are less influenced by hydrostatic pressure heads, but introduce difficulties with sterilisation (multiple-use item)
2. Rectal/vaginal: rectal or vaginal pressures (representing P_{abd}) are obtained using catheters with extracorporeal strain gauges
   a. Balloon: a small pressureless balloon at the end of the catheter is filled with water, with the lumen of the catheter communicating with the interior of the balloon
   b. Slow infusion: an open-ended catheter is infused at a rate of approximately 2 ml/min, in order to prevent pressure artifacts produced by faecal blockage or contact with rectal/vaginal mucosa.

iii. Volume transducers: employ mechanisms with electronic elements sensitive to deformation, which generate electrical impulses under load (force). The commonest configuration is a device which weighs the contents of a hanging bag of fluid. As filling occurs, the bag becomes lighter and fill volume is determined

iv. Fill rate controller

1. Infusion (roller) pump: Use of this device increases disposable item cost as a special pump-tube set is used. It also produces a pulsatile pressure artifact.
2. Pressure-cuff: This is cheaper as an ordinary IV-line can be used, and produces no pulsatile artifact, but fill rate control is less accurate

v. X-ray equipment

1. Fixed fluoroscopy unit
2. Mobile C-arm/image intensifier

vi. Amplifiers: amplify small signals produced by transducers. Many models available, with choice based on unit's requirements and budget.

vii. Signal processor and display hardware (PC) and software, user interface, printer. Importance of sampling rate: minimum 10 Hz for pressure/ flow [21].

4. Pressure-flow studies:
   - Description: urine flow rate provides only limited information regarding the underlying pathology that has resulted in voiding dysfunction. This is because flow rate depends on both the bladder outflow tract resistance and the contractility of the detrusor. For example, slow flow could be due associated with either high or low pressures, while normal flow could be associated with normal or high pressures. Pressure-flow studies are essential to describe the relationship between the bladder, bladder outlet, urethra, sphincter and pelvic floor during voiding. They are performed by asking the patient to void while simultaneously measuring flow rate and P_{det} (P_{ves} – P_{abd}). In some cases, concurrent fluoroscopy or EMG may be useful, or even essential adjuncts. Nomograms, such as the Abrams-Griffiths nomogram [28], are available to determine whether a patient has obstructed voiding or not. Many patients, however, fall into the "equivocal" category, and the use of other calculations, such as the Abrams-Griffiths (AG) number [29], may result in fewer uninterpretable results. The AG number is calculated thus: P_{det} x Q_{max} – (2 x Q_{max}). It is important to note that the aforementioned nomogram and calculation are only validated for males.
   - Equipment: as for pressure-studies, with the addition of

i. Flow transducer: different types exit, classified according to the mechanism by which flow is measured.

1. Spinning discs: flow rate is proportional to the amount of resistance to disc spin. Contamination on the disc causes false high readings, and the direction and point of impact of the stream of fluid can produce flow artifacts [30]. They are also expensive to repair.
2. Dipstick (capacitance): a metal strip capacitor is placed vertically in a straight-sided container. The solutes in urine conduct electricity across the capacitor, and as the urine level rises the effective capacitance falls. The change in capacitance give the volume voided, and the rate of change of volume give the flow rate. These flowmeters are affected by protein buildup and other contamination, which cause dielectric changes. They are also difficult to clean, and have largely been superseded by other mechanisms.
3. Weight: these devices measure the mass, and hence the volume of fluid voided, from which the flow can be calculated. These devices can produce error due to the inertia of urine falling into the container, and also depend on fluid density to calculate the flow. They therefore need separate calibration for urine, saline and saline/contrast mixtures. They are reliable and low-cost options.
4. Air displacement: calculate urine volume by measuring the amount of air leaving an enclosed chamber as it is displaced by urine. The advantages of these devices are the absence of moving parts, low cost,

ease of maintenance, and consistent calibration regardless of fluid density.

5. Electromyography:
    - Description: In UDS, EMG of the perineal floor is used to determine the degree of coordination between the external sphincter and detrusor contraction. It is a powerful tool in the correct circumstances (such as when neuropathic bladder outflow obstruction – detrusor-sphincter dyssynergia – is suspected) [23], otherwise it yields information that is interesting rather than essential.
    - Equipment:
        i. Electrodes
            1. Surface
            2. Needle
        ii. Amplifiers
        iii. Signal processor and display hardware (PC) and software, printer. Minimum sampling rate 20 kHz [21]

Preparation

- Patient
    - Pre-test information leaflet, which includes information on the study, what to bring with them, instructions to arrive with full bladder, etc.
    - Certain medication such as anti-cholinergic should be ceased to assess for detrusor overactivity
    - History: essential, to guide conduct of the test, but also to allow time for patient-clinician rapport to develop (necessary to allay anxiety and promote cooperation during study)
    - Clinical examination: focused on lower urinary tract, pelvic floor and neurological system
    - Briefing of patient
        - Aim of study
        - What to expect
        - What is required of patient (i.e. cooperation, communication, cough/Valsalva). Patients need to have a very clear understanding of the different sensory events they are required to report during filling. They also need to be completely relaxed (apart from when performing a manoeuvre at the clinician's request)
        - Time required (30 – 60min)
- Equipment
    - Switch on 1 hour prior to study, to allow electronics time to warm up and "settle"
    - 2-minute visual inspection
        - Front panel connections
        - Pressure transducers
        - Printer on, loaded with paper

- 3-minute functional test
- Consumables: in stock and laid out ready for use
- Enter patient details into UDS system

- Venue
  - Warm (prevents shivering)
  - Quiet
  - Privatc

The Study Phases

1. First void, for uroflowmetry and post-void residual measurement (ought to be performed as soon as patient arrives at unit – they were instructed to arrive with full bladder)
2. Insertion and connection of transducer probes and fill catheters
3. Urethral pressure measurement (may also be performed at various points in the filling phases
4. Fill phase with simultaneous pressure recordings and fluoroscopy. It is useful to obtain 5 seconds of quiet baseline recordings prior to starting fill
5. Cough/strain/Valsalva to test for leak-point pressures
6. It is important to ensure that the transducer is at patient level and both transducer measurements are "zero" to control pressure reading
7. Second void, during which the pressure-flow recordings taken
8. Throughout the measurement, cough test should be performed to ensure that the reading remain valid and accurate.

Phases 3 to 6 are usually performed supine, and then repeated in the erect position

Current Review on UDS

There is ongoing debate about the diagnostic utility of UDS in the management of men and women with urinary incontinence given the conflicting statements by various governing bodies. The National Institute for Clinical Excellence (NICE) in UK [31] has published a series of recommendations stating that history taking alone is sufficient to differentiate SUI from the other types of urinary incontinence and all patients should be trialed on conservative treatment. UDS should only be performed in women preoperatively if there is a clinical suspicion of detrusor overactivity (DO), previous surgery for SUI or pelvic organ prolapse, or if there are symptoms suggestive of coexisting voiding dysfunction. In contrast the International Consultation on Incontinence (ICS) [32] advocates the use of UDS in complicated cases of urinary incontinence, uncertain pathophysiology and the presence of neurogenic voiding dysfunction. The benefit of preoperative UDS also extends to women with prior history of extensive pelvic surgeries, radiation and persistent or recurrent of urinary incontinence [33]. On the other hand, the utility of UDS in men higher in differentiating DO from bladder outlet obstruction.

Free uroflowmetry, filling cystometry and a pressure flow study are essential components of UDS based on the recommendation by ICS Good Urodynamic Practice guideline [34]. The Urinary Incontinence Treatment Network has published extensively on the ideal reference urodynamic values and proposed standardised UDS protocol [35,36]. Unfortunately this practice has not been widely adopted and different UDS protocols and set-up continue to exist. Most patients with urinary incontinence will respond well to conservative measures and/or minimally invasive anti-incontinence surgery without the need for routine urodynamic testing. Systematic review by Martin [37] concluded that women with urodynamic evidence of SUI can be correctly identified based on history alone with a sensitivity of 92% and specificity of 56%. On the other hand, the Cochrane review by Glazener and Lapitan [38] reported more patients received pharmacological and surgical interventions following urodynamic testing, perhaps a reflection of the increased confidence among clinicians in advocating certain treatment pathways based on history and physical examintion.

Currently, many issues hinder the diagnostic accuracy of UDS such as the lack of protocol standardisation, numerous software programs, staff training and funding of the UDS unit, rectal line utilisation and concomitant EMG, handling of coexisting large pelvic organ prolapsed and technical and interpretation issues. Additionally, some experts believed that UDS is a poor investigative tool in detecting DO [39]. Unrecognised and under-detected DO may be due to the fact that DO is not always present during the filling phase, and UDS, being a transitory investigation, is not able to capture DO at its occurrence. Furthermore, conventional UDS employs antegrade filling instead of natural (orthograde) filling, thereby potentially limiting the occurrence of DO in these patients. On the other hand, ambulatory UDS has been shown to be more effective in identifying women with DO (69% vs 18% with conventional UDS) [40]. Several controversies continue to exist on the utility of UDS in the preoperative investigation value, degree of detrusor- or bladder neck-related voiding dysfunction, application of leak point pressures and urethral pressure profile, and the need on for UDS in healthy, treatment-naive woman with no history of prior incontinence or prolapsed surgery.

It is important to remember that UDS is a dynamic assessment tool attempting to replicate patient's symptoms and therefore has its limitations and the outcome needs to be interpreted with caution. Nonetheless UDS should be considered in patient with complex history, in women with prior stress-incontinent and/or large pelvic organ prolapsed, and in men and women with history of pelvic surgery or radiation, and underlying neurological conditions.

References

[1] Abrams, P., et al., Fourth International Consultation on Incontinence Recommendations of the International Scientific Committee: Evaluation and treatment of urinary incontinence, pelvic organ prolapse, and fecal incontinence. *Neurourology & Urodynamics,* 2010. 29(1): p. 213-40.

[2] Ek, A. and W.E. Bradley, History of cystometry. *Urology*, 1983. 22(3): p. 335-50.

[3] ROSE, D.K., DETERMINATION OF BLADDER PRESSURE WITH THE CYSTOMETER. *Journal of the American Medical Association*, 1927. 88(3): p. 151-157.

[4] Chancellor, M.B., et al., The invention of the modern uroflowmeter by Willard M. Drake, Jr at Jefferson Medical College. *Urology*, 1998. 51(4): p. 671-4.

[5] Von Garrelts, B., Analysis of micturition; a new method of recording the voiding of the bladder. *Acta Chirurgica Scandinavica,* 1957. 112(3-4): p. 326-40.

[6] Nyman, C.R., J. Boman, and A. Gidlof, Von Garrelts' uroflowmeter. A technical evaluation. *Urologia Internationalis*, 1979. 34(3): p. 184-9.

[7] Du Bois-Reymond, E., *Untersuchungen uber thierische Elektricitat [microform] / von Emil du Bois-Reymond.* 1848, Berlin :: G. Reimer.

[8] Helmholtz, H., *Messungen über Fortpflanzungsgeschwindigkeit der Reizung in den Nerven.* 1852.

[9] Franksson, C. and I. Petersén, Electromyographic Investigation Of Disturbances In The Striated Muscle Of The Urethral Sphincter. *British Journal of Urology*, 1955. 27(2): p. 154-161.

[10] Miller, E.R., X-ray movies. *Radiology*, 1954. 63(4): p. 571-2.

[11] Boyarsky, S., et al., *Neurogenic bladder.* 1967: Williams & Wilkins Co.

[12] Bates, C.P. and C.E. Corney, Synchronous cine-pressure-flow cystography: a method of routine urodynamic investigation. *British Journal of Radiology,* 1971. 44(517): p. 44-50.

[13] Bates, C.P., C.G. Whiteside, and R. Turner-Warwick, Synchronous cine-pressure-flow-cysto-urethrography with special reference to stress and urge incontinence. *British Journal of Urology,* 1970. 42(6): p. 714-23.

[14] Whiteside, G. and P. Bates, Synchronous video pressure-flow cystourethrography. *Urologic Clinics of North America*, 1979. 6(1): p. 93-102.

[15] Cole, E.E. and R.R. Dmochowski, Office urodynamics. *Urologic Clinics of North America*, 2005. 32(3): p. 353-70, vii.

[16] van Mastrigt, R. and D.J. Griffiths, ICS standard for digital exchange of urodynamic study data. *Neurourology & Urodynamics,* 2004. 23(3): p. 280-1.

[17] Haylen, B.T., et al., An International Urogynecological Association (IUGA) /International Continence Society (ICS) joint report on the terminology for female pelvic floor dysfunction. *International Urogynecology Journal,* 2010. 21(1): p. 5-26.

[18] Abrams, P., et al., The standardisation of terminology of lower urinary tract function: report from the Standardisation Sub-committee of the International Continence Society. *American Journal of Obstetrics & Gynecology,* 2002. 187(1): p. 116-26.

[19] Haylen, B.T., et al., An International Urogynecological Association (IUGA) / International Continence Society (ICS) joint terminology and classification of the complications related directly to the insertion of prostheses (meshes, implants, tapes) & grafts in female pelvic floor surgery. *International Urogynecology Journal*, 2011. 22(1): p. 3-15.

[20] Nordling, J., et al., Outcome measures for research in treatment of adult males with symptoms of lower urinary tract dysfunction. *Neurourology & Urodynamics*, 1998. 17(3): p. 263-71.

[21] Schafer, W., et al., Good urodynamic practices: uroflowmetry, filling cystometry, and pressure-flow studies. *Neurourology & Urodynamics,* 2002. 21(3): p. 261-74.

[22] Lose, G., et al., Standardisation of urethral pressure measurement: report from the Standardisation Sub-Committee of the International Continence Society. *Neurourology & Urodynamics,* 2002. 21(3): p. 258-60.
[23] Kelly, C.E. and R.J. Krane, Current concepts and controversies in urodynamics. *Current Urology Reports,* 2000. 1(3): p. 217-26.
[24] McGuire, E.J., J.R. Woodside, and T.A. Borden, Upper urinary tract deterioration in patients with myelodysplasia and detrusor hypertonia: a followup study. *Journal of Urology*, 1983. 129(4): p. 823-6.
[25] Bidair, M., et al., Transrectal ultrasound urodynamics. *Urology*, 1993. 42(6): p. 640-4; discussion 644-5.
[26] Koelbl, H. and G. Bernaschek, A new method for sonographic urethrocystography and simultaneous pressure-flow measurements. *Obstetrics & Gynecology*, 1989. 74(3 Pt 1): p. 417-22.
[27] Shabsigh, R., I.J. Fishman, and M. Krebs, Combined transrectal ultrasonography and urodynamics in the evaluation of detrusor-sphincter dyssynergia. *British Journal of Urology*, 1988. 62(4): p. 326-30.
[28] Abrams, P.H. and D.J. Griffiths, The assessment of prostatic obstruction from urodynamic measurements and from residual urine. *British Journal of Urology*, 1979. 51(2): p. 129-34.
[29] Lim, C.S. and P. Abrams, The Abrams-Griffiths nomogram. *World Journal of Urology*, 1995. 13(1): p. 34-9.
[30] Addla, S.K., et al., Avoid cruising on the uroflowmeter: evaluation of cruising artifact on spinning disc flowmeters in an experimental setup. *Neurourology & Urodynamics*, 2010. 29(7): p. 1301-5.
[31] NICE. *Urinary incontinence. The management of urinary incontinence in women.* National Institute of Clinical Excellence. 2006 available at: http://www.nice.org.uk/nicemedia/pdf/CG40fullguideline.pdf
[32] Griffiths D, Kondo A, Bauer S, Diamant N, Liao L, Lose G et al. Dynamic testing. *In Incontinence: Basics and Evaluation.* Eds Abrams P, L Cardozo, S Khoury and A Wein. Plymouth, United Kingdom: International Continence Society 2005:585-674
[33] Takacs EB, Zimmern PE. Recommendations for urodynamic assessment in the evaluation of women with stress urinary incontinence. *Nat Clin Pract Urol.* 2006;3(10);544-50
[34] Schafer W, Abrams P, Liao L, Mattiasson A, Pesce F, Spangberg A et al. Good urodynamic practices: uroflowmetry, filling cystometry, and pressure-flow studies. *Neurourol Urodyn* 2002;21:261-74
[35] Nager CW, Albo ME, Fitzgerald MP, McDermott SM, Kraus S, Richter HE et al. Process for development of multicenter urodynamic studies. *Urology* 2007;69:63-xx
[36] Nager CW, Albo ME, Fitzgerald MP, McDermott SM, Wruck L, Kraus S, Howden N, Norton P, Sirls, Varner E, Zimmern P for the Urinary Incontinence Treatment Network. Reference urodynamic values for stress incontinent women. *Neurourol Urodyn* 2007;26:333-40
[37] Martin JL, Williams KS, Sutton AJ, Abrams KR, Assassa RP. Systematic review and meta-analysis of methods of diagnostic assessment for urinary incontinence. *Neurourol Urodyn* 2006;25(7):674-83

[38] Glazener CMA, Lapitan MC. Urodynamic investigations for management of urinary incontinence in children and adults. *Cochrane Database Syst Rev* 2002;3:CD003195

[39] Caruso DJ, Kanagarajah P, Cohen BL, Ayyathurai R, Gomez C, Gousse AE. What is the predictive value of urodynamics to reproduce clinical findings of urinary frequency, urge urinary incontinence, and/or stress urinary incontinence? *Int Urogynecol J* 2010;21:1205-9

[40] Van Waalwijk, van Doorn ES, Remmers A, Janknegt RA. Conventional and extramural ambulatory urodynamic testing of the lower urinary tract in female volunteers. *J Urol* 1992;147(5):1319-25

In: Urinary Incontinence
Editor: Eric Chung
ISBN: 978-1-62618-482-4

Chapter 3

Imaging of Urethral Sphincter

Ángel Roberto Proaño Toro *
Department of Urology, Ecuadorian Institute of Social Security Hospital,
Guaranda, Ecuador

Abstract

Urinary incontinence (UI) is a common condition that causes a significant hygienic and psychosocial problem in an aging population. The intrinsic sphincter deficiency (ISD) in the context of effort urinary incontinence (EUI) has had difficulty in being evaluated in order to establish an effective medical or surgical treatment. Currently there is no single method of definitive diagnosis, but there are multiple tests to reach a consensus diagnosis based on clinical history, voiding history, and advanced studies. Urodynamic studies have been those which have tried to standardize the relation to changes in bladder and abdominal leak-point pressure, which combined with cystourethrography, has been considered the gold standard in diagnosis of ISD. With technological advancement, through ultrasound probes and endocavitary coils in magnetic resonance imaging (MRI), we can assess more accurately the structures related to the continence. More specifically, the special structure of the omega-shaped urethral rhabdosphincter (RS) and the bladder neck even correlated with their morphology and functional studies are the basis for research into new treatments.

Keywords: Rhabdosphincter, ultrasound, magnetic resonance imaging, autologous myoblasts-fibroblasts, urinary incontinence

* Correspondence: Name: Angel Roberto; Last name: Proaño Toro. E-mail: soninonino@hotmail.com; Home Address: Cruz Loma 200, Guaranda – Ecuador; Work Address: Augusto Chavez and Via Ambato, Guaranda, Ecuador.

Introduction

Over 200 million people worldwide suffer urinary incontinence (UI). [1] The prevalence varies due to the use of different definitions and heterogeneity of the populations studied, EPINCOT a Norwegian study showed prevalence in the female UI of 15 - 35%, in close relation to age and parity, being more frequent EUI; in men it can range from 10 to 30%. [2, 3]

The best studied risk factors are: age, obstetric history and obesity. During the childbirth, muscle lesions, connective tissue and nerves seem to be the most important factors in connection with EUI and mixed urinary incontinence, being more significant the first child birth than each of the following. [2, 4, 5]

EUI can be grouped into two categories: urethral hypermobility (UH) and intrinsic urethral sphincteric deficiency (ISD). Experimental data evidenced by Kamo et al., which was performed in female rats suggest that the mid-urethra and external urethral sphincter are critical to maintain continence and is the primary focus for the management of EUI. [6] In humans with advancing age there is a progressive decrease in the density of striated muscle cells in the rhabdosphincter (RS). This continuous loss due to apoptosis can lead to UI. These findings are the starting point for new therapeutic approaches that help delay the apoptosis or replace muscle cell in RS. [7]

According to the European Society of Urology, the initial diagnosis of incontinence includes the medical history, an abdominal and pelvic-perineal clinical examination, uro-analysis, post-void residual urine, urinary diary, renal function, cystourethroscopy, pressure flow studies with or without electromyography (EMG) and its impact on life quality, while imaging methods are not part of the initial routine, reserving for the study of complicated cases. [8]

This review focuses on the role of MRI and ultrasound in their different modalities for the evaluation of UI, especially in relationship to ISD and their potential uses in treatment.

Anatomy

Anatomical and functional studies have identified the structure and innervation of the urethral sphincter mechanism, leaving aside the old conception of a ring of striated muscle around the urethra. RE is a striated muscle loop in omega like shape, at level of the membranous urethra and innervated by branches of pudendal nerve. [9] While the proximal urethra and the layer of smooth muscle is innervated by autonomic nerves. [10]

In men, the membranous urethra of 1.5 cm in length receives autonomic innervation from the pelvic plexus through arms from the prostatic plexus and cavernous nerves (Figure 1). RS with its special configuration forms a cover on the sides and front of the membranous urethra and is inserted into the perineal body, continues with muscle bundles along the anterior and lateral prostate extending cranially to the neck bladder. [10]

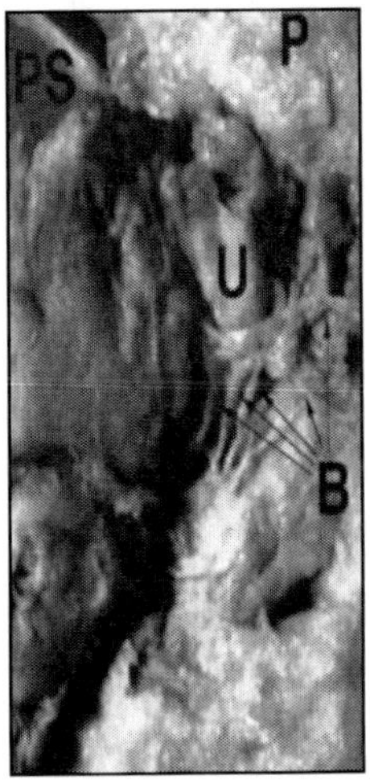

Figure 1. Fetal specimen, male, lateral view. PS= pubic symphysis, P= prostate, U= urethra, B= branches of the pelvic plexus innervating the urethra (marked by arrows).
Taken of Strasser H, Ninkovic M, Hess M, et al. *Anatomic and functional studies of the male and female urethral sphincter. World J Urol. 2000; 18: 324-329.10.*

In women, the proximal urethra and most of the middle third consists of three layers of smooth muscle, an external and internal are longitudinal and middle layer with circular fibers; the inner layer is very thin and is directed towards the external meatus. RS is identified in the middle and distal thirds, and its major portion is located at the ventral and lateral aspects of the urethra while the dorsal aspects predominates the collagen tissue (Figure 2). As in the male, the sphincter has an omega like shape in transverse sections, and innervation by the pudendal nerve branches into the inferior rectal nerves, perineal nerves and dorsal nerve of the clitoris. [10]

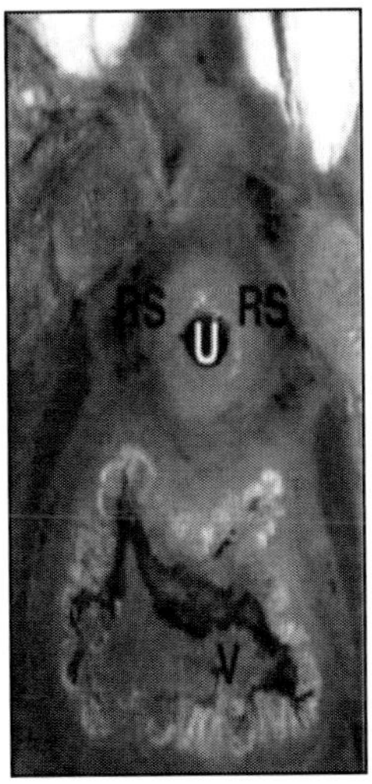

Figure 2. Female rhabdosphincter. RS= rhabdosphincter, U= urethra, V= vagina.
Taken of Strasser H, Ninkovic M, Hess M, et al. *Anatomic and functional studies of the male and female urethral sphincter. World J Urol. 2000; 18: 324-329* [10].

Videourodinamia

The combinations of cystourethrography and pressure flow studies have been considered the gold standard for diagnosis of UI due to ISD, but for its cost and low availability, have little practical application. However the diagnostic criteria correspond to the presence of "funneling" (an opening of the bladder neck and the proximal urethra) with subsequent leakage of contrast material caused by small increases in abdominal pressure in the absence of detrusor contraction. [11]

Nuclear Magnetic Resonance

Dynamic and static MRI, without exposure to ionizing radiation, provide a more accurate visualization of the pelvic floor structures, correlating laxity of the pelvic structures with specific dysfunctions [12], such as the mobility of the urethrovesical junction, connections of levator ani muscle, and "hammock" like configurations of the anterior vaginal wall. [13] MRI has shown no advantages in conventional colpocystorectography techniques to evaluate weakness of pelvic floor. MRI is recommended for patients that present UI with complex and high grade genital prolapse, divergent findings in clinical investigation and conventional imaging modalities in younger patients. [14] This diagnostics method has been attempted to identify women at "high risk" of developing pelvic floor disorders after their first child birth, and no differences were found in pelvimetry or the soft tissue, and there were no significant differences in intertuberous diameter, or in larger pelvic arches in women with UI. [15]

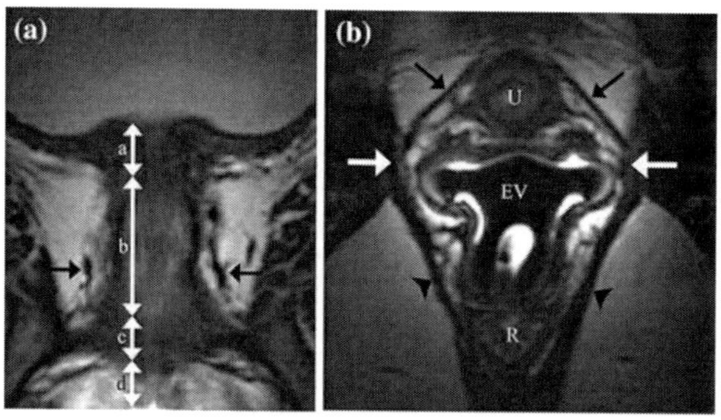

Figure 3. Continent woman. Images obtained with endovaginal MR coil. (a) Coronal T2-weighted image shows four segments of the urethra: (a) intramural, bladder neck level, 0.9cm long, (b) midurethra were urethral sphincter has a multilayered appearance, with the inner hyperintense smooth muscle and outer hypointense striated muscle, is 1.8cm, (c) urogenital diaphragm level, 0.9cm long, (d) distal urethra comprising fibrous tissue only, 0.9cm long. (b) Axial T2-weighted image at proximal urethra, 1cm from the internal meatus, shows a well-defined linear dark structure, anterior periurethral ligament (black arrows) attaching firmly together with the puborectalis muscle (arrowheads). Note symmetric vaginolevator attachments where the periurethral ligament and puborectalis muscle join (white arrows). U=urethra, R= rectum, EV= endovaginal coil.
Taken of Kim JK, Kim YJ, Choo MS, Cho KS. The urethra and its supporting structures in women with stress urinary incontinence: MR imaging using an endovaginal coil. AJR Am J Roentgenol. 2003; 180:1037-1044 [17].

As for evaluation of EUI associated with urethral hypermobility and ISD, the use of endocavitary coils allows better spatial resolution of urethral anatomy and supporting structures. [16] In urethra level can distinguish four segments related to continence, and various supporting structures (Figure 3) [17].

Endourethral coil, in axial plane, T2-weighted images of the midurethra show a multilayered target appearance. The inner muscle layer in a loose connective tissue matrix shows high signal intensity. The smooth muscle layer is thickest at the midurethal level and on the ventral side of the urethra. The outer layer of low-intensity tissue encircling the smooth muscle represents the striated urogenital sphincter muscle (rhabdosphicter) within a dense connective tissue layer. The striated muscle is thicker on the ventral and lateral side of the urethra, and thinner on the dorsal side (Figure 4). Therefore in patients with UI due to ISD, there is evidence of a thinning of the striated sphincter and opening of bladder neck and proximal urethra. [18]

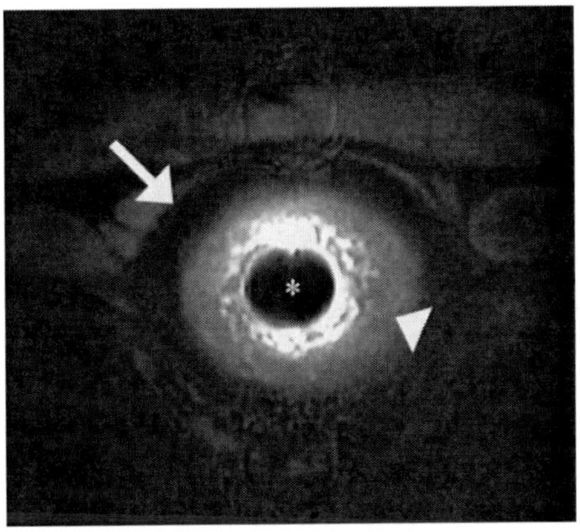

Figure 4. A 22 year old continent woman. Image obtained with 14F endourethral MR coil. Axial T2-weighted image of the midurethra, 1.5cm from the internal meatus, shows well-defined T2-dark outer striated muscle (arrow) and high signal inner smooth muscle (arrowhead). Asterisk represents 14 F endourethral coil.
Taken of Macura KJ, Genadry RR, Borman TL, et al. *Evaluation of the female urethra with intraurethral magnetic resonance imaging. J Magn Reson Imaging. 2004; 20: 153-159* [18].

Ultrasound

Ultrasound has proven to be an effective technique for evaluating the urethrovesical junction in EUI patients, with the advantage of being cheaper, easy to use and noninvasive without ionizing radiation exposure. It allows direct visualization of the urethra, the thickness, volume and the omega-shaped loop of striated urethral muscle, however urethral support mechanisms can only be evaluated indirectly (Figure 5). [19] Bladder neck mobility and competence at rest and with effort also may help in document bladder prolapse, urethral hypermobility and bladder neck insufficiency (Figure 6). [20]

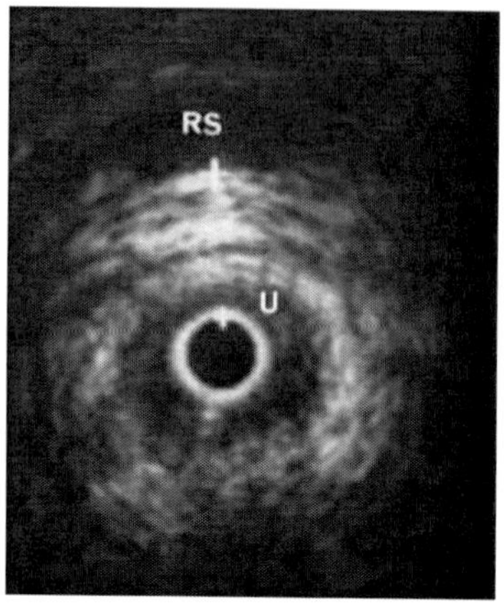

Figure 5. Transurethral ultrasound of the urethra (U) and the rhabdosphincter (RS) of the male urethra. *Taken of Strasser H, Ninkovic M, Hess M,* et al. *Anatomic and functional studies of the male and female urethral sphincter. World J Urol. 2000; 18: 324-329* [10].

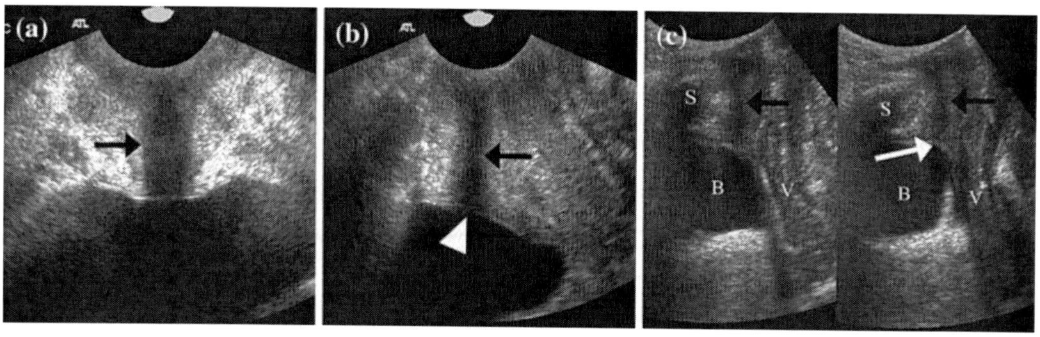

Figure 6. Ultrasound of the urethra in a 62 years old woman without a urinary incontinence. (a) Endovaginal ultrasound image of the urethra in coronal plane shows hypoechoic urethra (arrow). (b) Sagittal view shows urethra (arrow) and bladder neck (arrowhead) at rest. (c) Transperineal ultrasound image in sagittal plane during rest (left) and strain (right) shows minimal mobility of the urethra (black arrow) and intact bladder neck (white arrow). B= bladder V= vagina. S= symphysis pubis. Taken of Macura KJ, Genadry RR. Female urinary incontinence: pathophysiology, methods of evaluation and role of MR imaging. Abdom Imaging. 2008; 33: 371-380 [16].

Although in this methodology the sensitivity and specificity are low, the bladder neck funneling test is helpful to discard the existence of low Valsalva leak-point pressure with a negative predictive value of 92.8%. If bladder neck funneling does not exist, missing a diagnosis of ISD is uncommon. If the dilatation of the bladder neck is present it should be considered an additional evaluation of urethral sphincter (urodynamic investigation). Therefore trying to discard an ISD and identify urethral hypermobility. [20]

Pathological data obtained by different modes of ultrasound are directly related to aging; Strasser, et al., investigated the morphological changes and age-dependent functional level of the sphincter mechanism by the TUNEL technique (terminal deoxynucleotidyl transferase-mediated deoxyuridine triphosphate nick end-labeling) to determine rates of cellular apoptosis. It found a direct correlation between age and a decrease in volume and density of striated muscle cells; 87.6% in neonatal patients and 34.2% in women 92 years old of the rhabdosphincter consisted of striated muscle cells. [21] The transurethral ultrasonography can be used to detect these changes in vivo. The loss of urethral resistance as measured by the maximum urethral closure pressure is directly related to the thinning of RS, also a similar relationship was found with the thickness of the longitudinal smooth muscle layer, and replacement of skeletal muscle fibers by dense connective tissue or denervation injury may affect the function of a normally thick RS muscle (Figure 7). [22] For example, continent women show a striated muscle thickness of 3.5mm, women with EUI grade I 3.4mm, grade II EUI 3.3mm and a grade III EUI muscle thickness of 1.7mm. [23]

Digesu G, et al., found that through the use of 3D ultrasound, women with persistent EUI had significantly smaller urethral sphincter volumes preoperatively than those who had an objective cure, and this is a more useful diagnostic test than using traditional measures of urethral function such as maximum urethral closure pressure (MUCP), that women who have a smaller urethral sphincter might benefit from a more obstructive anti-incontinence procedure. [24]

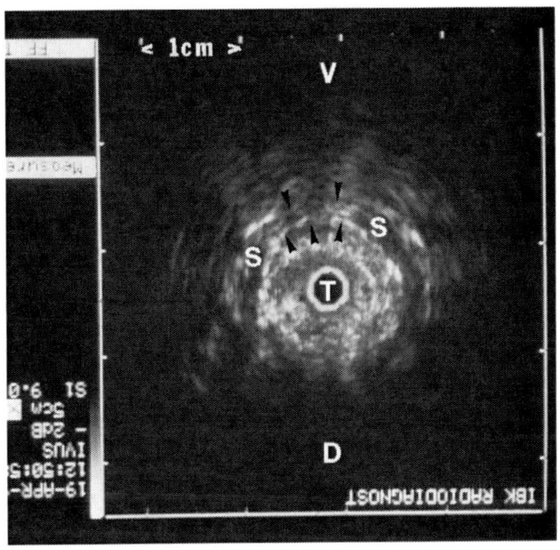

Figure 7. Intraurethral ultrasound of a grade-III stress urinary incontinent woman. The increased echogenicity of the sphincter muscle (arrows) is caused by atrophy. V= ventral, D= dorsal, S= sphincter, T= transducer.
Taken of Frauscher F, Helweg G, Strasser H, et al. *Intraurethral ultrasound: diagnostic evaluation of the striated urethral sphincter in incontinent females. Eur Radiol.1998; 8: 50-53* [23].

In addition to anatomical characteristics, the functionality of RS can be assessed by measuring contractile capacity. The distance between the ultrasound transducer and the inner aspect of the rhabdosphincter was measured while at rest and during voluntary contraction of the muscle; and the difference between these two readings served as a parameter for rhabdosphincter contractility by transurethral ultrasound (Figure 8). In continent women the contractility is 1.8mm, in grade I EUI it is 1.6mm, in grade 2 EUI it is 1mm, and grade III EUI it is 0.1mm. [23] In men with previous surgeries by three-dimensional transrectal ultrasound, it evaluates the distance between the inner aspect of the sphincter and the dorsal aspect of the membranous urethra (Figure 9). The contractility in continent patients is 1.42mm and in incontinent patients is only 0.59 mm; this suggests that in patients with contractility decreases less than 1.0mm are likely to suffer from postoperative urinary incontinence. [25]

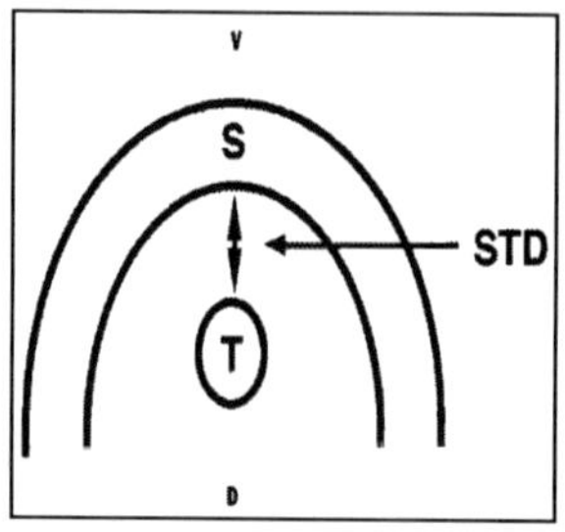

Figure 8. The measurement of the sphincter-transducer distance (STD). S= striated urethral sphincter; T= transducer, V= ventral, D= dorsal.
Taken of Frauscher F, Helweg G, Strasser H, et al. *Intraurethral ultrasound: diagnostic evaluation of the striated urethral sphincter in incontinent females. Eur Radiol.1998; 8: 50-53* [23].

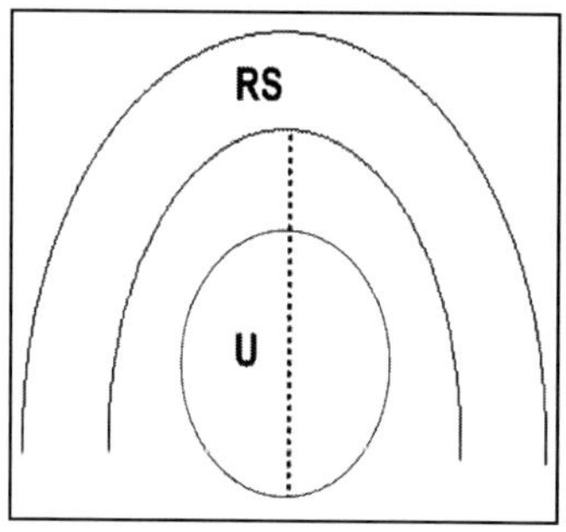

Figure 9. Schematic drawing of measurement of the rhabdosphincter-urethra distance. RS= rhabdosphincter, U= urethra.
Taken of Strasser H, Pinggera G, Gozzi C, et al. *Three-dimensional transrectal ultrasound of the male urethral rhabdosphincter. World J Urol. 2004; 22: 335-338* [25].

The direct visualization of the external urethral sphincter and the assessment of contractility offer new prospects for the management of EUI. [23]

Using a color Doppler translabial approach, Siracusano et al., published preliminary results comparing the urethral vasculature between continent and incontinent patients diagnosed with ISD through the urethral pressure profile and Valsalva leak-point pressure. All patients with ISD had minimal or poor blood flow in the urethral tissue. [26]

Therapeutic Implications

Transurethral and 3D ultrasounds were used as tools to assess the results, the research and the subsequent control of new treatments in urinary incontinence. Poon et al., studied the durability over time of periurethral collagen injection in women with EUI due to ISD. The authors showed that 97 + / - 33% of the volume of collagen injected was retained in tissues (Figure 10). [27]

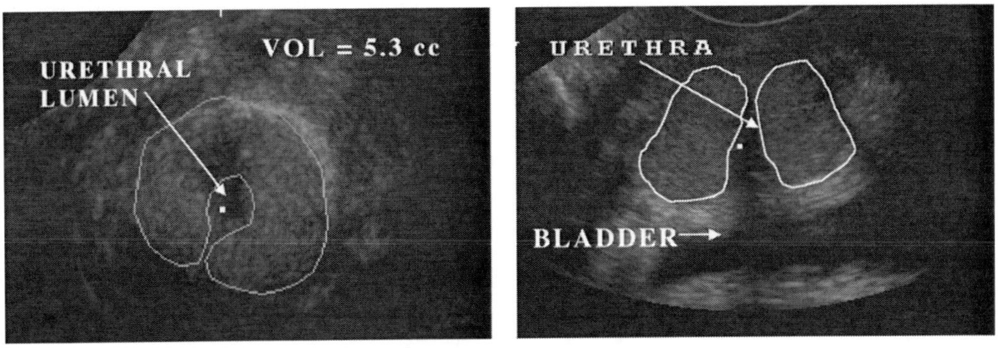

Figure 10. Circumferential periurethral collagen configuration on two-dimensional views from 3DUS study. Periurethral collagen outlined in axial (left) and coronal (right) planes through urethra and bladder.
Taken of Poon C, Zimmernen P, Wlson T, et al. *Three-dimensional ultrasonography to assess long-term durability of periurethral collagen in women with stress urinary incontinence due to intrinsic sphincter deficiency. Urology. 2005; 65: 60-64* [27].

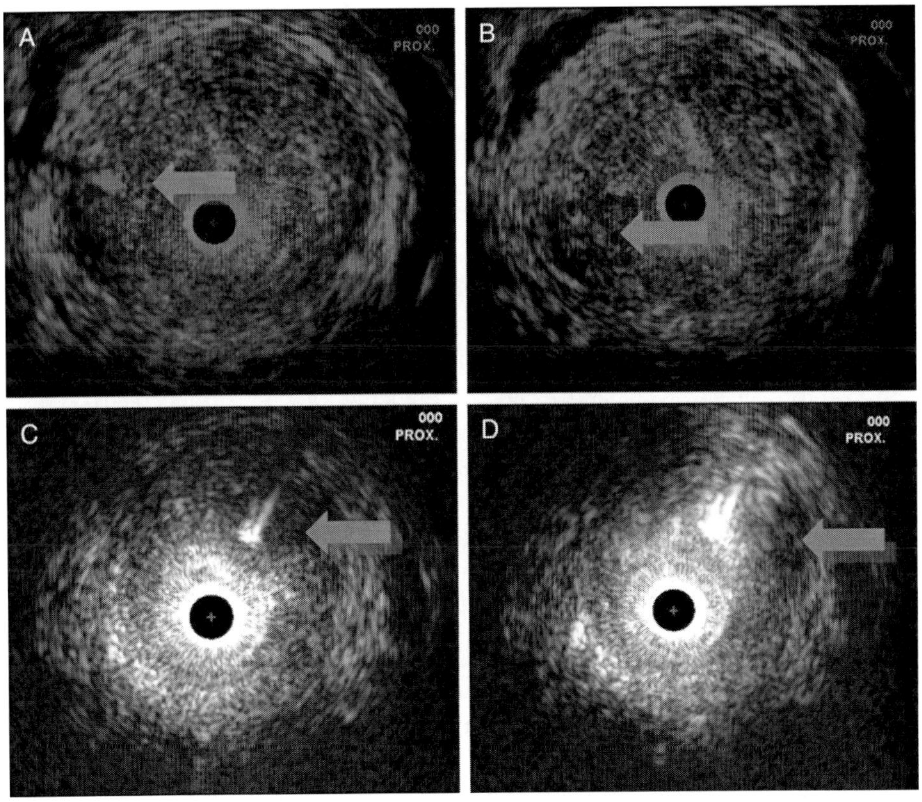

Figure 11. Ultrasound guided injection of autologous myoblasts and fibroblasts in incontinent patient. (a), tip of needle (arrow) is located at inner aspect of rhabdosphincter. (b), subsequently small depot of myoblasts is injected (arrow). (c), after injection of myoblasts, fibroblasts are injected into urethral submucosa. (d), small depots of fibroblasts can be visualized.
Taken of Mitterberger M, Marksteiner R, Margreiter E, et al. *Myoblasts and fibroblast therapy for post-prostatectomy urinary incontinence: 1-year follow up of 63 patients. J. Urol. 2008; 179: 226-231* [28].

In recent years doctors have developed an innovative therapeutic modality for EUI due to ISD by autologous myoblast and fibroblast cell transfer for structural and functional regeneration of the striated sphincter, using transurethral ultrasound. As for the application technique, the ultrasound guided application has a key role in this new treatment, it is not only crucial to inject the right types of cells, it is equally important to inject the cells into the right structure; ultrasonography allows precise and accurate injection of cells, which cannot be performed using standard endoscopic guidance (Figure 11). [28]

Conclusion

Urinary incontinence is a medical problem even though it is not life-threatening. It affects life quality in patients and incurs serious social and economic problems; therefore identifying the causes can indicate appropriate treatment. The new imaging techniques have a precise anatomical identification and the purpose is to investigate the structural and functional correlations in the sphincter muscle related to micturition and also to detect concomitant defects. These new imaging techniques are tools in the diagnosis and potential research protocols for therapeutic uses.

References

[1] Norton P, Brubaker L. Urinary incontinence in women. *Lancet.* 2006; 367: 57-67.

[2] Rortveit G, Hannestad YS, Daltveit AK, Hunskaar S. Age- and type-dependent effects of parity on urinary incontinence: the Norwegian EPINCONT study. Epidemiology of Incontinence in the County of Nord-Trondelag. *Obstet Gynecol.* 2001; 98:1004-1010.

[3] Hunskaar S, Burgio K, Clark A, et al. Epidemiology of urinary (UI) and faecal incontinence. In: Abrams P, Cardozo L, Khoury S, Wein A, editors. Incontinence, 3rd *International Consultation on Incontinence.* Plymouth: Health Publication Ltd; 2005. pp. 255–312.

[4] Meyer S, Schreyer A, De Grandi P, et al. The effects of birth on urinary continence mechanisms and other pelvic-floor characteristics. *Obstet. Gynecol.* 1998; 92: 613-618.

[5] Sampselle CM, Miller JM, Mims BL, et al. Effect of pelvic muscle exercise on transient incontinence during pregnancy and after birth. *Obstet. Gynecol.* 1998; 91: 406-412.

[6] Kamo T, Torimoto K, Chancellor MB, et al. Urethral closure mechanisms under sneeze-induced stress condition in rats: a new animal model for evaluation of stress urinary incontinence. *Am J Physiol Regul Integr Comp Physiol.* 2003; 285: 356-365.

[7] Strasser H, Tiefenthaler M, Steinlechner M, et al. Urinary incontinence in the elderly and age-dependent apoptosis of rabdosphincter cells. *Lancet.* 1999; 354: 918-919.

[8] Thüroff J, Abrams P, Andersson KE, et al. Guidelines on Urinary Incontinence. European Association of Urology. 2009. 11-34. http://www.uroweb.org/fileadmin/tx_eauguidelines/2009/Full/Incontinence.pdf Acceso en julio del 2009.

[9] Strasser H, Bartash G. Anatomy and innervation of the rhabdosphincter of the male urethra. *Semin Urol Oncol.* 2000; 18: 2-8.

[10] Strasser H, Ninkovic M, Hess M, et al. Anatomic and functional studies of the male and female urethral sphincter. *World J Urol.* 2000; 18: 324-329.

[11] Novara G, Artibani W. Imaging for urinary incontinence: a contemporary perspective. *Curr Opin Urol.* 2006; 16: 219-223.

[12] El Sayed RF, El Mashed S, Farag A, et al. Pelvic floor dysfunction: assessment with combined analysis of static and dynamic MR imaging findings. *Radiology.* 2008; 248: 518-530.

[13] Ansquer Y, Fernandez P, Aimot S, et al. MRI urethrovesical junction mobility is associated with global pelvic floor laxity in female stress incontinence. *Acta Obstet Gynecol Scand.* 2007; 29: 1-8.

[14] Treiber U, Hellerhoff P, Hanning C, et al. Dynamic MRI for evaluation of the female pelvis in urinary stress incontinence and pelvic organ prolapse. *Eur Urol Suppl.* 2004; 3: 202.

[15] Handa VL, Lockhart ME, Kenton KS, et al. Magnetic resonance assessment of pelvic anatomy and pelvic floor disorders after childbirth. *Int Urogynecol J.* 2009; 20: 133-139.

[16] Macura KJ, Genadry RR. Female urinary incontinence: pathophysiology, methods of evaluation and role of MR imaging. *Abdom Imaging.* 2008; 33: 371-380.

[17] Kim JK, Kim YJ, Choo MS, Cho KS. The urethra and its supporting structures in women with stress urinary incontinence: MR imaging using an endovaginal coil. *Am J Roentgenol.* 2003; 180:1037-1044.

[18] Macura KJ, Genadry RR, Borman TL, et al. Evaluation of the female urethra with intraurethral magnetic resonance imaging. *J Magn Reson Imaging.* 2004; 20: 153-159.

[19] Klauser A, Frauscher F, Strasser H, et al. Age-related rhabdosphincter function in female urinary stress incontinence: assessment of intraurethral sonography. *J Ultrasound Med.* 2004; 23: 631-637.

[20] Huang WC, Yang JM. Bladder neck funneling on ultrasound cystourethrography in primary stress urinary incontinence: a sign associated with urethral hypermobility and intrinsic sphincter deficiency. *Urology.* 2003; 61: 936-941.

[21] Strasser H, Tiefenthaler M, Steinlechner M, et al. Age dependent apoptosis and loss of rhabdosphincter cells. *J.Urol.* 2000; 164: 1781-1787.

[22] Heit M. Intraurethral ultrasonography: correlation of urethral anatomy with functional urodynamic parameters in stress incontinent women. *Int Urogynecol J.* 2000; 11: 204-211.

[23] Frauscher F, Helweg G, Strasser H, et al. Intraurethral ultrasound: diagnostic evaluation of the striated urethral sphincter in incontinent females. *Eur Radiol.*1998; 8: 50-53.

[24] Digesu G, Robinson D, Cardozo L, et al. Three-dimensional ultrasound of the urethral sphincter predicts continence surgery outcome. *Neurourol Urodyn.* 2009; 28: 90-94.

[25] Strasser H, Pinggera G, Gozzi C, et al. Three-dimensional transrectal ultrasound of the male urethral rhabdosphincter. *World J Urol.* 2004; 22: 335-338.

[26] Siracusano S, Bertolotto M, Silvestre G, et al. The feasibility of urethral color ultrasound imaging in the diagnosis of female intrinsic sphincter deficiency: preliminary results. *Spinal Cord.* 2002; 40: 192-195.

[27] Poon C, Zimmernen P, Wlson T, et al. Three-dimensional ultrasonography to assess long-term durability of periurethral collagen in women with stress urinary incontinence due to intrinsic sphincter deficiency. *Urology.* 2005; 65: 60-64.

[28] Mitterberger M, Marksteiner R, Margreiter E, et al. Myoblasts and fibroblast therapy for post-prostatectomy urinary incontinence: 1-year followup of 63 patients. *J. Urol.* 2008; 179: 226-231.

In: Urinary Incontinence
Editor: Eric Chung

ISBN: 978-1-62618-482-4

Chapter 4

A Review of Quality of Life Aspects and Physical Treatments in Female Urinary Incontinence

Daniela Oliveira, Cristina Jácome and Alda Marques
School of Health Sciences, University of Aveiro (ESSUA), Aveiro, Portugal

Abstract

Urinary Incontinence (UI), which is defined as an involuntary loss of urine, can be divided into three types: stress, urge and mixed UI. It is a common condition affecting 25% to 45% of women during the course of their lives, with a higher prevalence in adulthood. However, it affects younger women when specific conditions are present, e.g., practice of high impact sports. Despite its high prevalence, little attention has been given to the impact of UI on women's quality of life, namely on psychological, social, sexual and physical aspects. Furthermore, physical treatments, such as pelvic floor muscle training, vaginal cones, biofeedback and electrical stimulation, have been shown to be effective in the first-line management of this condition. Nevertheless, women experience a lack of information about these different methods available to prevent and treat UI. Therefore, this book chapter aims to increase awareness among women, professionals and general community, about UI impact on women's quality of life and available interventions to prevent and treat this condition.

1. Introduction

According to the International Continence Society, urinary incontinence (UI) is defined as the complaint of any involuntary loss of urine [1]. Urinary Incontinence is a common condition with a higher prevalence in adulthood [2, 3] however, it affects younger women when specific conditions are present, e.g., practice of high impact sports [4, 5]. The prevalence of this condition in women varies widely. A review by Buckley et al. reported that 25% to 45% of women suffer from UI [6].

Urinary incontinence can be classified in three types: stress, urge and mixed UI [1]. Stress UI is the complaint of an involuntary urine leakage on effort or physical exertion, or on sneezing or coughing [1]. In urge UI an involuntary urine leakage is accompanied by or immediately preceded by urgency [1]. The mixed UI is associated with both situations, as it is the complaint of an involuntary urine leakage associated with effort and also with urgency [1]. Stress UI is the most prevalent type of UI, affecting between 4% and 48% young and middle-aged women [3, 7, 8]. With increasing age, stress UI prevalence decreases and urge UI and mixed UI increases [3, 7]. These last two types are associated with more severe symptoms [7].

Urinary Incontinence is also a condition that profoundly affects women's quality of life. However, relatively little attention has been given to these aspects. Moreover, UI can be prevented and/or treated with several methods, e.g. physical, pharmacological and surgical [9, 10]. Physical treatments have been considered effective as a first-line management, however, women, different professionals and the community in general, lack of information regarding these interventions [4, 11]. These will be discussed in detail in this chapter.

2. Urinary Incontinence and Quality of Life Aspects

In a French cross-sectional study of 496 women, more than half (51.8%) considered that UI had a negative impact on their quality of life [12]. A Canadian study, aiming to compare the impact of 21 self-reported chronic conditions, found that UI has a severe impact on quality of life, similarly to the Alzheimer's disease and stroke [13]. The women's impaired quality of life due to UI involves a combination of the negative effects at different levels, such as psychological, social, sexual and physical [12, 14, 15].

2.1. Psychological

Several studies have shown a direct relationship between UI and indicators of psychological distress, such as depression and anxiety [15-17]. The prevalence of depression on women with UI has been reported in previous studies, with the estimates ranging from 15.5% to 43% [15-19]. A cross-sectional survey reported that women with UI were statistically significant more at risk of suffering from depression (15.5%) than continent women (9.2%) [19]. This study also found that younger women with UI (age 18–44) presented the highest prevalence of depression, almost three times more than women age 45 or older [19]. This has also been found in another cross-sectional study involving 338 incontinent women [17]. Moreover, the prevalence of depression in incontinent women differs by UI severity and frequency, i.e. women with severe and frequent UI symptoms are more likely to experience depression [17, 20-22]. In a population-based cross-sectional study of 5701 women it was verified that women with severe UI were 80% more likely to have depression compared with continent women, whereas women with mild-moderate UI presented a probability of 40% [21].

Anxiety is also a common problem among women with UI [18, 23]. Perry et al., in a prospective longitudinal postal survey, verified that the majority of the sample (57%) with UI experienced anxiety symptoms [18]. Urinary Incontinence is associated with feelings of loss of control due to the changes in function and therefore, probably, this is the main reason why incontinent women experience anxiety symptoms [24]. In terms of UI types and physiological aspects, the literature supports that mixed UI is the type of UI associated with higher levels of both depression and anxiety [23, 25].

2.2. Social

It is well documented in the literature that social aspects of life are disrupted by UI. Women suffering from UI experience embarrassment, frustration, loss of confidence and concern about urine leakage and odor [20, 24, 26]. To cope with these feelings, women tend to restrict their social relationships and avoid social activities [11, 26]. Social interactions are avoided mostly when occur in places with restricted toilet access, such as outdoor activities and sport events [27]. In a community-based descriptive cross-sectional study of 1718 women, aged from 15 to 49 years old, was observed that more than half of women (54.5%) reported that UI restricted their social activities, such as going out to a cinema or a park, visiting friends and relatives or going on picnics [26]. Fultz et al. studying 606 women with stress UI also found that a total of 36.5% perceived the impact of UI on their social activities [28].

In addition, UI can have a negative impact on women's occupational life. In a cross-sectional study of 2183 incontinent women, aged more than 18 years old, 38.1% reported that UI symptoms cause interruption of their work [12]. Fultz et al., in a large cross-section of 3364 employed women in the USA, observed that UI negatively impacts on several aspects of work, such as, concentration (45%), performance of physical activities (64%), self-confidence (77%) and completion of tasks without interruptions (74%) [29]. To manage UI symptoms, the most common strategies used by these workers were wearing pads (44%) and frequent bathroom breaks (47%) [29].

Urinary incontinence is also associated with absence from work [19, 29], however, according to our knowledge, no studies have objectively quantified this aspect. Nevertheless, considering the impact of UI on the work described above, it can be confirmed that UI greatly impacts on the productivity of women and on their professional well-being at workplace [12, 29, 30].

2.3. Sexual

Urinary Incontinence is also associated with adverse effects on female sexual function. The prevalence of female sexual dysfunction in incontinent women has been estimated to be from 25 to 50% [31-33]. According to the International Consensus Development Conference on Female Sexual Dysfunction, female sexual dysfunction includes problems such as sexual desire disorder, sexual arousal disorder, orgasmic disorder and sexual pain disorder [34]. Several studies have documented that women with UI have significantly lower scores of desire, arousal, lubrication, orgasm and satisfaction compared with control subjects [35-37].

These data suggest that incontinent women experienced sexual dysfunction in all phases of female sex response cycle [34].

Regarding UI types, sexual desire disorder has been shown to be more experienced by women with stress UI (47%), whilst orgasmic disorder has been mainly presented in women suffering from urge UI (46%) [36]. Mixed UI is the UI type that most impacts on women sexual function [36-39]. This happens, probably because mixed UI combines the causal factors of the other types of UI, which may cause more sexual problems [37]. Due to this sexual dysfunction, many women feel unattractive and experience fear of urine leakage during sexual intercourse, embarrassment due to urine odor and fear of the perception by the sexual partner [35, 36, 40]. These feelings lead to some women to avoid intimate sexual relationships [38]. Nilsson et al., in a research to assess the impact of UI on women's sexual life, found that almost half of the sample studied (43%) stated that the urinary symptoms impaired their sexual life and 49% expressed worries about having urine leakage during sexual activity [40].

Sexual dysfunction is therefore, a major problem among women with UI, impacting on women sexual quality of life and therefore in their interpersonal relationships.

2.4. Physical

Urinary Incontinence can be found in women who practice high-impact sports, specifically in athletes whose activities involve jumping [5, 41, 42]. In a study with 106 female athletes involved in athletics, basketball and indoor football, 41.5% had UI and its majority (61.4%) experienced stress UI symptoms [4].

The qualitative data of this study verified that activities requiring physical effort and jumping were those causing more restrictions in athletes' physical performance [4]. To deal with UI symptoms during physical activity, athletes use some strategies such as preventive urination and restriction of liquid intake [4, 43]. When these strategies are not sufficient, athletes perform physical activities in a restricted way, modifying their athletic technique [4]. These data provided significant evidence that UI affects negatively the physical and competitive performance of athletes. Furthermore, in other studies investigating the impact of UI on women practicing sport it was found that many women tend to abandon sports to avoid urine leakage during exercise [44, 45].

Nevertheless, UI do not only have an impact on the athletes' physical performance, the wellbeing associated with sports practice is also affected since athletes experience feelings of concern, fear that a new activity might trigger another leakage and frustration about the noticeability of urine leakage to others [4]. Furthermore, the impact of UI can be more concerning since it is being experienced by very young females. Carls, in a study with high school and college-age female athletes with ages between 14 and 21 years old, found that 38% suffer from stress UI [11]. In addition, the majority of athletes experiencing UI never talks to anyone about their leakage and do not seek help from health professionals [4]. Therefore, UI can be a stressful condition for young females and negatively influence their personal and competitive lifelong.

It can be more concerning when despite this marked evidence, health professionals, other professionals involved in athletes' performance and the general community experience lack of awareness of UI. This is reflected by pelvic floor muscle exercises not being routinely used in athletes' training plans, despite of being a preventive strategy for UI [4, 11, 41].

3. Conservative Treatment: Physical Therapies

Urinary Incontinence has multiple implications on women's quality of life. Its treatment is crucial for women to regain control of their lives. According to the Society of Obstetricians and Gynaecologists of Canada Clinical Practice Guideline [8], Scottish Intercollegiate Guidelines Network [10] and European Association of Urology [46], this condition should ideally be treated with conservative treatments in primary care settings prior to any specialized care, such as surgical procedures.

Conservative treatments are very well tolerated by women, vaginal bleeding or urinary infection, which are the adverse effects associated with these types of treatments, are rarely observed [47, 48]. Conservative treatments include lifestyle interventions, behavioral therapies, pharmacological treatments and physical therapies [9, 49].

There is a lack of evidence about lifestyle interventions and behavioral therapies and thus these interventions alone are not frequently recommended for UI management [9, 10]. Usually they are used in combination with other conservative treatments, such as pharmacological and physical [9]. Furthermore, the scarce literature about lifestyle interventions and behavioral therapies is only about UI treatment and not for its prevention [9, 10]. Pharmacological treatments, although may be effective, have some adverse effects and are also recommended to use as an adjuvant to other conservative or surgical treatments [50].

Physical therapies are the only interventions included in the conservative treatment with evidence not only to treat but also to prevent UI [50, 51]. Furthermore, these interventions not only can be applied in the clinical setting, but also at home [9]. Some evidence shows that physical therapies are associated with treatment high success rates when women are correctly instructed and advised [52, 53]. Physical therapies improve or restore pelvic floor function and bladder function control [54], increase women's understanding of lower urinary tract (dys)function [55] and improve women's quality of life [47], contributing to prevent and improve the urine leakage [47, 56]. The most recommended physical therapies for UI prevention and treatment, according to Scottish Intercollegiate Guidelines Network, National Collaborating Centre for Women's and Children's Health and European Association of Urology, are a combination or an individual application of pelvic floor muscle training, vaginal cones, biofeedback and electrical stimulation [8-10, 46].

3.1. Pelvic Floor Muscle Training

Pelvic floor muscle training includes the contraction of the pelvic floor musculature, i.e., the levator ani, the external anal sphincter and the striated urethral sphincter [57, 58]. Specifically, it is composed by two basic principles, the strength training and the skill training [59]. The first one involves gaining muscle hypertrophy by repeating specific exercises over weeks to months, improving urethral compression during activity, which consequently decreases the frequency of urine leakage episodes with time [59]. The second one involves learning how to contract the pelvic floor muscles during activities that cause urine leakage and therefore, decrease of losses occurs immediately [59]. The theory behind these two principals is that a strong and fast contraction of the pelvic floor muscles will compress the urethra. This compression will increase the maximal urethral closure pressure and the functional urethral length, and cause a significant improvement in the strength of the pelvic floor muscles [47, 56, 60], preventing urine leakage during an immediate pressure increase of the intra-abdominal area (e.g., coughing or jumping) [57, 61]. Hence, during an efficient contraction of the pelvic floor muscles, the urethra may be pressed against the pubic symphysis, which increases the urethral closure pressure, the stabilization of the pelvic floor muscles and the resistance to downward movement [61, 62]. Furthermore, the pelvic floor muscle training reduces the urine leakage [56, 60, 63, 64] and the number of pad changes [59, 63].

The idea of applying pelvic floor muscle training to treat stress UI has been introduced by Kegel in 1956 [65]. Over the years, several benefits were seen with this intervention on the number of urine leakage episodes in incontinent women [46, 56, 63] and on the pelvic floor muscle strength in continent and incontinent women [46, 47, 56, 66]. Currently, pelvic floor muscle training is recommended as a preventive strategy for women in their first pregnancy (grade of recommendation A) and as first-line management for women with all types of UI (grade of recommendation A) [46, 57].

Pelvic floor muscle training is a preventive strategy for asymptomatic women, such as natal and postnatal women [51, 66, 67] and in female elite athletes [41]. In a single-blind randomized controlled trial, which involved healthy nulliparous pregnant women, pelvic floor muscle strength was significantly higher in the women submitted to intensive pelvic floor muscle training [66]. However, other conservative treatments, such as vaginal cones, biofeedback and electrical stimulation, should also be available to women who are unable to contract their pelvic floor muscles correctly (approximately 30% of these women) [47, 68].

Pelvic floor muscle training has also been found to be associated with an improvement on the quality of life of incontinent women [47, 60, 64]. In a single-blind, randomized controlled trial, the quality of life increased significantly in 28.4% of the incontinent women treated with pelvic floor muscle training (after six months) [47]. However, the success of the pelvic floor muscle training often depends on women's motivation and cooperation, demonstrated by their adherence to the daily exercises, and on the physical therapist's enthusiasm and dedication [47, 69]. Furthermore, the efficacy of this intervention is also highly dependent on the women's education and instruction [70-74] and also on physical therapist's knowledge [69]. For these reasons, an intensive and supervised pelvic floor muscle training associated with an educative program is necessary, so women can prevent or understand their condition and choose the most adequate treatment [47, 60]. Only this way it will be possible to reduce the prevalence of UI in the long term [59, 64, 75].

Despite pelvic floor muscle training being considered a safe and simple intervention in the prevention and treatment of UI [51], it is not possible to determine whether muscle training is more effective than other treatments because of the limitations found in the studies design and methodology [76]. Some data suggest greater efficacy in the treatment of women suffering from stress UI when a combination of different methods is applied, i.e., pelvic floor muscle training with other conservative techniques, such as pharmacological therapy [59], biofeedback [60] and vaginal cones [54, 69].

3.2. Vaginal Cones

In 1985, Plevnik proposed the use of pelvic floor muscle training by retraining a cone in the vagina, which provides a positive feedback, helping women with stress UI or mixed UI to become aware of the pelvic floor muscles [46, 77]. The idea was to reduce the degree of difficulty in learning the exercise and facilitate the performance of the exercises in the correct way [54, 63].

The vaginal cones (grade of recommendation A [57] or B [46]) are positioned in the vagina above the level of the pelvic floor muscles [57]. Passive and active contractions of these muscles are necessary to avoid the cones from slipping out of the vagina [57]. The sets of vaginal cones consist of cones of equal volume but different weights (Figure 1) [78]. Thus, women insert a cone of increasingly heavier weight as they are able to retain it [57, 69]. The feeling of "losing the cone" from the vagina is thought to initiate a powerful sensory biofeedback response, causing the pelvic floor muscles to contract around the cone to retrain it against gravity [54, 69].

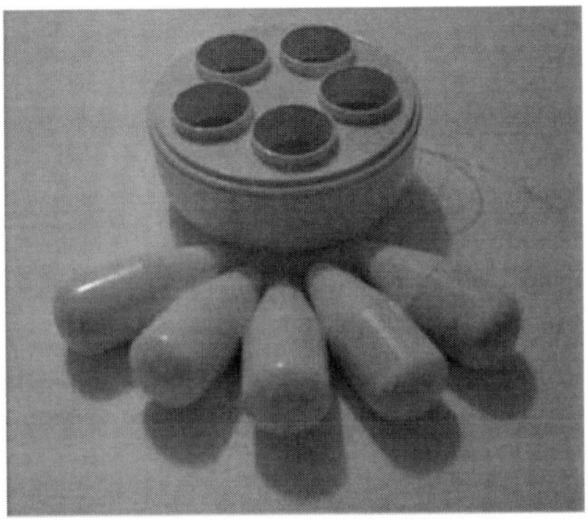

Figure 1. Vaginal cones.

Herbison, Plevnik and Mantle in a systematic review about vaginal cones for pelvic floor muscle training applied to UI treatment, conclude that the use of the vaginal cones is more effective than no active treatment in women with stress UI [79]. It is recommended as an easy and cost-effective method of UI treatment that can be added to other options of treatment such as to pelvic floor muscle training [54, 69]. After vaginal cones being applied in the treatment of women with stress UI it was verified a significant decrease in the amount and frequency of urine leakage [54, 63, 69] and in the pad weight [47]; an increase of the pelvic floor muscles strength as well as an improvement on physical activities [54, 77]. However, significant improvements have not been found when using vaginal cones to treat UI regarding sexual life, daily life limitations, interpersonal relationships and avoidance of particular places [54]. Furthermore, the side-effects and discomfort of vaginal cones lead to a low patient compliance which limits the clinical applicability of the cones in the long term [46, 54, 63].

In an attempt to solve these disadvantages, a similar conservative treatment with vaginal balls has been tested recently [56]. There is some evidence that this approach is an effective treatment in increasing the pelvic floor muscle strength and in improving urine leakage [54,

56, 63, 69]. However, there is a need for further randomized controlled trials to evaluate the real benefits of vaginal balls comparatively to vaginal cones for the treatment of incontinent women [75].

3.3. Biofeedback

The research using biofeedback (Figure 2) as a treatment for re-education of the pelvic floor muscles began with Kegel's early studies through the use of a perineometer, which have demonstrated a 90% improvement in urinary symptoms [65]. Biofeedback (grade of recommendation A [46, 57]) can promote awareness of the physiological action of the pelvic floor muscles by visual, tactile or auditory resources and thus, increase the success rate of pelvic floor exercises [1, 54, 60, 78].

The primary component of the biofeedback applied to UI is teaching women how to identify and exercise the pelvic floor muscles; and how to use these muscles to prevent urine leakage by aborting detrusor contractions and occluding the urethra during contractions that cannot be inhibited (during an increase in the intra-abdominal pressure) [60, 80]. Thereby, biofeedback allows women to gain or regain control over the contractions of their pelvic floor muscles, maximizing force and sustaining contractions, which is crucial to build strength [54, 80].

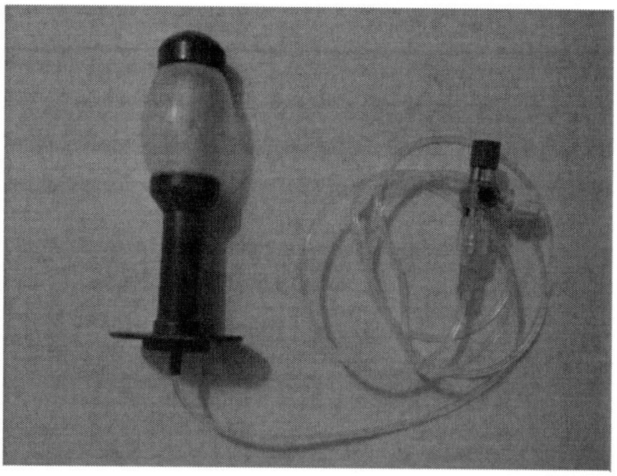

Figure 2. Vaginal probe for biofeedback.

Several studies have been encouraging the use of biofeedback and suggest that adding biofeedback to pelvic floor muscle training might be more effective than pelvic floor muscle training alone [81, 82]. The use of biofeedback has shown to contribute to i) an increase of maximal pelvic floor muscle contractile power and ii) an improvement in the degree of UI and in the pad test results [54]. Seo, Yoon and Kim, 2004, in a randomized prospective trial, reported that the tendency of women to avoid particular places due to urinary leakage, the effect of urinary leakage on physical activities and the quality of life showed significant improvements after treatments with biofeedback [54]. This type of conservative treatment seems to improve motivation in an exercise program and allows progress to be monitored [60].

In spite of the contribution of biofeedback to improve pelvic floor muscle strength, there is a persistent essential disadvantage of vaginal biofeedback [60]. Intra-vaginal pressure increases not only due to contractions of the pelvic floor muscles, but also due to an increase in the abdominal pressure and consequently, if women contract the abdominal muscles (instead of contracting pelvic floor muscles), the perineometer may give misleading information on the intensity of the pelvic floor muscles contraction [60]. Furthermore, because of diversity of treatment protocols, the findings concerning the role of biofeedback on UI treatment are inconclusive [76]. Further research is therefore, needed to analyze the effectiveness of pelvic floor muscle exercises and adjunctive biofeedback on UI treatment [81].

3.4. Electrical Stimulation

Electrical Stimulation of the pelvic floor muscles (grade of recommendation C [46, 57]) was originally proposed in 1963 to treat fecal incontinence [83], stress UI, urge UI or mixed UI [46]. It has been performed in three different ways: percutaneously using a needle or surface electrode, intra-anally using an anal electrode and intravaginally using a vaginal probe (Figure 3) [84]. The type and the characteristics of electrical stimulation may be adapted to the clinical situation [53], e.g., to treat stress UI a frequency of approximately 50 Hz [46, 53], twice a day, during 6 months is recommended [46] and for treating mixed UI [53] and urge UI low frequencies [46, 53] from 4-10 Hz, twice a day, during 9 weeks are recommended [46].

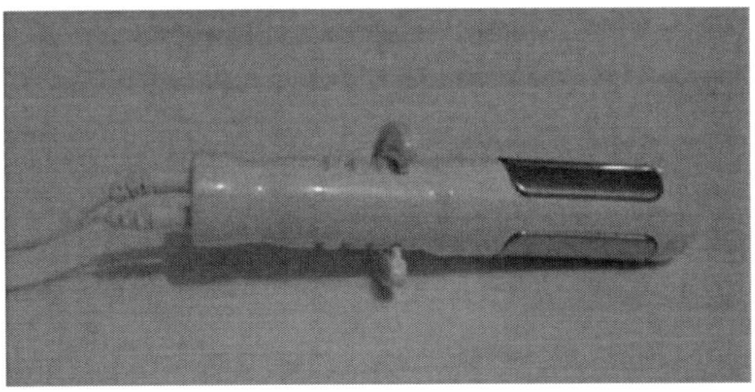

Figure 3. Vaginal probe for electrical stimulation.

This conservative treatment refers to electric current, usually by the use of vaginal electrodes, to stimulate the pelvic floor muscles through their nerve supply or to normalize the reflex activity [1, 85]. Therefore, electrical stimulation induces a reflex contraction of the striated para-urethral and peri-urethral muscles, accompanied by a simultaneous reflex inhibition of the detrusor muscle, stimulating afferents fibers of the pudendal nerve [55].

Numerous clinical trials have reported on the safety and efficacy of electrical stimulation in treating stress UI and mixed UI [53, 61]. Specifically, it has been shown to improve pelvic floor muscles strength and endurance [86-88]; to reduce the number of leakage episodes and the amount of urine losses in pad testing and to improve quality of life in incontinent women [47]. Furthermore, Luber and Wolde-Tsadik, in a study aiming to explore the effectiveness of electrical stimulation in women with stress UI, found that this physical treatment assists incontinent women to become conscious of their pelvic floor muscles function and concluded that electrical stimulation should be used to facilitate biofeedback-enhanced pelvic floor muscles rehabilitation in these women [48]. However, other studies reported no differences between the electrical stimulation treatment group and the control group regarding the number of urine leakage, pelvic floor muscles strength and quality of life [89, 90]. On the other hand, the majority of the studies that reported good results using electrical stimulation to treat stress UI were performed without a control group [48, 90, 91]. Therefore, the electrical stimulation as a monotherapy in treating UI has been questioned [91].

4. Safety of Physical Treatments

The practice of UI physical interventions should be encouraged because it is associated with minimal adverse outcomes, unlike pharmacological and surgical treatments [57]. The use of drugs for UI treatment produces many side-effects such as dry mouth and inability to void in particular, compromising compliance and causing the recurrence of UI [92]. Furthermore, the risks of surgical treatment, such as infection, urethral injuries, hemorrhage, are not always accepted by women [47, 50].

Adverse events, such as vaginal bleeding, vaginal erosions or urinary infection, were rarely associated with physical treatments [47, 48]. In a single-blind randomized controlled trial which compare different physical treatments in the management of women with stress UI verified that this type of interventions were very well tolerated by women and no adverse events could be correlated with any treatment [47]. Moreover, these strategies are non-invasive and do not exclude future options that may be necessary to treat UI [55].

5. Treatment-Seeking for UI

Despite the multiple implications of UI on women's quality of life and the number of UI physical treatments available, with high grades of recommendation, it is uncommon to find professionals using these strategies to prevent the condition [4, 11, 41]. Furthermore, many incontinent women do not seek help from health professionals. In the Norwegian EPINCONT Study, only 26% of the incontinent women consulted a physician because of their UI [93]. This is in line with the data from a review where it has been reported that fewer than 50% of women with UI discuss their symptoms with health professionals [94].

One of the major barriers for women to seek treatment for UI is their belief that is a normal phenomenon associated with aging and childbirth, instead considering UI as a pathological condition [25, 26]. The shame and the embarrassment experienced due to the negative social stigma of UI may also restrict the discussion of this topic with their health professionals [4, 26]. Another reason explaining the low treatment-seeking rates among UI women are the lack of knowledge regarding the available treatment options and places [4]. Carls, in a study with 86 young athletes found that 91% of these athletes had no knowledge of pelvic muscle exercises and that 83% of the athletes with stress UI would perform the exercises it if they knew how to [11].

Primary care health professionals involved in women's health, aware of the barriers for women to seek UI treatment and of the potential adverse effects of UI on women's quality of life, should assess the presence of UI symptoms during women contacts [9]. In women reporting risk factors associated with UI, health professionals should recommend pelvic floor muscle exercises as a preventive intervention [50]. Specifically, professionals involved in athletes' performance should be aware that sport practice is a risk factor for UI and therefore, should include a regimen of pelvic floor muscle exercises in athletes' training plans. Women suffering from UI should be offered information about treatment options available and respective places. Furthermore, health professionals should also promote a greater understanding about the potential improvements achieved through these interventions, when if applied to prevent or treat the condition [10]. The implementation of these recommendations could help to encourage women to seek and adhere to UI treatments.

Conclusion

Urinary Incontinence is a prevalent condition among young and adult women [2-5] which can have greatly negative effects on various dimensions of their lives, namely, psychological, social, sexual and physical [12, 14, 15]. Due to these adverse effects, interventions for UI prevention and treatment are essential. This condition can be managed through conservative and surgical treatments however, conservative are recommended as first-line management [9]. Physical therapies are a group of conservative interventions which have shown that can be implemented as a UI preventive strategy and/or as a treatment intervention. These therapies are safe, non-invasive, very well tolerated by women and do not exclude future treatment options [55].

Despite these available interventions, many women do not seek help for their UI and prefer their own ways to cope with this problem. Thus, more attention regarding UI should be given by all health professionals involved in women's health. Specifically, health professionals should increase awareness about UI among women and general public, provide information about prevention, available treatments and different possible delivering settings.

References

[1] Abrams P, Cardozo L, Fall M, Griffiths D, Rosier P, Ulmsten U, et al. The standardisation of terminology of lower urinary tract function: Report from the standardisation sub-committee of the International Continence Society. *Neurourology and Urodynamics*. 2002;21(2):167-78.

[2] Nitti VW. The Prevalence of Urinary Incontinence. *Reviews in Urology*. 2001;3(1):S2-S6.

[3] Hunskaar S, Lose G, Sykes D, Voss S. The prevalence of urinary incontinence in women in four European countries. *British Journal of Urology International*. 2004;93(3):324-30.

[4] Jácome C, Oliveira D, Marques A, Sá-Couto P. Prevalence and impact of urinary incontinence among female athletes. *International Journal of Gynecology & Obstetrics.* 2011;114(1):60-3.

[5] Thyssen HH, Clevin L, Olesen S, Lose G. Urinary Incontinence in Elite Female Athletes and Dancers. *International Urogynecology Journal.* 2002;13(1):15-7.

[6] Buckley BS, Lapitan MCM. Prevalence of Urinary Incontinence in Men, Women, and Children-Current Evidence: Findings of the Fourth International Consultation on Incontinence. *Urology.* 2010;76(2):265-70.

[7] Hannestad YS, Rortveit G, Sandvik H, Hunskaar S. A community-based epidemiological survey of female urinary incontinence:: The Norwegian EPINCONT Study. *Journal of Clinical Epidemiology.* 2000;53(11):1150-7.

[8] Robert M, Ross S. SOGC Clinical Practice Guideline: Conservative Management of Urinary Incontinence. *Journal of obstetrics and gynaecology Canada.* 2006;28(12):1113-8.

[9] National Collaborating Centre for Women's and Children's Health. Urinary incontinence: the management of urinary incontinence in women. London: Royal College of Obstetricians and Gynaecologists Press; 2006. Available from: http://www.nice.org.uk/nicemedia/live/10996/30281/30281.pdf.

[10] Scottish Intercollegiate Guidelines Network. Management of urinary incontinence in primary care - A national clinical guideline 2004. Available from: *http://www.sign.ac.uk/guidelines/fulltext/79/index.html.*

[11] Carls C. The Prevalence of Stress Urinary Incontinence in High School and College-Age Female Athletes in the Midwest: Implications for Education and Prevention. *Urologic Nursing.* 2007;27(1):21-4.

[12] Lasserre A, Pelat C, Guéroult V, Hanslik T, Chartier-Kastler E, Blanchon T, et al. Urinary Incontinence in French Women: Prevalence, Risk Factors, and Impact on Quality of Life. *European Urology.* 2009;56(1):177-83.

[13] Schultz SE, Kopec JA. Impact of chronic conditions. *Health Reports.* 2003;14(4):41-53.

[14] Broome B. The impact of urinary incontinence on self-efficacy and quality of life. *Health and Quality of Life Outcomes.* 2003;1(1):1-3.

[15] Knorst M, Resende T, Goldim J. Clinical profile, quality of life and depressive symptoms of women with urinary incontince attending a university hospital. *Revista Brasileira de Fisioterapia.* 2011;15(2):109-16.

[16] Dugan E, Cohen SJ, Bland DR, Preisser JS, Davis CC, Suggs PK, et al. The association of depressive symptoms and urinary incontinence among older adults. *Journal of the American Geriatrics Society.* 2000;48(4):413-6.

[17] Sung VW, West DS, Hernandez AL, Wheeler Ii TL, Myers DL, Subak LL. Association between urinary incontinence and depressive symptoms in overweight and obese women. *American Journal of Obstetrics and Gynecology.* 2009;200(5):557.e1-e5.

[18] Perry S, McGrother CW, Turner K. An investigation of the relationship between anxiety and depression and urge incontinence in women: Development of a psychological model. *British Journal of Health Psychology.* 2006;11(3):463-82.

[19] Vigod SN, Stewart DE. Major Depression in Female Urinary Incontinence. *Psychosomatics.* 2006 April 1, 2006;47(2):147-51.

[20] Lose G. The Burden of Stress Urinary Incontinence. *European Urology Supplements.* 2005;4(1):5-10.

[21] Nygaard I, Turvey C, Burns TL, Crischilles E, Wallace R. Urinary incontinence and depression in middle-aged United States women. *Obstetrics & Gynecology*. 2003;101(1):149-56.
[22] Melville J, Delaney K, Newton K, Katon W. Incontinence severity and major depression in incontinent women. Obstetrics & Gynecology. 2005;106(3):585-92.
[23] Lim JR, Bak CW, Lee JB. Comparison of anxiety between patients with mixed incontinence and those with stress urinary incontinence. *Scandinavian Journal of Urology & Nephrology*. 2007;41(5):403-6.
[24] Bogner HR, O'Donnell AJ, de Vries HF, Northington GM, Joo JH. The temporal relationship between anxiety disorders and urinary incontinence among community-dwelling adults. *Journal of Anxiety Disorders*. 2011;25(2):203-8.
[25] Coyne KS, Kvasz M, Ireland AM, Milsom I, Kopp ZS, Chapple CR. Urinary Incontinence and its Relationship to Mental Health and Health-Related Quality of Life in Men and Women in Sweden, the United Kingdom, and the United States. *European Urology*. 2012;61(1):88-95..
[26] Hemachandra NN, Rajapaksa LC, Manderson L. A "usual occurrence:" Stress incontinence among reproductive aged women in Sri Lanka. *Social Science & Medicine*. 2009;69(9):1395-401.
[27] Yip S-K, Cardozo L. Psychological morbidity and female urinary incontinence. *Best Practice & Research Clinical Obstetrics & Gynaecology*. 2007;21(2):321-9.
[28] Fultz NH, Burgio K, Diokno AC, Kinchen KS, Obenchain R, Bump RC. Burden of stress urinary incontinence for community-dwelling women. *American Journal of Obstetrics and Gynecology*. 2003;189(5):1275-82.
[29] Fultz N, Girts T, Kinchen K, Nygaard I, Pohl G, Sternfeld B. Prevalence, management and impact of urinary incontinence in the workplace. *Occupational Medicine*. 2005 October 2005;55(7):552-7.
[30] Tubaro A. Defining overactive bladder: Epidemiology and burden of disease. *Urology*. 2004;64(Supplement 1):2-6.
[31] Sutherst JR. Sexual Dysfunction and Urinary Incontinence. *BJOG: An International Journal of Obstetrics & Gynaecology*. 1979;86(5):387-8.
[32] Ellerkmann RM, Cundiff GW, Melick CF, Nihira MA, Leffler K, Bent AE. Correlation of symptoms with location and severity of pelvic organ prolapse. *American Journal of Obstetrics and Gynecology*. 2001;185(6):1332-8.
[33] Temml C, Haidinger G, Schmidbauer J, Schatzl G, Madersbacher S. Urinary incontinence in both sexes: Prevalence rates and impact on quality of life and sexual life. *Neurourology and Urodynamics*. 2000;19(3):259-71.
[34] Basson R, Berman J, Burnett A, Derogatis L, Ferguson D, Fourcroy J, et al. Report of the International Consensus Development Conference on Female Sexual Dysfunction: Definitions and Classifications. *The Journal of Urology*. 2000;163(3):888-93.
[35] Aslan G, Koseoglu H, Sadik O, Gimen S, Cihan A, Esen A. Sexual function in women with urinary incontinence. *International Journal of Impotence Research*. 2004;17(3):248-51.
[36] Salonia A, Zanni G, Nappi RE, Briganti A, Dehò F, Fabbri F, et al. Sexual Dysfunction is Common in Women with Lower Urinary Tract Symptoms and Urinary Incontinence: Results of a Cross-Sectional Study. *European Urology*. 2004;45(5):642-8.

[37] Sen I, Onaran M, Aksakal N, Acar C, Tan M, Acar A, et al. The impact of urinary incontinence on female sexual function. *Advances in Therapy*. 2006;23(6):999-1008.

[38] Coksuer H, Ercan CM, Haliloglu B, Yucel M, Cam C, Kabaca C, et al. Does urinary incontinence subtypes affect sexual function? *European Journal of Obstetrics & Gynecology and Reproductive Biology*. 2011;159(1):213-217.

[39] Ozkan S, Ogce F, Cakir D. Quality of life and sexual function of women with urinary incontinence. *Japan Journal of Nursing Science*. 2011;8(1):11-9.

[40] Nilsson M, Lalos O, Lindkvist H, Lalos A. Impact of female urinary incontinence and urgency on women's and their partners' sexual life. *Neurourology and Urodynamics*. 2011;30(7):1276-80.

[41] Bø K. Urinary Incontinence, Pelvic Floor Dysfunction, Exercise and Sport. *Sports Medicine*. 2004;34(7):451-64.

[42] Nygaard IE. Does prolonged high-impact activity contribute to later urinary incontinence? A retrospective cohort study of female olympians. *Obstetrics & Gynecology*. 1997;90(5):718-22.

[43] Eliasson K, Nordlander I, Mattsson E, Larson B, Hammarström M. Prevalence of urinary leakage in nulliparous women with respect to physical activity and micturition habits. *International Urogynecology Journal*. 2004;15(3):149-53.

[44] Salvatore S, Serati M, Laterza RM, Uccella S, Torella M, Bolis P. The impact of urinary stress incontinence in young and middle-age women practicing recreational sport activity: an epidemiological study. *British journal of sports medicine*. 2009;43(14):1115-8.

[45] Eliasson K, Edner A, Mattsson E. Urinary incontinence in very young and mostly nulliparous women with a history of regular organised high-impact trampoline training: occurrence and risk factors. International *Urogynecology Journal*. 2008;19(5):687-96.

[46] Schröder A, Abrams P, Andersson K-E, Artibani W, Chapple CR, Drake MJ, et al. Guidelines on Urinary Incontinence. European Association of Urology,2010.

[47] Castro RA, Arruda RM, Zanetti MRD, Santos PD, Sartori MGE, Girão MJBC. Single-blind, randomized, controlled trial of pelvic floor muscle training, electrical stimulation, vaginal cones, and no active treatment in the management of stress urinary incontinence. *Clinics*. 2008;63(4):465-72.

[48] Luber KM, Wolde-Tsadik G. Efficacy of functional electrical stimulation in treating genuine stress incontinence: a randomized clinical trial. *Neurourology and Urodynamics*. 1997;16(6):543-51.

[49] Dmochowski R, Miklos J, Norton P, Zinner N, Yalcin I, Bump R. Duloxetine versus placebo for the treatment of North American women with stress urinary. *Journal of Urology*. 2004;170(4 Pt 1):1259-63.

[50] Wilson PD. Incontinence International Continence Society; 2005. Available from: *http://www.icsoffice.org/Publications/ICI_3/book.pdf.*

[51] Hay-Smith J, Mørkved S, Fairbrother K, Herbison G. Pelvic floor muscle training for prevention and treatment of urinary and faecal incontinence in antenatal and postnatal women . *The Cochrane Database of Systematic Reviews*. 2009(1).

[52] Aukee P, Immonen P, Laaksonen DE, Laippala P, Penttinen J, Airaksinen O. The effect of home biofeedback training on stress incontinence. *Acta Obstetricia et Gynecologica Scandinavica*. 2004;83(10):973-7.

[53] Barroso JVC, Ramos JGL, Martins-Costa S, Sanches PRS, Muller AF. Transvaginal electrical stimulation in the treatment of urinary incontinence. *British Journal of Urology International*. 2004;93(3):319-23.

[54] Seo JT, Yoon H, Kim YH. A randomized prospective study comparing new vaginal cone and FES-Biofeedback. *Yonsei Medical Journal*. 2004;45(5):879-84.

[55] Berghmans LCM, Hendriks HJM, Bie RAD, Doorn ESCVWV, Bo K, Kerrebroeck PEVV. Conservative treatment of urge urinary incontinence in women: a systematic review of randomized clinical trials. *British Journal of Urology International*. 2000;85(3):254-63.

[56] Arvonen T, Fianu-Jonasson A, Tyni-Lenné R. Effectiveness of Two Conservative Modes of Physical Therapy in Women With Urinary Stress Incontinence. *Neurourology and Urodynamics*. 2001;20(5):591-9.

[57] Robert M, Ross S. Society of Obstetricians and Gynaecologists of Canada Clinical Practice Guideline: Conservative Management of Urinary Incontinence. *Journal of obstetrics and gynaecology Canada*. 2006;28(12):1113-8.

[58] Dumoulin C, Hay-Smith J. Pelvic floor muscle training versus no treatment, or inactive control treatments, for urinary incontinence in women. *Cochrane database systematic reviews*. 2010(1).

[59] Ghoniem GM, Leeuwen JSV, Elser DM, Freeman RM, Zhao YD, Yalcin I, et al. A randomized controlled trial of duloxetine alone, pelvic floor muscle training alone, combined treatment and no active treatment in women with stress urinary incontinence. *The Journal of Urology*. 2005;173(5):1647-53.

[60] Wong KS, Fung KY, Fung SM, Fung CW, Tang CH. Biofeedback of Pelvic Floor Muscles in the Management of Genuine Stress Incontinence in Chinese Women: Randomised controlled trial. *Physiotherapy*. 2001;87(12):644-8.

[61] Bø K. Physiotherapy to treat genuine stress incontinence. *Survey MIIC*, editor1996.

[62] Bø K. Pelvic floor muscle training is effective in treatment of female stress urinary incontinence, but how does it work? *International Urogynecology Journal*. 2004;15(2):76-84.

[63] Cammu H, Nylen MV. Pelvic floor exercises versus vaginal weight cones in genuine stress incontinence. *European Journal of Obstretics & Gynecology and Reproductive Biology*. 1998;77(1):89-93.

[64] Dumoulin C, Hay-Smith J. Pelvic floor muscle training versus no treatment for urinary incontinence in women: A Cochrane systematic review. *European Journal of Physical and Rehabilitation Medicine*. 2008;44(1):47-63.

[65] Kegel A. Stress incontinence of urine in women: physiologic treatment. *Journal - International College of Surgeons*. 1956;25(4 Part 1):487-99.

[66] Mørkved S, Bø K, Schei B, Salvesen KÅ. *Pelvic Floor Muscle Training During Pregnancy to Prevent Urinary Incontinence: A Single-Blind Randomized Controlled Trial*. The American College of Obstetricians and Gynecologists. 2003;101(2):313-9.

[67] Reilly ETC, Freeman RM, Waterfield MR, A.E. Waterfield, Steggles P, Pedlar F. Prevention of postpartum stress incontinence in primigravidae with increased bladder neck mobility: a randomised controlled trial of antenatal pelvic floor exercises. *BJOG: an International Journal of Obstetrics and Gynaecology*. 2002;109(1):68-76.

[68] Bø K. Pelvic floor muscle strength and response to pelvic floor muscle training for stress urinary incontinence. *Neurourology and Urodynamics*. 2003;22(1):654-8.

[69] Oláh KS, Bridges N, Denning J, Farrar DJ. The conservative management of patients with symptoms of stress incontinence: A randomized, prospective study comparing weighted vaginal cones and interferential therapy. *American Journal of Obstetrics & Gynecology*. 1990;162(1):87-92.

[70] Tapp A, Cardozo L, Hills B, Barnick C, editors. Who benefits from physiotherapy? *18th annual meeting of the international continence society; 1986; Boston.*

[71] Bump R, Hurt W, Fantl A, Wyman J. Assessment of Kegel pelvic muscle exercise performance after brief verbal instruction. *American Journal of Obstetrics & Gynecology*. 1991;165(2):327-9.

[72] Hahn I, Milson I, Fall M, Ekelund P. Long-term results of pelvic training in female stress urinary incontinence. *British Journal of Urology*. 1993;72(4):421-7.

[73] Hong J. The efficacy of pelvic floor muscle exercise in patients with genuine stress incontinence. *Korean Journal of Urology*. 1997;38(6):639-43.

[74] Hendriks C, Michelle V. Pelvic floor muscle exercises: 5 years later. *Urology* 1995;45(1):113-7.

[75] Wilson PD, Herbison GP. A randomized controlled trial of pelvic floor muscle exercises to treat postnatal urinary incontinence. *International Urogynecology Journal.* 1998;9(5):257-64.

[76] Hay-Smith E, Bø K, Berghmans L, Hendriks H, de Bie R, van Waalwijk van Doorn E. Pelvic floor muscle training for urinary incontinence in women. *The Cochrane Database of Systematic Reviews*. 2003(1).

[77] Plevnik S, editor. New method for testing and strengthening of pelvic floor muscles. *15th annual meeting of the international continence society*; 1985.

[78] Thakar R, Stanton S. Regular review: management of urinary incontinence in women. *British Medical Journal*. 2000;321(7272):1326-31.

[79] Herbison G, Dean N. Weighted vaginal cones for urinary incontinence. *The Cochrane Database of Systematic Reviews*. 2002(1).

[80] Burgio KL, Goode PS, Locher JL, Umlauf MG, Roth DL, Richter HE, et al. Behavioral Training With and Without Biofeedback in the Treatment of Urge Incontinence in Older Women. *Journal of American Medical Association*. 2002;288(18):2293-9.

[81] Burns PA, Pranikoff K, Nochajski TH, Hadley EC, Levy KJ, Ory MG. A comparison of effectiveness of biofeedback and pelvic muscle exercise treatment of stress incontinence in older community-dwelling women. *Journal of Gerontoloy: medical sciences*. 1993;48(4):M167-M74.

[82] Berghmans LCM, Frederiks CMA, Bie RAd, Weil EHJ, Smeets LWH, Doorn ESCvWv, et al. Efficacy of Biofeedback, When Included With Pelvic Floor Muscle Exercise Treatment, for Genuine Stress Incontinence. *Neurourology and Urodynamics*. 1996;15(1):37-52.

[83] Caldwell K. The electrical control of sphincteric incontinence. *Lancet*. 1963;2:174-5.

[84] Yamanishi T, Yasuda K, Sakakibara R, Hattori T, Suda S. Randomized, double-blind study of electrical stimulation for urinary incontinence due to detrusor overactivity. *Urology*. 2000;55(3):353-7.

[85] Berghmans LCM, Hendriks HJM, Bo K, Hay-Smith E, De Bies R, Van Waalwijk, et al. Conservative treatment of stress urinary incontinence in women: a systematic review of randomized clinical trials. *British Journal of Urology* 1998;82(2):181-9.

[86] Amaro J, Gameiro M, Padovani C. Treatment of urinary stress incontinence by intravaginal electrical stimulation and pelvic floor physiotherapy. *International Urogynecology Journal*. 2003;14(3):204-8.

[87] Jeyaseelan S, Haslam E, J W, Roe B, Oldham J. An evaluation of a new pattern of electrical stimulation as a treatment of urinary stress incontinence: a randomized, double-blind, controlled trial. *Clinical Rehabilitation*. 2000;14(6):631-40.

[88] Wang A, Wang Y, Chen M. Single-blind, randomized trial of pelvic floor muscle training, biofeedback-assisted pelvic floor muscle training, and electrical stimulation in the management of overactive bladder. *Urology*. 2004;63(1):61-6.

[89] Spruijt J, Vierhout M, Verstraeten R, Janssens J, Burger C. Vaginal electrical stimulation of the pelvic floor: a randomized feasibility study in urinary incontinence elderly women. *Acta Obstetricia et Gynecologica Scandinavica*. 2003;82(11):1043-8.

[90] Sand P, Richardson D, Staskin D, ea. Pelvic floor electrical stimulation in the treatment of genuine stress incontinence: A multicenter, placebo controlled trial. *American Journal of Obstetrics & Gynecology*. 1995;173(1):72-9.

[91] Amaro JL, Gameiro MO, Padovani CR. Effect of intravaginal electrical stimulation on pelvic floors muscle strength. *International Urogynecology Journal* 2005;16(5):355-8.

[92] Resnick N. Improving treatment of urinary incontinence. *JAMA: the Journal of the American Medical Association*. 1998;280(23):2034-5.

[93] Hannestad YS, Rortveit G, Hunskaar S. Help-seeking and associated factors in female urinary incontinence. The Norwegian EPINCONT Study. *Scandinavian Journal of Primary Health Care*. 2002;20(2):102-7.

[94] Koch LH. Help-Seeking Behaviors of Women with Urinary Incontinence: An Integrative Literature Review. *Journal of Midwifery & Women's Health*. 2006;51(6):e39-e44.

Treatment Options

In: Urinary Incontinence
Editor: Eric Chung
ISBN: 978-1-62618-482-4

Chapter 5

Preventive Factors for Urinary Incontinence

***Fumi Hirayama*[1] *and Andy H. Lee*[*2]**
[1]Medical Network Group, Innovation Center for Medical Redox Navigation, Kyushu University, Fukuoka, Japan
[2]School of Public Health, Curtin Health Innovation Research Institute, Curtin University, Perth, WA, Australia

Abstract

Urinary incontinence (UI) is a distressing condition for middle aged and older adults. The prevalence of UI varies substantially worldwide, depending on the definition adopted, the population being studied, and the instrument used for assessing leakage. Established risk factors are the female gender, obesity, advanced age and cigarette smoking. The main treatments include pharmacological prescriptions, conservative therapies (such as pelvic floor muscle exercise, biofeedback, electrical stimulation), and surgery. This chapter reviews the epidemiological evidence on emerging factors which may protect against the disease. Increasing green tea consumption appears to reduce the prevalence of UI among women. Low alcohol intake particularly beer is inversely associated with male UI, whereas the corresponding relationship for women remains inconsistent. Moreover, physical activity in daily life may mediate against the development of UI. Further research is required to understand the biological mechanisms concerning these factors, especially by gender and incontinence subtype, in order to prevent this bothersome condition for the aging population.

* Corresponding author: Professor Andy H. Lee, School of Public Health, Curtin University, GPO Box U 1987, Perth, WA, 6845, Australia, Phone: +61 8 92664180, Fax: +61 8 92662958, Email: Andy.Lee@curtin.edu.au.

Definition and Prevalence

Urinary incontinence (UI) is a distressing condition and costly problem in middle-aged and older people. The International Continence Society has defined UI as "a condition where involuntary loss of urine is a social or hygienic problem and is objectively demonstrable" [1]. The leakage of urine occurs when intra-vesical pressure exceeds urethral closure pressure in the absence of a detrusor contraction, or due to bladder neck hyper-mobility or poor urethral closure pressure [2]. However, the prevalence of UI varies substantially worldwide, depending on the definition of UI adopted, methodology used (face-to-face interview, telephone interview or postal survey), study design (facility-based or population-based), age of target population, and the instrument used for assessing leakage [1, 3].

According to the latest report from the European Association of Urology with UI defined as "occurring once within the last 12 months to several times per day or week", the prevalence of UI is estimated to be 1%-39% for men and 5%-69% for women [3]. A systematic review of 14 longitudinal studies indicated that the prevalence of UI varied between 0.8% and 19% [4], but another recent systematic review observed a even wider range of 16.2% to 81.9% from seven cross-sectional studies, two prospective studies and one experimental study, noting the non-uniformity of definition of UI across studies [5].

Risk Factors

Besides advanced age and the female gender, body mass index and neurologic diseases are established risk factors of UI [1, 3, 6]. For people who are overweight or obese, their large abdominal wall weight increases intra-abdominal pressure and intra-vesical pressure, as well as inducing changes to urethral mobility [7]. Moreover, diabetes mellitus, pregnancy and childbirth, family history, cigarette smoking, lower urinary tract symptoms, cognitive and functional impairment, and prostatic resection have been identified as risk factors of UI, despite inconsistent reports [1, 3, 6].

Several dietary risk factors have been investigated in the literature. In a study involving 5454 men residing in the United Kingdom, potato consumption of eight times or more per week was associated with an increased risk of overactive bladder; the odds ratio (OR) being 1.40, 95% confidence interval (CI) 1.00-1.97, when compared to men with low consumption $\leq$ 5 times per week [8]. A prospective longitudinal study of 5816 women in the United Kingdom found total fat, saturated fat, and vitamin B12 could increase the risk of stress UI [9], whereas a population-based cross-sectional study conducted in the USA showed no relation between total fat and UI [10]. The USA study, however, suggested a positive association for total energy intake (OR 2.86, 95% CI 1.56-5.23 for the highest versus lowest quintile) [10].

Caffeine intake (including coffee, tea, caffeinated soda, and chocolate) was another potential risk factor because research has shown that caffeine intake can lead to a rise in detrusor pressure upon bladder filling [11]. A large prospective cohort study of 65176 women aged 37 to 79 years in the USA observed a slight increase in risk of UI for the highest versus lowest level of caffeine intake (relative risk 1.19, 95% CI 1.06-1.34) [12]. The finding was consistent with a cross-sectional population-based study of 27936 Norwegian women, in which tea drinkers experienced a higher risk of UI than non-drinkers [13]. A cohort study of 6424 women aged 40 years or over in the United Kingdom suggested carbonated drinks could increase the risk of stress incontinence [14]. However, total beverage intake (including soda, juice, water, tea, coffee, milk, punch and alcohol) was unrelated to UI according to a recent cohort study [15].

Evidence for new risk factors has also emerged. A community-based study of 700 Japanese males aged 40 years or above found men with UI had lower forced expiratory volume in one second (FEV1) and lower forced vital capacity (FVC) than others without the condition [16]. Respiratory functions appeared to be inversely associated with UI; the OR were 0.67 (95% CI 0.43-1.04) for FEV1 and 0.63 (95% CI 0.40-0.98) for FVC [16]. The study further revealed that men presented with respiratory symptoms, especially breathlessness, had higher prevalence of UI than others without such symptoms (OR 2.11, 95% CI 1.10-4.06 for breathlessness), but the increase in risk was not evident among women [17]. Further studies are required to ascertain the relationship between lung function, respiratory symptoms and UI.

Protective Factors

Green Tea

Green tea is a non-fermented product and its health benefits are well known. A cross-sectional study of 300 community-dwelling Japanese women aged 40 to 75 years found that women with UI had lower intake of green tea than those without UI. Relative to non-drinkers, the OR of UI was 0.37 (95% CI 0.15-0.91) for drinking at least 700 ml daily, and 0.34 (95% CI 0.13-0.88) for drinking four or more cups per day [18]. Therefore, a higher consumption of green tea was inversely associated with the risk of UI. Tea is the second most popular beverage in the world after water [19]. Green tea contains polyphenols (especially catechins), minerals and vitamins which possess antioxidant properties [19] and responsible for its beneficial effect [18]. Although high caffeine intake is related to detrusor instability [11], unlike black tea and coffee, the amount of caffeine present in green tea leaves is very small [20] and green tea has practically no side effects.

Alcohol Consumption

A large prospective cohort study of men in the United Kingdom showed significant negative association between beer intake at baseline and subsequent onset of overactive bladder, with reduced risk at all levels of intake compared with those who seldom/never drank beer [8]. Similarly, a community-based study in Japan reported inverse association between male UI and low levels of alcohol consumption in middle-aged and older men. Compared to non-drinkers, the OR of UI was 0.43 (95% CI 0.19-0.96) for low ethanol intake at 0.1 to 32 g per day, and 0.53 (95% CI 0.22-1.28) for drinking one can of beer (350 ml) daily [21].

It has been suggested that the protective role of beer in the development of overactive bladder may be due to its non-alcoholic ingredients as well as the alcoholic content. Some of these ingredients can affect the contractile properties of the urethra and detrusor muscle [8]. Moreover, experimental studies have shown that ethanol causes transient changes in sex hormones, which can relax the contractility of the detrusor muscle by suppressing calcium influx through the calcium channels of smooth muscle membrane [22]. On the other hand, high levels of alcohol intake produced no significant benefit probably due to the diuretic effect when large amount is consumed. Unlike men, the effect of alcohol consumption on UI appeared to be inconsistent for women. Sex differences in pathophysiological mechanisms for UI may explain the contrasting results between men and women.

Physical Activity

Physical activity is a modifiable lifestyle factor for many chronic diseases with established health benefits. A cross-sectional study of 1000 Japanese older adults with mean age 66.2 years showed that habitual walking levels were lower among incontinent subjects than others without the condition. The adjusted OR of UI was 0.36 (95% CI 0.14-0.92) for men and 0.43 (95% CI 0.20-0.96) for women, when comparing frequent walkers with over 1000 metabolic equivalent tasks (MET) minutes of walking per week to completely sedentary participants [23]. The prevalence of UI also decreased with total and moderate activity levels, but the corresponding reductions in risk were not statistically significant. Therefore, regular walking of at least 1000 MET min per week, or equivalently 5 hours per week, appeared to be protective against UI [23].

A randomized controlled trial in 27 USA centers similarly recommended walking or low intensity activities [24]. A cross-sectional population-based study in Norway found that low-impact physical activity (not sweating or out of breath) of 3 or more hours weekly was associated with a reduced risk of UI for women, OR 0.8 (95% CI 0.7-0.9), when compared to less than one hour of walking per week [13]. Another cross-sectional survey conducted in Japan linked physical activity to a lower prevalence of UI among elderly men and women [25]. According to a prospective study in the USA, long walking durations could reduce the risk of developing UI, the OR being 0.74 (95% CI 0.63-0.88) for the highest versus the lowest levels of walking [26]. Therefore, physical activity in daily life may mediate against the development of UI.

Weight Reduction and Cesarean Section

Because body mass index is a risk factor for UI, reducing body weight appears to be a logical way to prevent UI. Indeed, evidence from both systematic review [7] and a randomized control trial suggested that weight reduction is a sufficient treatment for overweight or diabetes women with UI [24].

Two cross-sectional studies have reported cesarean section had a protective effect on UI compared with vaginal delivery, OR 0.5 (95% CI 0.3-0.9) [27] and OR 0.52 (95% CI 0.35-0.78) [28]. However, more scientific evidence is needed to substantiate the claim.

Dietary Protective Factors

The prevalence of UI can be affected by certain foods. A cross-sectional study in Finland reported that daily vegetable intake and butter consumption were associated with decreased lower urinary tract symptoms [29]. A cohort study of women aged 40 years or more in the United Kingdom revealed that a high intake of bread could reduce the risk of stress UI [14], which may be due to the good vitamins contained in bread.

Treatment

The main treatments include surgery, conservative behavioral therapies and pharmacological prescriptions. Surgery is recommended to treat stress UI and may be suitable for appropriately selected patients who are unable to comply with other non-surgical therapies [30]. Behavioral therapies include toilet assistance, bladder training, and pelvic floor muscle training such as vaginal cones, electrical stimulation, and biofeedback. These behavioral treatments have little side effects and should be considered as a first-line treatment for UI [3]. In particular, pelvic floor muscle training and bladder inhibition with biofeedback therapy are recommended for any type of UI [30].

Although pharmacological treatment is the least invasive, drugs are normally prescribed as an adjunct therapy. Hormonal therapy such as oestrogen and desmopressin are available for women [3]. Moreover, nutritional therapy for UI has gained some credibility since the recognition of complementary and alternative medicine by governments as part of the integrated health care. Anecdotal evidence has suggested that certain vitamin and mineral supplements, plant extracts and herbs, taken as an adjunct to standard treatment, may produce an enhanced, synergistic activity similar to the drugs used to treat UI [31]. However, scientific evidence is still lacking and claims concerning their effectiveness have not been substantiated [32].

Conclusion

UI is a distressing condition and costly problem for middle aged and older adults. This chapter has briefly reviewed the risk factors and treatment for the disease. Several lifestyle and behavioral factors have also been identified based on emerging epidemiological evidence. Further research is required to understand the biological mechanisms concerning these factors, especially by gender and incontinence subtype, in order to prevent this bothersome condition for the aging population. It is also hopeful that these preventive factors could slow down the progression of UI and improve the quality of life for those with UI.

References

[1] Hunskaar, S, Burgio, K, Diokno, AC, Herzog, AC, Hjälmaás, K and Lapitan, MC. 2002. *Incontinence: Second International Consultation on Incontinence Paris, July 1-3, 2001,* Health Publication Ltd, Plymouth.

[2] Neumann, PB, Grimmer, KA and Deenadayalan, Y. 2006, 'Pelvic floor muscle training and adjunctive therapies for the treatment of stress urinary incontinence in women: a systematic review'. *BMC Womens Health,* vol. 6, no. 11, pp. 1-28.

[3] Thuroff, JW, Abrams, P, Andersson, KE, Artibani, W, Chapple, CR, Drake, MJ, Hampel, C, Neisius, A, Schroder, A and Tubaro, A. 2011, 'EAU guidelines on urinary incontinence'. *Eur Urol,* vol. 59, no. 3, pp. 387-400.

[4] Irwin, DE, Milsom, I, Chancellor, MB, Kopp, Z and Guan, Z. 2010, 'Dynamic progression of overactive bladder and urinary incontinence symptoms: a systematic review'. *Eur Urol,* vol. 58, no. 4, pp. 532-43.

[5] Kwon, BE, Kim, GY, Son, YJ, Roh, YS and You, MA. 2010, 'Quality of life of women with urinary incontinence: a systematic literature review'. *Int Neurourol J,* vol. 14, no. 3, pp. 133-8.

[6] National Institutes of Health. 2007, 'NIH state-of-the-science conference statement on prevention of fecal and urinary incontinence in adults'. *NIH Consens State Sci Statements,* vol. 24, no. 1, pp. 1-37.

[7] Hunskaar, S. 2008, 'A systematic review of overweight and obesity as risk factors and targets for clinical intervention for urinary incontinence in women'. *Neurourol Urodyn,* vol. 27, no. 8, pp. 749-57.

[8] Dallosso, HM, Matthews, RJ, Mcgrother, CW, Donaldson, MM and Shaw, C. 2004, 'The association of diet and other lifestyle factors with the onset of overactive bladder: a longitudinal study in men'. *Public Health Nutr,* vol. 7, no. 7, pp. 885-91.

[9] Dallosso, H, Matthews, R, Mcgrother, C and Donaldson, M. 2004, 'Diet as a risk factor for the development of stress urinary incontinence: a longitudinal study in women'. *Eur J Clin Nutr,* vol. 58, no. 6, pp. 920-6.

[10] Maserejian, NN, Giovannucci, EL, Mcvary, KT, Mcgrother, C and Mckinlay, JB. 2010, 'Dietary macronutrient and energy intake and urinary incontinence in women'. *Am J Epidemiol,* vol. 171, no. 10, pp. 1116-25.

[11] Creighton, SM and Stanton, SL. 1990, 'Caffeine: does it affect your bladder?'. *Br J Urol,* vol. 66, no. 6, pp. 613-4.

[12] Jura, YH, Townsend, MK, Curhan, GC, Resnick, NM and Grodstein, F. 2011, 'Caffeine intake, and the risk of stress, urgency and mixed urinary incontinence'. *J Urol,* vol. 185, no. 5, pp. 1775-80.

[13] Hannestad, YS, Rortveit, G, Daltveit, AK and Hunskaar, S. 2003, 'Are smoking and other lifestyle factors associated with female urinary incontinence? The Norwegian EPINCONT Study'. *BJOG,* vol. 110, no. 3, pp. 247-54.

[14] Dallosso, HM, Mcgrother, CW, Matthews, RJ and Donaldson, MM. 2003, 'The association of diet and other lifestyle factors with overactive bladder and stress incontinence: a longitudinal study in women'. *BJU Int,* vol. 92, no. 1, pp. 69-77.

[15] Townsend, MK, Jura, YH, Curhan, GC, Resnick, NM and Grodstein, F. 2011, 'Fluid intake and risk of stress, urgency, and mixed urinary incontinence'. *Am J Obstet Gynecol,* vol. 205, no. 73, pp. e1-6.

[16] Hirayama, F, Lee, AH, Binns, CW, Nishimura, K and Taniguchi, H. 2009, 'Association of impaired respiratory function with urinary incontinence'. *Respirology,* vol. 14, no. 5, pp. 753-6.

[17] Hirayama, F, Lee, AH, Hiramatsu, T and Tanikawa, Y. 2010, 'Breathlessness is associated with urinary incontinence in men: A community-based study'. *BMC Pulm Med,* vol. 10, no. 2, pp. 1-5.

[18] Hirayama, F and Lee, AH. 2011, 'Green tea drinking is inversely associated with urinary incontinence in middle-aged and older women'. *Neurourol Urodyn,* vol. 30, no. 7, pp. 1262-5.

[19] Cabrera, C, Artacho, R and Gimenez, R. 2006, 'Beneficial effects of green tea--a review'. *J Am Coll Nutr,* vol. 25, no. 2, pp. 79-99.

[20] Ministry of Education, Culture, Sports Science and Technology, Japan. 2005, *Standard tables of food composition in Japan, fifth revised and enlarged edition. ttp://www.mext.go.jp/b_menu/shingi/gijyutu/gijyutu3/toushin/05031802.htm.*

[21] Lee, AH and Hirayama, F. 2011, 'Is alcohol consumption associated with male urinary incontinence?'. *Lower Urinary Tract Symptoms,* vol. 3, no. 1, pp. 19-24.

[22] Ratz, PH, Mccammon, KA, Altstatt, D, Blackmore, PF, Shenfeld, OZ and Schlossberg, SM. 1999, 'Differential effects of sex hormones and phytoestrogens on peak and steady state contractions in isolated rabbit detrusor'. *J Urol,* vol. 162, no. 5, pp. 1821-8.

[23] Lee, AH and Hirayama, F. 2011, 'Physical Activity and Urinary Incontinence in Older Adults: A Community-Based Study'. *Curr Aging Sci,* vol. 4, pp. 1-6.

[24] Brown, JS, Wing, R, Barrett-Connor, E, Nyberg, LM, Kusek, JW, Orchard, TJ, Ma, Y, Vittinghoff, E and Kanaya, AM. 2006, 'Lifestyle intervention is associated with lower prevalence of urinary incontinence: the Diabetes Prevention Program'. *Diabetes Care,* vol. 29, no. 2, pp. 385-90.

[25] Kikuchi, A, Niu, K, Ikeda, Y, Hozawa, A, Nakagawa, H, Guo, H, Ohmori-Matsuda, K, Yang, G, Farmawati, A, Sami, A, Arai, Y, Tsuji, I and Nagatomi, R. 2007, 'Association between physical activity and urinary incontinence in a community-based elderly population aged 70 years and over'. *European Urology,* vol. 52, no. 3, pp. 868-74.

[26] Danforth, KN, Shah, AD, Townsend, MK, Lifford, KL, Curhan, GC, Resnick, NM and Grodstein, F. 2007, 'Physical activity and urinary incontinence among healthy, older women'. *Obstet Gynecol,* vol. 109, no. 3, pp. 721-7.

[27] Burgio, KL, Borello-France, D, Richter, HE, Fitzgerald, MP, Whitehead, W, Handa, VL, Nygaard, I, Fine, P, Zyczynski, H, Visco, AG, Brown, MB and Weber, AM. 2007, 'Risk factors for fecal and urinary incontinence after childbirth: the childbirth and pelvic symptoms study'. *Am J Gastroenterol,* vol. 102, no. 9, pp. 1998-2004.

[28] Goldberg, RP, Kwon, C, Gandhi, S, Atkuru, LV, Sorensen, M and Sand, PK. 2003, 'Urinary incontinence among mothers of multiples: the protective effect of cesarean delivery'. *Am J Obstet Gynecol,* vol. 188, no. 6, pp. 1447-50; discussion 50-3.

[29] Koskimaki, J, Hakama, M, Huhtala, H and Tammela, TL. 2000, 'Association of dietary elements and lower urinary tract symptoms'. *Scand J Urol Nephrol,* vol. 34, no. 1, pp. 46-50.

[30] Wound Care Information Network. 1996. *Summary of the Agency for Health Care Policy and Research (AHCPR) Clinical Practice Guideline.* http://www.medicaledu.com/ahcpr.htm.

[31] Bottomley, JM. 2000, 'Complementary nutrition in treating urinary incontinence'. *Top Geriatr Rehabil,* vol. 16, no. 1, pp. 61-77.

[32] Shamliyan, TA, Kane, RL, Wyman, J and Wilt, TJ. 2008, 'Systematic review: randomized, controlled trials of nonsurgical treatments for urinary incontinence in women'. *Ann Intern Med,* vol. 148, no. 6, pp. 459-73.

In: Urinary Incontinence
Editor: Eric Chung

ISBN: 978-1-62618-482-4

Chapter 6

Behavioral Therapy for Urinary Incontinence

Hunkyung Kim
Tokyo Metropolitan Institute of Gerontology, Japan

Abstract

Background

Urinary incontinence among the elderly is a common problem that leads to loss of independence, decreased quality of life, social restrictions, and increased risk of hospitalization. Several treatments are currently available for elderly people with urinary incontinence including surgery, drug therapies, and behavioral interventions. Recently, much attention has been placed on the behavioral treatments for UI, including pelvic floor muscle (PFM) exercise and bladder training, weight loss exercise, and thermal therapy, as they have few risks, no side effects, and are effective.

Treatment

Pelvic floor muscle exercise: PFM exercises, which were first initiated by Kegel in 1948, has been found to be effective in reducing stress urinary incontinence with improvement rates ranging from 17%-80%. However, current focus has extensively been on treatment of stress urinary incontinence with little attention on the effects of behavioral treatments on other types of urinary incontinence, such as urge or mixed urinary incontinence. Previous research has found that PFM exercise reduced urine leakage in people with urge and mixed urinary incontinence because of the inhibition of the bladder reflex associated with PFM contractions. While further investigation is still needed, there is evidence indicating that exercise interventions may be equally effective in treating stress, urge, and mixed urinary incontinence.

Weight loss exercise: Several factors such as obesity and high body mass index (BMI) have been associated with higher risk of urinary incontinence. Surgically induced weight loss in morbidly obese women has been found to reduce stress and urge urinary incontinence. Hence, fitness exercises focused on strengthening the abdominal muscles and reducing abdominal fat as well as BMI may also decrease the risk of urinary incontinence in the elderly. An 8% weight reduction in obese women has been reported to decrease weekly incontinence episodes by 47%. In light of such recent information, weight loss has been suggested as a first-line treatment for obese women with urinary incontinence.

Thermal therapy: Recent studies have expanded the focus of urinary incontinence interventions to thermal therapy as well. Previous research has indicated that abdominal and lower back heating may have positive effects on renal function via renal sympathetic nerve activity suppression, promotion of bladder voiding, and increasing urination frequency. Moreover, the combination of both heat therapy and exercise has shown to be effective in the treatment of stress, urge, and mixed urinary incontinence.

Conclusions

Behavioral treatments for urinary incontinence, especially PFM and fitness exercises along with combinations of other therapies, are effective in reducing incontinence in the elderly population. These treatments are often recommended as first line treatment because they are considerably safe with no risks and no side effects.

This chapter will discuss the benefits of behavioral treatments on different types of urinary incontinence, as well as the rationale behind how and why weight loss can reduce the risk of urinary incontinence. The chapter will present and examine in detail the effects of PFM exercise, biofeedback, pelvic floor electrical stimulation, vaginal cones, and thermal therapy on improving urine leakage episodes in people with urinary incontinence. While further research is still necessary, the combinations of behavioral interventions seem to be promising in the treatment of urinary incontinence.

1. Introduction

Urinary incontinence, particularly in the elderly, is considered to be an important determining factor for admission into long-term care and has been associated with loss of independence, reduced quality of life, restricted social activities, and increased anxiety and social isolation. Thus, prevention and treatment of urinary incontinence in its early stages are important strategies in maintaining health and independence among the elderly.

There is general agreement on the multifactorial nature of incontinence. Permanent incontinence is typically the result of neurological damage, intrinsic bladder or urethral pathology. However, incontinence is also associated with several potentially reversible conditions. Lower urinary tract function, environmental factors, physical and cognitive function, psychological distress, mobility, manual dexterity, medical conditions, and medications may all have an effect on urinary incontinence status in the elderly (Landi et al., 2003). The incidence of urinary incontinence is typically higher in women than men, and those who experience incontinence are usually older with a lower functional fitness level for both sexes. Although there is a large amount of information regarding the mechanisms and treatment options for urinary incontinence, little is known about the potentially reversible causes of this condition in community-dwelling elderly people. Several of the known causes that may be reversible include urinary tract infections, as they can cause the urge to void quite frequently, physical restraints and drastic limits of mobility, and environmental hazards.

Obesity, lifestyle (such as smoking status and social activity), and functional fitness are significantly associated with the onset of urinary incontinence in community-dwelling elderly people (Kim et al., 2004) (Table 1).

Table 1. Multiple logistic regression model of risk factors associated with the onset of urinary incontinence

Sex	Variable		OR	95%CI
Male	Age (per 1 yr)		1.23	1.11-1.38
	Plasma albumin (per 0.1 g/dl)		0.70	0.54-0.88
	Smoking status	non-smoker	1.00	
		previous smoker	1.53	0.56-4.59
		current smoker	2.33	0.82-7.61
Female	Grip strength (per 1 kg)		0.92	0.86-0.98
	Social role (per 1 point)		1.81	1.19-2.73
	BMI (per 1 kg/m^2)		1.10	1.01-1.20
	Smoking status	non-smoker	1.00	
		current smoker	7.53	1.36-41.63

2. Treatment

Urinary incontinence is often differentiated into stress, urge, and mixed urinary incontinence. Stress incontinence is defined as urine leakage associated with coughing, sneezing, laughing, heavy lifting, standing, running, or other types of physical activity that increase abdominal pressure. Leakage associated with running water or an urge to void and not being able to reach the toilet in time is urge incontinence. Mixed urinary incontinence shows symptoms of both stress and urge incontinence.

Surgery, drug and behavioral therapies are common treatments for urinary incontinence. Behavioral treatments such as pelvic floor muscle (PFM) exercises and bladder training are often recommended for the management of stress urinary incontinence, because they are non-invasive, have potential benefits, few risks and no side effects. While until recently, treatments have varied according to incontinence type, with an emphasis on stress incontinence, results of research have suggested that behavioral treatments are not only more effective than drug treatments, they are also safe, effective conservative treatments for urge and mixed incontinence as well (Burgio et al., 1998). The recommended conservative treatments for the prevention of urinary incontinence are behavioral treatments involving PFM exercises and various different combinations of other treatments including bladder training, biofeedback, electrical stimulation, vaginal cones, and/or thermal therapy.

Table 2. Summaries of different interventions targeting reductions in urinary incontinence episodes.

Table 2. Summarizes several research trials that have investigated the effects of these behavioral treatments on urinary incontinence

Study	Participants	Intervention	Outcomes	Conclusion
Kegel (1951)	500+women with stress urinary incontinence (UI)	PFM exercise 20 minutes a day, 3 times a day, or a total of 300 contractions using a Perineometer	Continence improved in 84% of patients with stress UI	Physiological therapy for stress UI is useful and successful
Burns et al. (1993)	123 women, age 55 and older with stress UI	8 week treatment, 3 month, 6 month follow-up Biofeedback(n=40) PFM exercise(n=43) Control(n=40)	Improvement in urine loss frequency Biofeedback=61% PFM exercise=43% Control=6%	Biofeedback and PFM exercise are effective and benefits are maintained for 6 months
Bo et al. (1999)	107 women, age range 24-70 years with stress UI	6 month trial PFM exercise(n=25) Electrical stimulation(ES)(n=25) Vaginal cones(n=27) Control group(n=30)	Reduction in leakage PFM exercise =-30.2g ES=-7.4g Cones=-14.7g Control=-12.7g	PFM exercise is most effective
Goode et al. (2003)	200 women, age range 40-78 with stress UI	8 weeks PFM exercise(n=66) PFM=ES(n=67) Self-help booklet(n=67)	Reduction in weekly episodes PFM exercise=68.6% PFM=ES71.9% Self-help booklet 52.5%	PFM+ES did not increase effectiveness in treating UI
Kim et al. (2007)	70 women, age 70 and older with stress UI	3 month trial, 1 year follow up PFM and fitness (n=35) Control (n=35)	Cure rate of urine leakage Exercise=54.5% Control=9.4%	↓ in BMI and ↑ in walking speed may contribute to improvement of UI
Fantl et al. (1991)	123 women, age 55 and older with UI	6 weeks, 6 months follow up Bladder training(n=60) Control(n=63)	Bladder training reduced UI episodes by 57%. Urine loss volume was reduced by 54%	Bladder training recommended as an intial step in UI treatment
Goode et al. (2011)	208 men, age range 51-84 with UI persisting after radial prostatectomy	8 weeks Behavior(PFM exercise+bladder training(n=70) Behavior+biofeedback and ES(n=70) Control (n=68)	Reduction in weekly UI episodes Behavior=55% Behavior+biofeedback and ES=51% Control=24%	Additional biofeedback and ES did not increase effectiveness in treating post prostatectomy incontinence
Burgio et al. (2002)	222 women, age range 55-92 years with urge or mixed UI	8 weeks PFM exercise(n=74) PFm and Biofeedback(n=73) Self-help booklet(n=75)	Reduction in weekly UI episodes	Improvement in urge UI was seen in all interventions
Kim et al. (2011a)	127 women, age 70 and older with stress urge, and mixed UI	3 month trial, 7 month follow up PFM and fitness(n=63) Control(n=64)	Cure rate of urine leakage PFM and fitness=44.1% Stress UI=63.2% Urge UI=35.0% Mixed UI=40.1% Control=1.6%	Multidemsional exercise may be effective for all tree types of UI
Kim et al. (2011b)	147 women, age 70 and older with stress urge, and mixed UI	3 month trial PFM and fitness +heat and steam generating sheet (HSGS) (n=37) PFM and fitness (n=37) (HSGS) (n=37) Education (n=36)	Cure of urine leakage PFM and fitness+HSGS=54.1% PFM and fitness=34.3% HSGS=21.6 Education=2.9%	HSGS can be used in addition to PFM and fitness exercise to reduce incontinence
Stubak et al. (2005)	40 obese women, age range 46-62, with UI	3 month, 6 months follow-up Liguid diet weight reduction program(n=24) Weight-list control(n=24)	Reduction in weekly UI episodes Weightloss program=60% Control=15%	Weight reduction is effective in treating UI for obese women
Stubak et al. (2009)	338 overweight and obese women with IU	6 months Intervention (diet and excercise weight-loss program with behavior modification) (n=22) Education (n-112)	Reduction in weekly UI episodes Intervention=47% Education=28%	Behavioral intervention targeting weight loss reduced UI episodes among overweight and obese women

2.1. Pelvic Floor Muscle Exercise

PFM exercises (Figure 1), were first initiated by Kegal in 1948. These exercises are hypothesized to enhance urethral resistance by increasing the strength and endurance of the periurethral and perivaginal muscles as well as by improving the anatomic support to the bladder neck and proximal urethra (Kegel, 1948). The effectiveness of PFM exercises for the improvement of urine leakage has been validated by many investigators, with improvement rates ranging widely from 17 to 84% (Bo, 1995). PFM exercises have been the preferred treatment for stress incontinence; however, recently they have been recommended for urge or mixed incontinence as well, due to the reflex bladder inhibition associated with pelvic floor muscle contraction (Kim, 2012).

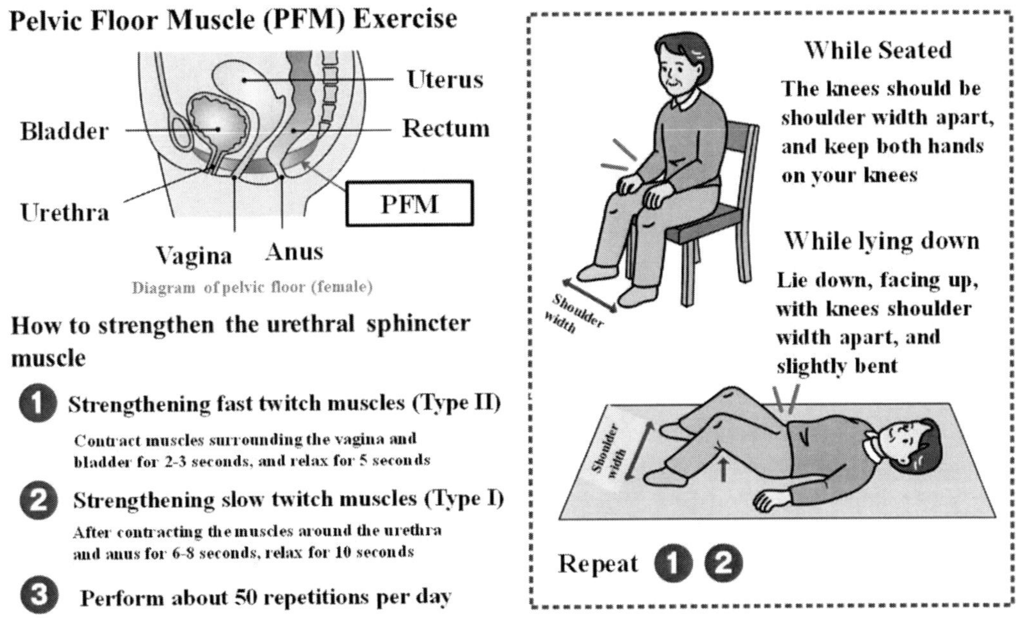

Figure 1. Pelvic floor muscle exercise for the treatment of urinary incontinence.

Elderly people participating in PFM training programs should be educated in the structure of the pelvic floor muscles (Figure 1) in order to gain awareness, and ultimately for proper execution of the exercises (Kim, 2012). Particularly, participants should be informed that straining the abdomen and increasing abdominal pressure would exert an added load on the PFMs. Training should focus on isolated force exertion of the PFMs without excessively straining the abdomen. Commonly, exercise programs include strengthening of both the fast and slow-twitch muscle fibers located at the pelvic floor. PFM exercise programs often incorporate alternations of: fast contractions, usually held for about three seconds followed by five second relaxation periods; sustained contractions, where the participants would hold the contraction for about six to eight seconds; and ten-second relaxation periods between the contractions. The PFM exercises can be performed in the seated, lying, and standing positions with the legs shoulder-width apart, and the emphasis placed on isolated training of the PFMs

(Figure 1). Regardless of the positions the exercises are performed (seated, lying, standing), the beneficial effects are equal (Borello-France et al., 2006).

Kegel (1948) also introduced a device known as the Perineometer to monitor PFM strength progress by measuring the strength of perineal muscular contraction, and is now widely used as a biofeedback instrument (described in further detail below). The Perineometer consists of a pneumatic vaginal chamber (8 cm in length, and 2 cm in diameter), which is inserted into the vaginal cavity, connected to an external pressure gauge. Women can watch the dial on the gauge as they contract their PFMs as instructed and monitor their progress. In the study conducted by Kegel (1948), the initial measurements (the first five days of starting PFM training) showed weak muscular contractions of about 20 mm of mercury resistance. Over the course of 25 days of progressive PFM training (20 minutes, three times a day), stronger muscular contractions were detected, at 80 mm of mercury resistance.

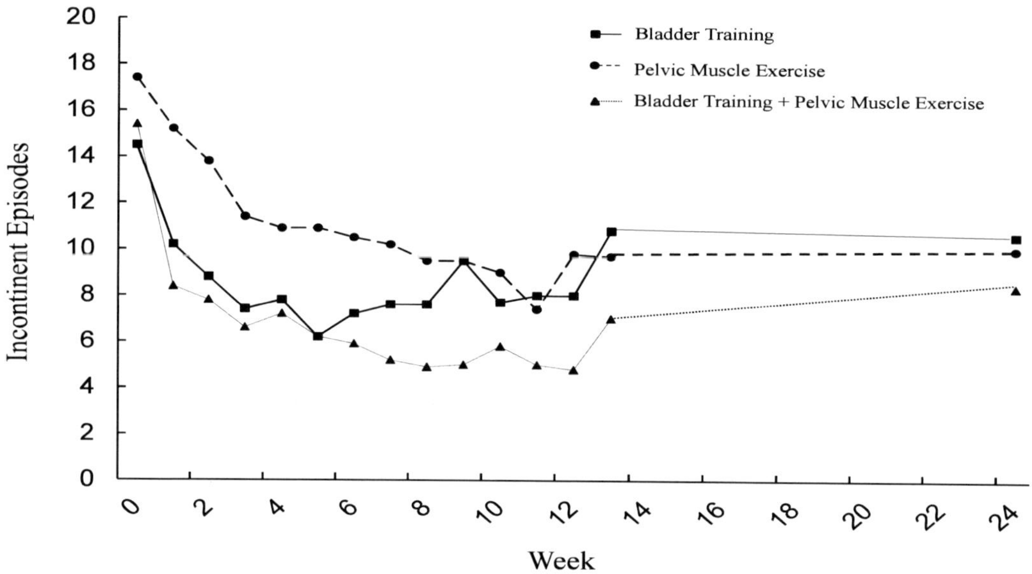

Figure 2. Change in mean weekly number of incontinent episodes over time by treatment group. (Wyman, J.F.; Fantl, J.A.; McClish, D.K. & Bump, R.C. (1998). Comparative efficacy of behavioral interventions in the management of female urinary incontinence. Continence Program for Women Research Group. *American Journal of Obstetrics and Gynecology, 179,* 999-1007, with permission from Elsevier).

Exercise training periods vary between 3 weeks and 6 months. The greatest effect is seen at 6 weeks for bladder training; between 11 to 12 weeks for PFM exercise; and combined bladder training and PFM exercise seems to be most effective between 8 to 12 weeks of training (Wyman et al., 1998) (Figure 2).

2.2. Fitness Exercise

Previous studies have reported that urinary incontinence is associated with obesity and high body mass index (BMI). These studies suggest that increases in body weight causes increases in abdominal-wall weight, which in turn increases intra-abdominal pressure and intra-vesicular pressure (Bo, 2004). Therefore, abdominal fat reduction from exercise may decrease intra-abdominal pressure, perhaps causing improvements in urethral sphincter contraction; hence, decreasing urinary incontinence risk (Figure 3). Bump et al. (1992) found that surgically induced weight loss in obese women significantly reduces weekly incontinence episodes. Weight reduction is desirable for obese women with urinary incontinence (Subak et al., 2009).

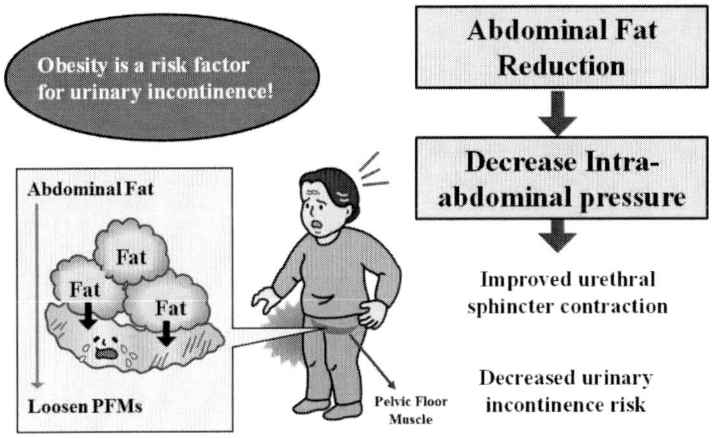

Figure 3. Relationship between abdominal fat and loosened pelvic floor muscles.

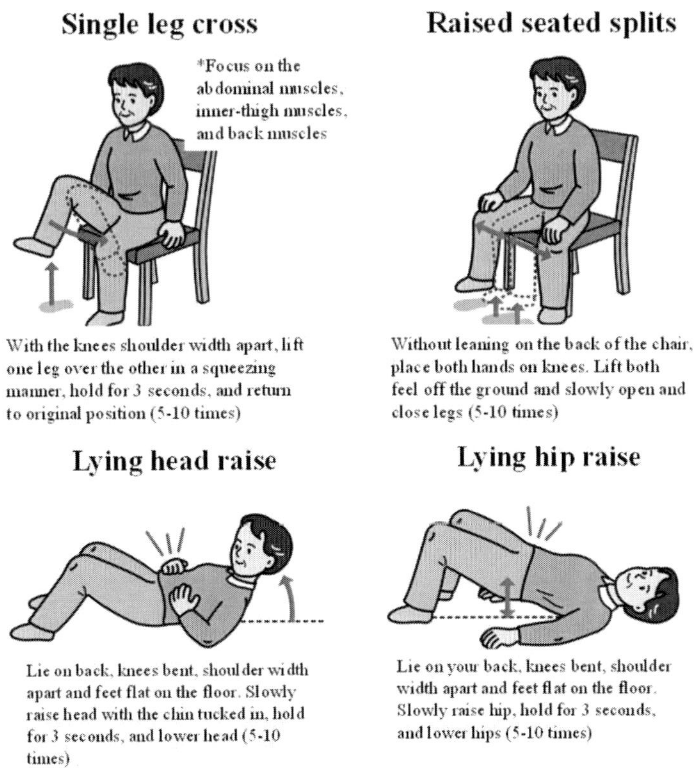

Figure 4. Examples of exercises aimed to reduce abdominal fat and increase mobility.

While a direct cause-effect relationship has not been established between obesity and incontinence, weight reduction or decrease in BMI may be beneficial for treatment of incontinence. Kim et al. (2007) investigated the distribution of subjects cured from urinary incontinence according to tertiles of changes in BMI, maximum walking speed, and adductor muscle strength, and found that a significantly higher proportion among those who were cured of incontinence episodes, demonstrated improvements in BMI and walking speeds. Therefore, decrease in BMI and increase in walking speed are desirable outcomes for the treatment of stress urinary incontinence (Kim, 2012) (Table 3).

Table 3. Cured of urine leakage according to body mass index (BMI), maximum walking speed, and adductor muscle strength tertiles. (Kim, H.; Suzuki, T.; Yoshida, Y. & Yoshida, H. (2007). Effectiveness of multidimensional exercises for the treatment of stress urinary incontinence in elderly community-dwelling Japanese women: a randomized, controlled, crossover trial. *Journal of the American Geriatrics Society, 55,* 1932-1939, with permission from the American Geriatrics Society)

Variable Changes Compared with Baseline		Cured of Urine Leakage n(%)	Cochran's Q value	*p*- value	Post-hoc †
3-month exercise (n=33)					
BMI	Decreased (D)	16 (48.5)	7.091	0.029	D,N>I
	No change (N)	13 (39.4)			
	Increased (I)	4 (12.1)			
Maximum walking speed	Increased	17 (51.5)	6.545	0.038	I>D
	No change	11 (33.3)			
	Decreased	5 (15.2)			
Adductor muscle strength	Increased	11 (33.3)	4.545	0.103	
	No change	6 (18.2)			
	Decreased	16 (48.5)			
1-Year Follow-up (n=20)					
BMI	Decreased	10 (50.0)	3.700	0.157	
	No change	3 (15.0)			
	Increased	7 (35.0)			
Maximum walking speed	Increased	10 (50.0)	6.100	0.047	I>D
	No change	8 (40.0)			
	Decreased	2 (10.0)			
Adductor muscle strength	Increased	9 (45.0)	3.100	0.212	
	No change	8 (40.0)			
	Decreased	3 (15.0)			

2.3. Other Treatments

Commonly, PFM exercises are recommended for people with stress urinary incontinence, and fitness exercises have been effective in reducing incontinence episodes in the obese. Several other incontinence treatments have been developed apart from PFM and fitness exercises, and they have been the focus of recent investigation in order to determine the efficacy and validity of these treatment methods.

The use of an educational or retraining program as an intervention was introduced by Jeffcoate and Francis in 1966. The therapy, known as bladder training or sometimes as bladder discipline or drill, consists of three components: patient education, scheduled voiding, and positive reinforcement. Patient education includes teaching patients about the bladder and how continence is normally maintained; scheduled voiding is a fixed or flexible time table for voiding aimed to increase the interval between voids; and positive reinforcement offers encouragement and support provided by a healthcare professional. Bladder training is often prescribed to those experiencing urge urinary incontinence, with uninhibited bladder contractions, as well as those with stress or mixed incontinence. The purpose of bladder training is to inhibit involuntary bladder contractions, increase the interval between voids, and/or induce unspecified psychological benefits. The mechanism of bladder training remains unclear: one hypothesis is that the capacity of the bladder increases by lengthening the interval between voids, which may lead to the reduction in urinary incontinence (Wallace et al., 2009). While research has shown that bladder training can reduce the number of incontinence episodes and the volume of urine loss, this treatment method seems to be more effective as a supplement to PFM exercises, than as a stand-alone treatment (Wyman et al., 1998).

Unlike bladder training, which is very difficult to implement in those with cognitive impairment, other forms of toileting assistance methods such as prompted voiding and timed voiding can be used for elderly people with cognitive impairments. Prompted voiding is used to teach elderly people who may or may not be cognitively impaired to initiate toileting through the requesting of help, or notifying the urge to void to caregivers, and in turn receiving positive reinforcement from the caregivers, a form of operant conditioning. This therapy also requires more mobility in the elderly by having caregivers assist them to the toilet instead of simply changing urinary pads after each incontinence episode. The distinction between prompted voiding and other toileting assistance interventions is that prompted voiding is not initiated and controlled by caregivers, but the individuals with urinary incontinence themselves. The disadvantages with prompted voiding are that it requires a significant amount of commitment and motivation from caregivers, and there are major resource implications which may make this therapy inconvenient. While there has been evidence suggesting that prompted voiding is more effective than no therapy, the evidence is quite weak and further validation is necessary (Eustice et al., 2000).

Timed voiding sometimes referred to as scheduled, routine, or regular toileting is a therapy where the intervals between voiding are fixed. This program is considered a passive toileting assistance program initiated by caregivers, and is often provided to elderly people in long-term residential care facilities with cognitive or motor impairments. In contrast to bladder training, the intervals between voids are not lengthened or shortened, and the aim of this method is to avoid incontinence episodes and not to improve bladder function. Timed voiding is different from prompted voiding in that the caregivers initiate and maintain the program without participation from the elderly patients or residents, and there are no positive reinforcements. However like prompted voiding, evidence of the efficacy of timed voiding toileting assistance programs is inconclusive, and the evidence is insufficient (Ostaszkiewicz et al., 2004). There are also limited investigations where toileting assistance interventions are combined with other forms of behavioral urinary incontinence treatments.

Biofeedback is a training technique aimed to reduce urinary incontinence. Biofeedback can be defined as "augmented, concurrent or terminal feedback of biological signals that enables a person to identify and modify a bodily function of which they are usually unaware" (Herderschee et al., 2011). Augmented feedback refers to any supplementary information given, such as verbal feedback on performance, which can be given during muscle contraction (concurrent) or after (terminal). Kegel first published a report of biofeedback for stress urinary incontinence, where he developed the perineometer (1948), which as previously described, is an instrument now regarded as a biofeedback devise. A perineometer measures the strength of PFM contractions in women using an intravaginal balloon attached to an external manometer. Biofeedback is not only limited to squeeze pressure. Other devices are also used to measure different biological signals such as electrical activity or movement with ultrasound. Whether or not biofeedback is essential for behavioral treatment of urinary incontinence remains uncertain. Several researchers have investigated the role of biofeedback on the treatment of incontinence. Burgio et al.,(1986) indicated that biofeedback is more effective than verbal feedback for teaching selective sphincter control, and only those who had biofeedback treatment demonstrated increases in sphincter strength with training. These results however, were obtained from a very small sample size. Burns et al.,(1993) conducted a randomized controlled trial to assess the efficacy of biofeedback and PFM exercise for the treatment of stress incontinence in older community-dwelling women showing that biofeedback and PFM exercise are effective for treating stress incontinence. Although there were no significant differences in treatment effects between PFM exercise and biofeedback, the results suggest that there is a possibility that biofeedback may be more effective for incontinence of moderate and severe frequency. Burgio et al., (2002) evaluated the effects of training with and without biofeedback for urge incontinence. Behavioral training with biofeedback yielded a mean 63.1% reduction and verbal feedback a mean 69.4% reduction in incontinence episodes. Biofeedback showed less improvement in urinary incontinence compared with verbal feedback alone. A recent randomized controlled trial conducted to evaluate the effectiveness of behavioral therapy for reducing persistent post-prostatectomy incontinence found that the combination of biofeedback with pelvic floor electrical stimulation did not result in greater effectiveness (Goode et al., 2011).

PFM exercise is the most common conservative treatment of urinary incontinence. The correct execution of these exercises is an essential factor for the improvement of incontinence, as improper PFM contractions may reduce the force of urethral contraction (Bump, 1991). Therefore, there have been attempts to make it easier for women to train their PFMs. One method that has been developed is using a set of graded weighted vaginal cones (Peattie et al., 1988). The vaginal cone is placed in the vagina so that the PFMs must contract in order to prevent the cone from slipping out. Research has shown that cones were better than no active treatment; however, there is not enough evidence to show that adding cones to PFM exercise is more effective than cones or PFM exercise alone (Herbison and Dean, 2002).

Pelvic floor electrical stimulation has been suggested as an effective and safe therapy for treatment of stress urinary incontinence (Sand et al., 1995). Electrical stimulation consists of brief electrical impulses administered via needle or surface electrodes and is used to inhibit detrusor overactivity or to cause contraction of PFMs, providing passive exercise. A randomized controlled trial found that the addition of pelvic floor electrical stimulation to an extensive PFM exercise program did not significantly reduce the frequency of episodes, but pelvic floor stimulation group had significantly better patient self-perception of outcomes and satisfaction with progress (Goode et al., 2003).

Table 4. Cured of urine leakage after the 3-month exercise between the intervention and control groups. (Kim, H.; Yoshida, H. & Suzuki, T. (2011a). The effects of multidimensional exercise treatment on community-dwelling elderly Japanese women with stress, urge, and mixed urinary incontinence: A randomized controlled trial. *International Journal of Nursing Studies, 48,* 1165-1172, with permission from Elsevier)

Variables[a]	G[b]	Baseline	3-month exercise	7-month follow-up	ANOVA[c] G×T	p Value
Body Weight (kg)	I	52.0 ± 8.9	51.9 ± 8.8	50.9 ± 8.9	F=5.78	0.018
	C	53.9 ± 8.2	53.9 ± 8.2	53.9 ± 8.1		
BMI (kg/m^2)	I	23.7 ± 3.4	23.5 ± 3.0	23.2 ± 3.1	F=11.49	0.001
	C	24.1 ± 2.9	24.0 ± 2.7	24.4 ± 3.4		
WC (cm)	I	78.8 ± 10.3	77.8 ± 9.7	77.7 ± 9.9	F=4.06	0.041
	C	79.3 ± 10.4	79.2 ± 10.5	78.9 ± 9.6		
UWS (m/sec)	I	1.2 ± 0.2	1.2 ± 0.2	1.2 ± 0.2	F=2.79	0.099
	C	1.1 ± 0.3	1.1 ± 0.3	1.1 ± 0.2		
MWS(m/sec)	I	1.7 ± 0.4	1.8 ± 0.4	1.8 ± 0.4	F=5.10	0.027
	C	1.7 ± 0.4	1.6 ± 0.3	1.6 ± 0.4		
GS (kg)	I	19.0 ± 4.7	20.7 ± 5.0	19.8 ± 5.7	F=0.37	0.547
	C	19.0 ± 4.2	20.2 ± 3.5	19.5 ± 3.8		
AMS (kg)	I	20.5 ± 7.1	24.1 ± 7.7	24.3 ± 7.9	F=11.00	0.001
	C	21.2 ± 4.8	22.1 ± 4.8	21.8 ± 4.9		
ULS (point)	I	5.0 ± 1.0	3.0 ± 2.0	3.6 ± 2.2	F=7.64	0.007
	C	5.1 ± 1.0	4.4 ± 1.6	4.8 ± 1.6		
Cure of urine leakage	I	0.0	44.1	39.3	21.96	<0.001
	C	0.0	1.6	1.6		
Cure of urine leakage in intervention group	Stress	0.0	63.2[d]	66.7[e]	15.77	<0.001
	Urge	0.0	35.0[d]	26.1[e]	7.49	0.032
	Mixed	0.0	40.0[d]	30.0[e]	9.56	0.016

[a] Data are presented as mean and standard deviation.

WC=waist circumference; UWS=usual walking speed; MWS=maximum walking speed; GS=Grip strenghth; AMS=adductor muscle strength; ULS=urine leakage score.

[b] G=group, I=intervention group, C=control group.

[c] ANOVA=analysis of variance, T=time. Chi-square and p values from generalized estimating equation. Cochran's Q-value.

[d] Kruskal-Wallis test; chi-square=1.99, p =0.391

[e] Kruskal-Wallis test; chi-square=10.28, p = 0.008

(scheffes post-hoc=stess>urge, mixed urinary incontinence)

Previous research has not shown convincing evidence that biofeedback, electrical stimulation, and vaginal cones together with PFM exercise have significant effects on improving urinary incontinence compared with PFM exercise alone. Furthermore, several problems arise with the use of electrical stimulation and vaginal cones. Electrical stimulation, while offering passive exercise of the PFMs, is not as effective as voluntary contraction of the muscles, and most patients have low tolerance for electrical stimulation. Many women have also reported that electrical stimulation as well as vaginal cones was difficult to use (Bo et al., 1999).

Despite the aforementioned limitations of pelvic floor electrical stimulation and vaginal cones, these methods of treatment may be helpful for elderly people who have difficulty with voluntary contraction of the PFMs whether from weakness or decline in cognitive and motor function. Elderly people who cannot identify and isolate their PFMs can benefit greatly from pelvic floor electrical stimulation and vaginal cones without having to resort to more invasive treatments with greater risks.

One recent trial suggested that PFM and fitness exercises are beneficial for all three types of urinary incontinence after a training period of three months; however, the mechanisms of these positive effects have not been made clear. This study did find that the effects of combined PFM and fitness exercises are maintained more in those with stress incontinence compared to those with urge or mixed incontinence (Kim et al., 2011a) (Table 4).

Among the different combinations of treatments previously described, the combination of PFM exercises with a fitness exercise program is recommended. By repeating PFM exercises with fitness exercises aimed to reduce abdominal fat, improvements in cure rates of urinary incontinence can be expected (Figure 5).

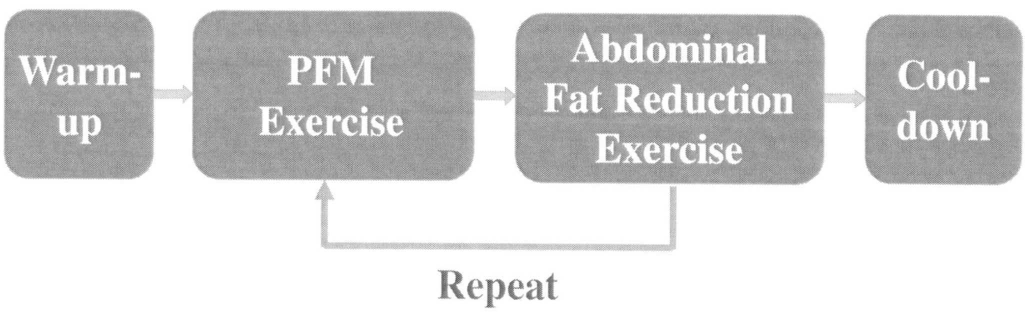

Figure 5. Recommended flow of combined PFM and abdominal fat reduction exercise.

Performing both PFM and fitness exercises may lead to greater physical function in elderly adults with urinary incontinence, which in turn may lead to a more active social lifestyle, increasing their quality of life. In fact, Kim et al. (2007), who investigated the effects of a combined PFM and fitness exercise intervention on cure rates of stress urinary incontinence as well as correlations between functional fitness measures and cure rates of incontinence, found that 54% of women who completed a 3 month PFM and fitness exercise class were cured of urine leakage (Table 5).

Moreover, as depicted in Tables 3 and 5, the PFM and fitness exercise program increased maximum walking speed in community-dwelling elderly women. Not only is this increase in walking speed an indicator of improved function, maximum walking speed may be correlated with being cured from urine leakage. Kim et al. (2007) suggested that an increase of 10.0% or more in walking speed may lead to improvements in urinary incontinence, and increased walking speeds can be maintained for at least one year after an exercise program (Table 3).

Table 5. Comparison of functional fitness and incontinence variables between the intervention and control groups after the 3-month exercise program. (Kim, H.; Suzuki, T.; Yoshida, Y. & Yoshida, H. (2007). Effectiveness of multidimensional exercises for the treatment of stress urinary incontinence in elderly community-dwelling Japanese women: a randomized, controlled, crossover trial. *Journal of the American Geriatrics Society, 55,* 1932-1939, with permission from the American Geriatrics Society)

Variable	Group	Baseline	3-Month Exercise	Analysis of Variance (Group ×Time)	*P*-Value
Body Weight, kg, mean±SD	I	52.2 ± 9.2	50.8 ± 9.2	$F(1, 63)=9.1$	0.004
	C	53.1 ± 9.4	52.9 ± 9.1		
BMI, kg/m^2, mean±SD	I	24.5 ± 4.2	23.8 ± 4.0	$F(1, 63)=5.9$	0.019
	C	24.2 ± 3.8	24.1 ± 3.6		
Usual walking speed, m/s, mean±SD	I	1.1 ± 0.3	1.1 ± 0.2	$F(1, 63)=1.0$	0.312
	C	1.1 ± 0.2	1.1 ± 0.3		
Maximum walking speed, m/s, mean±SD	I	1.6 ± 0.4	1.7 ± 0.4	$F(1, 63)=4.7$	0.035
	C	1.7 ± 0.3	1.6 ± 0.3		
Grip strength, kg, mean±SD	I	17.5 ± 4.3	18.2 ± 4.0	$F(1, 63)=0.1$	0.729
	C	18.5 ± 4.8	18.9 ± 4.8		
Adductor muscle strength, Nm, mean±SD					
Seated	I	48.6 ± 14.4	59.4 ± 14.7	$F(1, 63)=13.4$	0.001
	C	50.2 ± 12	51.5 ± 13.1		
Supine	I	42.3 ± 14.6	49.2 ± 17.3	$F(1, 63)=10.8$	0.002
	C	39.8 ± 10.1	40.7 ± 11.2		
Frequency score of urine leakage, point,	I	3.4 ± 1.3	1.5 ± 1.8	$F(1,63)=6.0$	0.018
mean±SD	C	3 ± 1.4	2.4 ± 1.4		
Cured of urine leakage (%)	I	0	54.5	Z=3.863	<0.001
	C	0	9.4		

SD = standard deviation; I = intervention group; C = control group.

2.4.3. PFM and Thermal Therapy

Recently, abdominal and lower back heating have been introduced as treatments for urinary incontinence (Kim, 2012). Heating may have positive effects on renal function by suppressing renal sympathetic nerve activity, promoting bladder voiding, and increasing frequency of urination (Tsai and Chen, 1993).

One previous study used a heat and steam generating sheet (HSGS), a thin, flexible filmed sheet that generates heat and steam immediately after unsealing, as a thermal treatment (Kim, 2011b). The sheet increases the temperature of the skin surface to 38 to 40℃ as it generates heat and steam for over 5 hours. This particular study showed that the HSGS combined with exercise yielded the highest incontinence cure rates compared with exercise or the HSGS alone. The HSGS also seems to have beneficial effects for different urinary incontinence types. Research reveals higher cure rates in those with stress urinary incontinence with the combination of both exercise and HSGS; however, there is strong evidence that the HSGS can be used as a supplementary treatment method in order to enhance the effects of behavioral therapy on those with stress, as well as urge and mixed urinary incontinence (Kim et al., 2011b) (Table 6).

Table 6. Cure rate of urinary incontinence according to urinary incontinence type and intervention group. (Kim, H.; Yoshida, H. & Suzuki, T. (2011b). Effects of exercise treatment with or without heat and steam generating sheet on urine loss in community-dwelling Japanese elderly women with urinary incontinence. *Geriatrics and Gerontology International*, *11*, 452-459, with permission from the Japan Geriatrics Society)

Type of UI	Ex+HSGS n=37	Ex n=35	HSGS n=37	GE n=34	χ^2 value	*P*-value*
Stress UI, %(n)	61.5(8)	53.8(7)	25.0(3)	9.1(1)	8.94	0.03
Urge UI, %(n)	50.0(7)	16.7(2)	13.3(2)	0.0(0)	12.88	0.005
Mixed UI, %(n)	40.0(4)	30.0(3)	30.0(3)	0.0(0)	3.02	0.389
Total cure rate	51.4(19)	34.3(12)	21.6(1)	2.9(1)	21.89	<0.001

UI=urinary incontinence; Ex=exercise group; HSGS=heat and steam generating sheet group; GE=general education group.

* Kruskal-Wallis test.

3. Predictor Variables

Several characteristics that may influence treatment outcomes have been examined, including age, gender, urine loss frequency and amount, incontinence type, duration of urinary incontinence, chronic conditions, medications, and functional fitness as well as compliance to the prescribed exercise therapy. Compliance to exercise is the key factor to long-term success (Lagro-Janssen & van Weel., 1998; McDowell et al., 1999), BMI reduction also has positive influences on urge, mixed and stress UI treatment (Kim et al., 2011a) (Table 7), and weight loss may be an effective treatment in obese women (Subak et al., 2005, 2009).

Behavioral treatments are effective in reducing urinary incontinence episodes; however, in some cases, the treatments described in this chapter may be insufficient. When the behavioral methods do not successfully reduce incontinence episodes in the elderly, other medical treatments such as surgery and pharmacological therapies may be necessary to alleviate the symptoms of urinary incontinence.

Table 7. Adjusted odds ratios for cure of urine leakage after intervention and the 7-month follow-up. (Kim, H.; Yoshida, H. & Suzuki, T. (2011a). The effects of multidimensional exercise treatment on community-dwelling elderly Japanese women with stress, urge, and mixed urinary incontinence: A randomized controlled trial. *International Journal of Nursing Studies, 48,* 1165-1172, with permission from Elsevier)

	After 3-month exercise			After 7-month follow-up		
	Adjusted			Adjusted		
Variable	OR *	95%CI	*p* Value	OR *	95%CI	*p* Value
Amount of urine leakage	0.69	0.39-0.98	0.049	0.78	0.26-1.88	0.600
Frequency of urine leakage	1.16	0.24-5.79	0.856	1.63	0.73-4.01	0.248
Compliance to exercise	1.03	1.01-1.16	0.048	1.13	1.02-1.29	0.031
Decreased of BMI	0.67	0.48-0.89	0.011	0.78	0.60-0.96	0.028
Increased of walking speed	0.97	0.91-1.04	0.414	0.99	0.94-1.06	0.913
Period of urine leakage	1.01	0.91-1.13	0.919	1.01	0.91-1.14	0.913

Conclusion

Urinary incontinence is highly prevalent in the elderly population and associated with morbidity and poor outcomes. Many factors contribute to the development of urinary incontinence in the elderly including sex, chronic disease, obesity, low sphincter muscle strength, lifestyle (smoking, alcohol, sedentariness), impaired mobility, and aging itself, some of which are preventable and/or modifiable. The benefits of behavioral treatments such as PFM and weight or BMI reduction exercises are that they are safe with few risks and no side effects. These therapies are often recommended as first line treatments for elderly people with urinary incontinence.

Evidence reveals that PFM training and fitness exercise targeted at reducing modifiable risk factors are effective strategies for treating urinary incontinence in elderly people, regardless of urinary incontinence type.

References

Bo, K. (1995). Pelvic floor muscle exercise for the treatment of stress urinary incontinence: an exercise physiology perspective. *International Urogynecology Journal, 6,* 282-291.

Bo, K. (2004). Pelvic floor muscle training is effective in treatment of female stress urinary incontinence, but how does it work? *International Urogynecology Journal, 15,* 76-84.

Bo, K.; Talseth, T. & Holme, I. (1999). Single blind, randomized controlled trial of pelvic floor exercises, electrical stimulation, vaginal cones, and no treatment in management of genuine stress incontinence in women. *British Medical Journal, 318,* 487-493.

Borello-France, D.F.; Zyczynski, H.M.; Downey, P.A.: Rause, C.R. & Wister, J.A. (2006). Effect of pelvic-floor muscle exercise position on continence and quality-of-life outcomes in women with stress urinary incontinence. *Physical Therapy, 86,* 974-986.

Bump, R.C.; Hurt, W.G.; Fantl, A. & Wyman, J.F. (1991). *American Journal of Obstetrics and Gynecology, 165,* 322-329.

Bump, R.C.; Sugerman, H.J.; Fantl, JA. & McClish, D.K. (1992). Obesity and lower urinary tract function in women: effect of surgically induced weight loss. *American Journal of Obstetrics and Gynecology, 167* 392-397.

Burgio, K.L.; Goode, P.S.; Locher, J.L.; Umlauf, M.G.; Roth, D.L.; Richter, H.E.; Varner, R.E. & Lloyd, I.K. (2002). Behavioral training with and without biofeedback in the treatment of urge incontinence in older women. A randomized controlled trial. *The Journal of the American Medical Association, 288,* 2293-2299.

Burgio, K.L.; Locher, J.L.; Goode, P.S.; Hardin, J.M.; McDowell, B.J.; Dombrowski, M. & Candib, D. (1998). Behavioral vs drug treatment for urge urinary incontinence in older women: a randomized controlled trial. *The Journal of the American Medical Association, 280,* 1995-2000.

Burgio, K.L.; Robinson, J.C. & Engel, B.T. (1986). The role of biofeedback in Kegel exercise training for stress urinary incontinence. *American Journal of Obstetrics and Gynecology, 154,* 58-64.

Burns, P.A.; Pranikoff, K.; Nochajski, T.H.; Hadley, E.C.; Levy. K.J. & Ory, M.G. (1993). A comparison of effectiveness of biofeedback and pelvic muscle exercise treatment of stress incontinence in older community-dwelling women. *The Journals of Gerontology. Series A, Biological Sciences and Medical Sciences, 48,* M167-174.

Eustice, S.; Roe, B. & Paterson, J. (2000). Prompted voiding for the management of urinary incontinence in adults. *Cochrane Database of Systematic Reviews, Issue 2,* CD002113.

Fantl, J.A.; Wyman, J.F.; McClish, D.K.; Harkins, S.W.; Elswick, R.K.; Taylor, J.R. & Hadley, E.C. (1991). Efficacy of bladder training in older women with urinary incontinence. *The Journal of the American Medical Association, 265,* 609-613.

Goode, P.S.; Burgio, K.L.; Johnson, T.M.,II.; Clay, O.J.; Roth, D.L.; Markland, A.D.; Burkhardt, J.H.; Issa, M.M. & Lloyd, L.K. (2011). Behavioral therapy with or without biofeedback and pelvic floor electrical stimulation for persistent postprostatectomy incontinence: a randomized controlled trial. *The Journal of the American Medical Association, 305,* 151-159.

Goode, P.S.; Burgio, K.L.; Locher, J.L.; Roth, D.L.; Umlauf, M.G.; Richter, H.E.; Varner, R.E. & Lloyd, L.K. (2003). Effect of behavioral training with or without pelvic floor electrical stimulation on stress incontinence in women: a randomized controlled trial. *The Journal of the American Medical Association, 290,* 345-352.

Herbison, G.P. & Dean, N. (2002). Weighted vaginal cones for urinary incontinence. *Cochrane Database of Systematic Reviews, Issue 1,* CD002114.

Herderschee, R.; Hay-Smith, E.J.C.; Herbison, G.P; Roovers, J.P & Heineman, M.J. (2011). Feedback or biofeedback to augment pelvic floor muscle training for urinary incontinence in women. *Cochrane Database of Systematic Reviews, Issue 7,* CD009252.

Jeffcoate, T.N. & Francis, W.J. (1966). Urgency incontinence in the female. *American Journal Obstetrics and Gynecology, 94,* 604-618.

Kegel, A.H. (1948). Progressive resistance exercise in the functional restoration of the perineal muscles. *American Journal of Obstetrics and Gynecology, 56,* 238-248.

Kegel, A.H. (1951). Physiologic therapy for urinary stress incontinence. *The Journal of the American Medical Association, 146,* 915-917.

Kim, H.; Suzuki, T.; Yoshida, Y. & Yoshida, H. (2007). Effectiveness of multidimensional exercises for the treatment of stress urinary incontinence in elderly community-dwelling Japanese women: a randomized, controlled, crossover trial. *Journal of the American Geriatrics Society, 55,* 1932-1939.

Kim, H.; Yoshida, H.; Hu, X.; Yukawa, H.; Shinkai, S.; Kumagai, S.; Fujiwara, Y.; Yoshida, Y.; Furuna, T.; Sugiura, M.; Ishizaki, T. & Suzuki, T. (2004). Risk factors associated with onset of urinary incontinence in community-dwelling elderly population: a 4-year follow-up study. *Nihon Koshu Eisei Zasshi, 51,* 612-622 [Article in Japanese].

Kim, H.; Yoshida, H. & Suzuki, T. (2011a). The effects of multidimensional exercise treatment on community-dwelling elderly Japanese women with stress, urge, and mixed urinary incontinence: A randomized controlled trial. *International Journal of Nursing Studies, 48,* 1165-1172.

Kim, H.; Yoshida, H. & Suzuki, T. (2011b). Effects of exercise treatment with or without heat and steam generating sheet on urine loss in community-dwelling Japanese elderly women with urinary incontinence. *Geriatrics and Gerontology International, 11,* 452-459.

Kim, H (2012). Behavioral Treatment for Geriatric Syndrome, Geriatrics, Craig S. Atwood (Ed.), ISBN: 978-953-51-0080-5, InTech, DOI: 10.5772/33556. Available from: http://www.intechopen.com/books/geriatrics/behavioral-treatment-for-geriatric-syndrome.

Lagro-Janssen, T. & van Weel, C. (1998). Long-term effect of treatment of female incontinence in general practice. *British Journal of General Practice, 48,*1735-1738.

Landi, F.; Cesari, M.; Russo, A.; Onder, G.; Lattanzio, F. & Bernabei, R. (2003). Potentially reversible risk factors and urinary incontinence in frail older people living in community. *Age and Ageing, 32,*194-199.

McDowell, B.J.; Engberg, S.; Sereika, S.; Donovan, N.; Jubeck, M.E.; Weber, E. & Engberg, R. (1999). Effectiveness of behavioral therapy to treat incontinence in homebound older adults. *Journal of the American Geriatrics Society, 47,*309-318.

Ostaszkiewicz, J.; Johnston, L. & Roe, B. (2004). Timed voiding for the management of urinary incontinence in adults. *Cochrane Database of Systematic Reviews, Issue 1,* CD002802.

Peattie, A.B.; Plevnik, S. & Stanton, S.L. (1988). Vaginal cones: a conservative method of treating genuine stress incontinence. *British Journal of Obstetrics and Gynecology, 95,*1049-1053.

Sand, P.K.; Richardson, D.A.; Staskin, D.R.; Swift, S.E.; Appell, R.A.; Whitmore, K.E. & Ostergard, D.R. (1995). Pelvic floor electrical stimulation in the treatment of genuine stress incontinence: A multicenter, placebo-controlled trial. *American Journal of Obstetrics and Gyencology, 173,* 72-79.

Subak, L.L.; Whitcomb, E.; Shen, H.; Saxton, J.; Vittinghoff, E. & Brown, J.S. (2005). Weight loss: A novel and effective treatment for urinary incontinence. *The Journal of Urology, 174,* 190-195.

Subak, L.L.; Wing, R.; West, D.S.; Franklin, F.; Vittinghoff, E.; Creasman, J.M.; Richter, H.E.; Myers, D.; Burgio, K.L.; Gorin, A.A.; Macer, J.; Kusek, J.W. & Grady, D. (2009). Weight loss to treat urinary incontinence in overweight and obese women. *The New England Journal of Medicine, 360,*481-490.

Tsai, T.J. & Chen, C.F. (1993). Effects of heat therapy on renal hemodynamics, compensatory hypertrophy and glomerulonephritis in rats. *Nephron, 63,* 207-213.

Wallace, S.A.; Roe, B.; Williams, K. & Palmer, M. (2004). Bladder training for urinary incontinence in adults. *Cochrane Database of Systematic Reviews, Issue 1,* CD001308.

Wyman, J.F.; Fantl, J.A.; McClish, D.K. & Bump, R.C. (1998). Comparative efficacy of behavioral interventions in the management of female urinary incontinence. Continence Program for Women Research Group. *American Journal of Obstetrics and Gynecology*, Vol.179, No.4, pp. 999-1007.

In: Urinary Incontinence
Editor: Eric Chung

ISBN: 978-1-62618-482-4

Chapter 7

The Role of Physical Therapies in Urinary Incontinences

Renata Teles Buere[1], Ericka Kirsthine Valentin[1], Gisele Silva Ribeiro[1], José Anacleto Dutra De Resende Júnior[2], Danilo Souza Lima Da Costa Cruz[2], João Luiz Schiavini[2] and Ronaldo Damião[2]

[1]Department of Physical Therapy,
Pedro Ernesto University Hospital (HUPE),
Polyclinic Piquet Carneiro, Rio de Janeiro State University,
Rio de Janeiro, Brazil
[2]Department of Urology, Pedro Ernesto University Hospital (HUPE),
Rio de Janeiro State University, Rio de Janeiro, Brazil

Abstract

Urinary incontinence is a common problem with high prevalence that cause serious economic, social and psychological problems, besides that affecting significantly the quality of life. Its prevalence varies widely from 3% to 55% depending on the definition used and population studied. It is estimated that approximately 29.5 million Americans suffer from UI and expenses generated by this issue revolves around 26.4 billion dollars (Dmochowski et al., 2003; Wagner; Hu, 1998).

A recent study (EPIC) on the epidemiology of UI, the largest population-based study carried out so far, in five countries and over 19 000 women, showed a 11.8% prevalence of overactive bladder, and this rate increased with age (Irwin et al., 2006).

Urinary incontinence is an important component of health care expenditure, and an important and neglected cause of morbidity in women. Studies evaluating management of this condition show that the majority of women respond to simple measures such as pelvic floor exercises.

Common treatments for UI include surgery, drug therapies, and behavioral interventions. Behavioral interventions such as pelvic floor muscle (PFM) exercises and bladder training have potential benefits with few risks and no side effects. PFM exercises, initiated by Kegel in 1948 have been found to be efficacious for stress incontinence (Kegel, 1948) Many investigators have validated the effectiveness of the short-term effect of PFM exercises in reducing urine leakage, with improvement rates reported to range from 17% to 84% (Kegel, 1951) (Bo, 1995).

Physical therapies continue to play an important conservative role in the management of UI. Unfortunately it require strong commitment from the patients, constant reinforcement from the health care physicians and many patients will require re-educated and re-train to adhere to the plan and ultimately benefit from this treatment option.

Introduction

Urinary incontinence (UI) is a common problem and causes major economic, social and psychological problems resulting in poor quality of life. The prevalence of UI varies widely from 3% to 55% depending on the definition used and population studied. It is estimated that approximately 29.5 million Americans suffer from UI and more than 20 billion dollars were spent on issues related to UI (Dmochowski et al., 2003; Wagner; Hu, 1998). The recent EPIC study, the largest population-based epidemiology study on UI, was conducted in five countries and involved over 19 000 women, showed an 11.8% prevalence of overactive bladder, and this rate increased with age (Irwin et al., 2006).

The management of UI forms an important component of health care expenditure. Many published literature showed that the majority of women respond to simple measures such as lifestyle modification and pelvic floor exercises.

Behavioral interventions such as pelvic floor muscle training (PFMT) and bladder retraining have potential benefits with few risks and no side effects. PFMT was first proposed by Kegel in 1948 and has been found to be highly effective in the treatment of stress urinary incontinence (Kegel, 1948). Many investigators have validated the short-term efficacy PFMT in reducing the amount of urine leakage, with improvement rates reported to range from 17% to 84% (Kegel, 1951) (Bo, 1995).

Lower Tract Voiding Physiology

The pelvic floor is responsible for supporting the pelvic organs and forms part of the mechanisms of urinary and fecal continence. As a striated skeletal muscle, it can be trained to increase its muscle tone and strength. The pelvic floor musculature consists of 70% slow or tonic fibers (Type I) that is responsible for the action of the anti-gravity muscles, and 30% phasic or fast fibers (Type II) that play a key part in urethral closure against sudden increase the intra-abdominal pressure.

The lower urinary tract is innervated by both parasympathetic and sympathetic autonomic nervous system and also the somatic nervous system. The parasympathetic innervations are derived from pelvic nerve S2-4 while the sympathetic innervations arise from hypo gastric nerve T11, T12, L1 and L2.

Table 1. Muscles of the Pelvic Floor (Adapter from Moreno and Spence) (MORENO, 2004) (SPENCE, 1991)

Muscles of the Pelvic Floor				
Levator ani, puborectalis muscle, pubococcygeus muscle, Muscle iliococcygeal				
Muscles	Origin	Insertion	Innervation	Action
Puborectalis	The inner surface of the pubis	Around the anorectal junction	Sacral (S3 and S4)	Supports the pelvic viscera, resists the increase of intra-abdominal pressure, raises the floor of the pelvis, assists and / or prevents defecation, childbirth supports the head of the fetus during the dilatation of the cervix
Pubococcygeus	The inner surface of the pubis, ischial spine	Coccyx and ligament anococcígeo		
Iliococcygeal	Arch tendon of the m. ischial spine and internal obturator	Coccyx and ligament anococcígeus		
Muscles	Origin	Insertion	Innervation	Action
Muscles	Origin	Insertion	Innervation	Action
Isquiococcígeus (m coccygeal)	Ischial spine and sacrospinal ligament	Sacrum and coccyx, laterally	Sacral (S3 and S4)	It strengthens the pelvic floor and helps the levator ani muscle to support the pelvic viscera
External anal sphincter	Central tendon of perineum	Dermis and subcutaneous tissue around the anus and ligament anococcígeus	Pudendal {S2 and S4)	Fecal continence
Superficial and deep transverse perineal	Ischial tuberosity and inferior ramus of the ischium	Central tendon of perineum	Pudendal {S2 and S4)	Protection of the levator ani muscle and tendon fixed the center of the perineum
External urethral sphincter	Muscular ring around the membranous urethra (ostium external)	Muscular ring around the membranous urethra (ostium external)	Pudendal{S2 and S4)	Urinary continence
Ischiocavernosus	Ischial tuberosity and ramus of the ischium	At the root of the clitoris or penis (corpus cavernosum)	Pudendal {S2 and S4)	Fixed branches of the lower branches of the clitoris to the pubis and the ischium and the urogenital diaphragm. Slows the return of blood to the veins, keeping the erection of the clitoris or penis.
Bulbospongiosus	In women: central tendon of the perineum. In men: median raphe in the root of the penis.	In women, side of the vagina to the base of the clitoris and the urogenital diaphragm. In men, circulating the root of the penis and attaches on the the opposite side.	Pudendal {S2 and S4)	In women: helps the erection of the clitoris and fixing the bulb of the vestibule in the urogenital diaphragm. In men: channel empties the urethra and helps penis erection.

Conservative Management of Urinary Incontinence

Several conservative approaches have been proposed for the treatment of urinary incontinence. PFMT in conjunction with vaginal cones, electrical stimulation, biofeedback, or electromyography are utilized widely and effectively in the management of UI (Berghmans et al., 2000). This physical therapy simple, affordable and has minimal morbidity. All patients are advised to keep a voiding diary and a 24 hour pad weight to document the degree of UI.

The Pelvic Floor Muscles Training (PFMT)

PFMT was first developed in 1948 and is defined by International Continence Society (ICS) as a repetitive selective voluntary contractions and relaxations of pelvic floor muscles. The PFMT should be performed according to the principles of exercise physiology (standardize frequency, intensity and duration) and it is recommended that PFMT should be carried out over a three to six months period and incorporated into the daily activities. In order to achieve better outcomes, it should be patient driven. Physiotherapist input has been shown to improve the outcomes (Inside; International; Journal, 1995; Kegel, 1948, 1951).

The PFMT can be accomplished in several positions. We suggest you start by lying down and evolve into a sitting position and the standing position. It is important that the muscles are trained in isolation without the use of accessory muscles such as abdominals, gluteus, adductors and rotators of the thigh. In a comprehensive manner, a systematic review by Cochrane provides support for recommending the training of the pelvic floor muscles as a first line of conservative treatment programs for women with stress urinary incontinence, urgency or mixed (Level A evidence) (Dumoulin, 2010).

A focused pelvic floor examination should be conducted as part of the assessment for UI (Figure 1). It is important to observe the tropism, color, asymmetry, scarring and urethral position. When performing vaginal examination, Bivalve speculum should be used and patient should be asked to perform Valsalva maneuver to exclude pelvic organ prolapse.

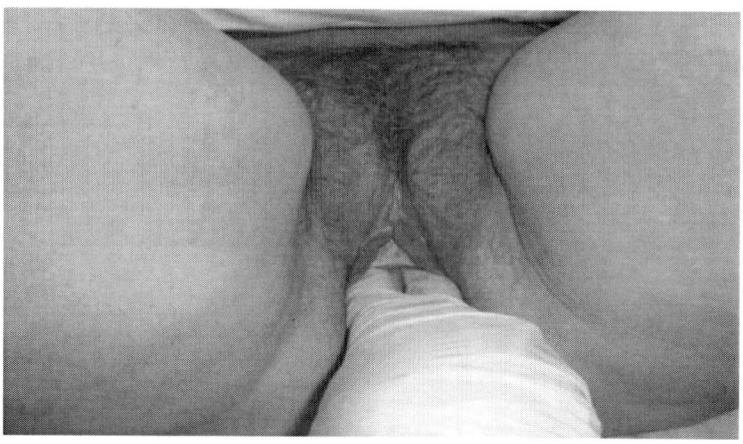

Figure 1. Specific examination for Pelvic floor muscles.

Advantages of the pelvic floor muscle training PFMT:

- Improvement in the tropism of muscle fibers
- Better awareness of muscle groups
- Increasing the connective tissue
- Increased recruitment of motor neurons
- Minimally invasive treatment
- Low cost / easy acceptance
- Degree of success of moderate to high
- Can be applied individually or in groups in almost all patients

Vaginal Cones

Plevnik (1985) introduced exercises using vaginal cones to assist women to train the pelvic floor musculatures (Bø; Talseth; Holme, 1999; Kato; Kondo, 1997; Plevnik, 1985). The patients are encouraged to try to retain various cones of increasing weight in the vagina to increase the pelvic muscle tone. This technique consists of using a set of cones of equal size but of increasing weight, with anatomical shape which allows its introduction into the vagina. The reflex action of the pelvic floor muscles provides an internal strengthening that quickly restores muscle tone. Recovery will be noticed after two to three weeks, at which point it is recommended to use higher weights, in order to continue improving the process (Cammu; Van Nylen, 1998).

The cones (Figure 2) act by recruiting the muscle fibers of types I and II, and improve proprioception perineal muscles of these patients, resulting in increased strength. The favorable results in the treatment of stress urinary incontinence (Sui) using vaginal cone varies from 60% to 80% of cases (Kegel, 1951; Peattie, A.B., Plevnik, S., Station, 1988; Plevnik, 1985; Schubler, 1994).

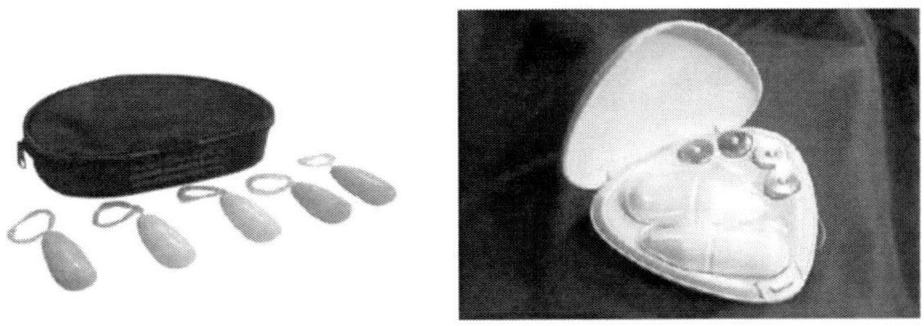

Figure 2. Vaginal Cones.

Electrical Stimulation

Electrical stimulation (ES) is designed to strengthen the pelvic floor muscles and improve proprioception and promote inhibition of detrusor muscle.

The electrical discharge generates a nerve stimulation applied to the motor unit action potential that generates the form of muscle contraction. The ES can be performed with surface electrodes via posterior tibia (Figure 3), sacral (Figure 4), perirectal (Figure 5), perivaginal (Figure 6), intra-rectal (Figure 7) or intra-vaginal (Figure 8) areas using specific probes for each individual cases.

The evidence for the efficacy of the use of ES in the literature is lacking (Shamliyan et al., 2008). However, ES and magnetic stimulation have been approved for use in many Western countries. The type of electrical current utilized is preferably an asymmetric biphasic current depolarized. The frequency of the electrical current depends on the goal of treatment, and 4 to 80 Hz is the recommended intensity as the tolerable pain threshold in many patients.

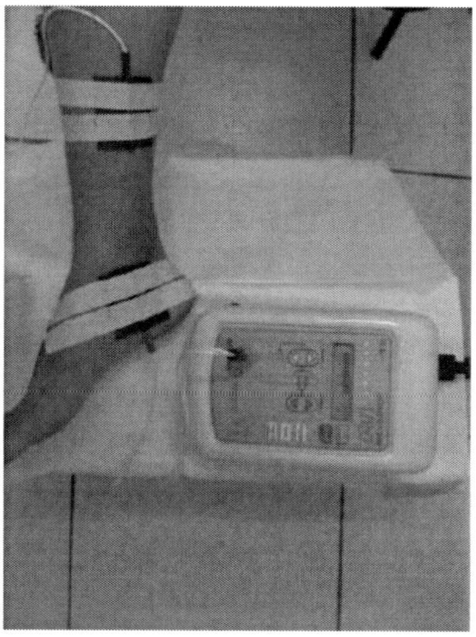

Figure 3. Electrical stimulation posterior tibiae using surface electrodes.

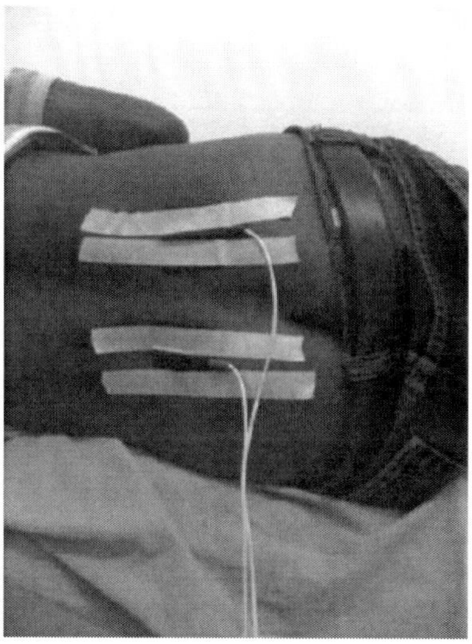

Figure 4. Electrical stimulation in sacral region.

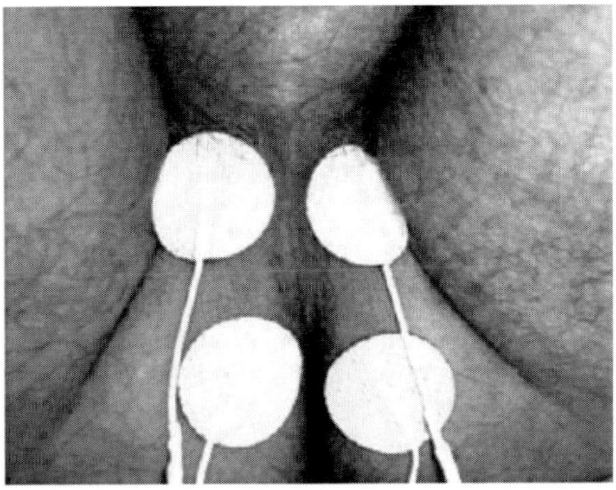

Figure 5. Perirectal electrical stimulation.

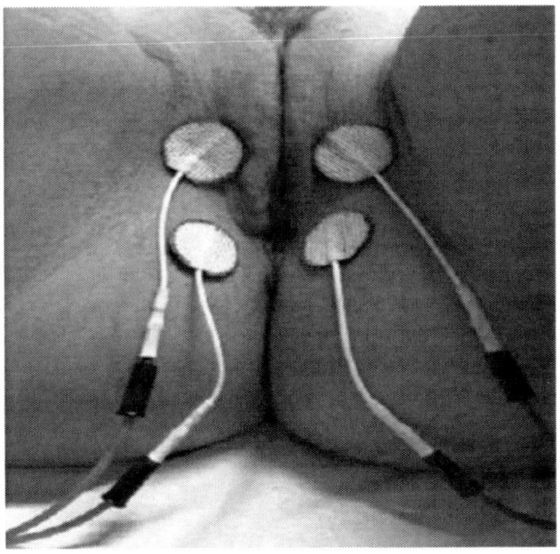

Figure 6. Peri vaginal electrical stimulation.

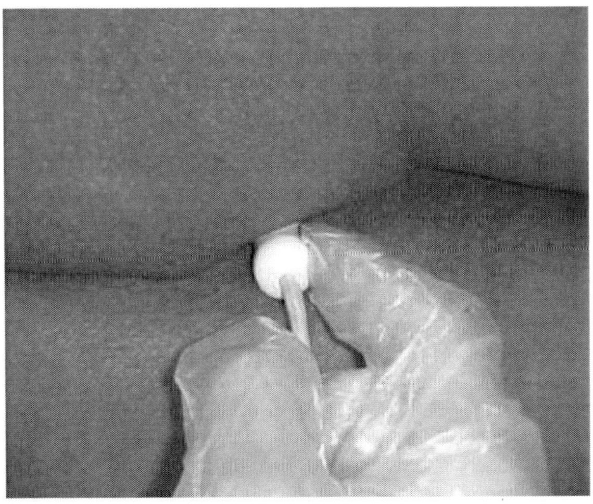

Figure 7. Intra rectal electrical stimulation.

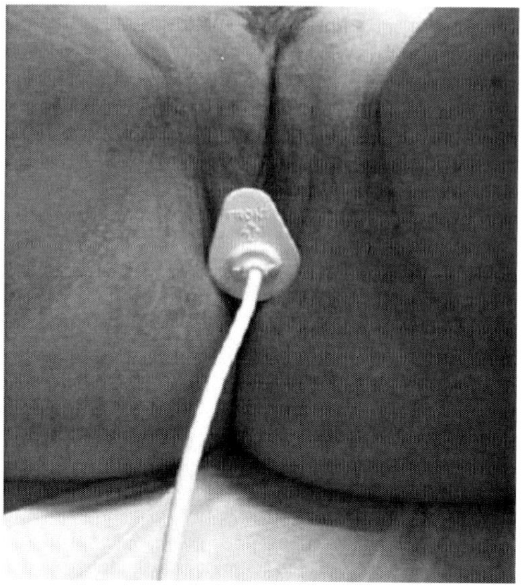

Figure 8. Intra vaginal electrical stimulation.

Biofeedback

The biofeedback by pressure was developed by Kegel and is mainly used as a research tool. Electromyography biofeedback is the preferred option. The goal of biofeedback is to stimulate the sphincteric activity and makes it perceptible to the patient either by visual or auditory stimuli. Biofeedback aims to improve the learning of muscle contraction, isolate the specific pelvic floor muscles, and increases the pelvic muscle reflex contraction.

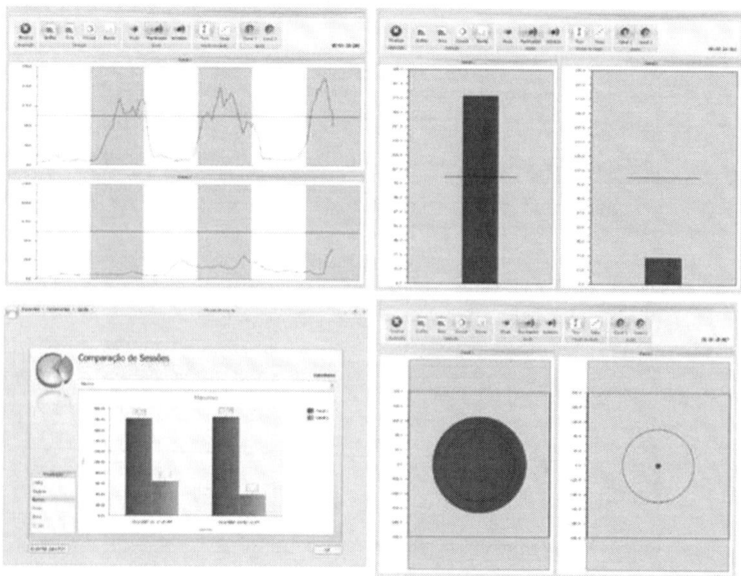

Figure 9. Patient Training Pelvic Floor Muscles using Biofeedback.

Behavior Therapy

Behavioral therapy for UI consists of educating patients on their condition and assisting the patients to develop strategies to minimize or eliminate incontinence (Payne, 2000). Behavioral therapy includes changing the toileting behavior and habits of daily life that can potentially contribute to the worsening of urinary incontinence. The following are suggestions on behavioral modification:

- Delayed urination: Guidance is given to the patient to urinate at pre-determined intervals, usually 2 to 4 hourly. This ensures that the patient will be emptying the bladder at intervals with planned objectives of preventing urinary frequency increased or decreased in an attempt to avoid involuntary detrusor contractions and urinary incontinence.
- Bladder training provides guidance of urination with scheduled intervals, with the intervention to reduce leakage episodes; it is intended with this training retrain functional bladder capacity.
- Bladder diary consists of documenting all voiding events in the last 24 hours. The patient must record the time of day when void in the toilet and the quantity of the voiding. Record if you have leakage and what kind of activity were relationated with the leakage. Record if had urge or urge-incontinence. Record the quantity and a kind of liquid was intake.

Day:			Date:			
Name:						
Time	Toilet	Leakage	Was there an urge?	Activity	Intake	Bowel movement

Conclusion

Physical therapies continue to play an important conservative role in the management of UI. Unfortunately it require strong commitment from the patients, constant reinforcement from the health care physicians and many patients will require re-educated and re-train to adhere to the plan and ultimately benefit from this treatment option.

References

Berghmans, L. C. et al. Conservative treatment of urge urinary incontinence in women: a systematic review of randomized clinical trials. *BJU international,* v. 85, n. 3, p. 254-63, fev. 2000.

Bo, K. Pelvic Floor Muscle Exercise for the Treatment of Stress Urinary Incontinence: *An Exercise Physiology Perspective.* p. 282-291, 1995.

BØ, K.; Talseth, T.; Holme, I. Single blind, randomised controlled trial of pelvic floor exercises, electrical stimulation, vaginal cones, and no treatment in management of genuine stress incontinence in women. 1999.

Cammu, H.; Van Nylen, M. Pelvic floor exercises versus vaginal weight cones in genuine stress incontinence. *European journal of obstetrics, gynecology, and reproductive biology*, v. 77, n. 1, p. 89-93, mar. 1998.

Dmochowski, R. R. et al. Duloxetine versus placebo for the treatment of North American women with stress urinary incontinence. *The Journal of urology,* v. 170, n. 4 Pt 1, p. 1259-63, out. 2003.

Dumoulin, C. Pelvic floor muscle training versus no treatment, or inactive control treatments, for urinary incontinence in women . p. 1-2, 2010.

Inside, L.; International, G.; Journal, U. Pelvic floor muscle exercise for the treatment of stress urinary incontinence: An exercise physiology perspective. *International Urogynecology Journal,* v. 6, n. 5, p. 282-291, 1995.

Irwin, D. E. et al. Population-based survey of urinary incontinence, overactive bladder, and other lower urinary tract symptoms in five countries: results of the EPIC study. *European urology,* v. 50, n. 6, p. 1306-14; *discussion* 1314-5, dez. 2006.

Kato, K.; Kondo, A. Clinical value of vaginal cones for the management of female stress incontinence. *International Urogynecology Journal And Pelvic Floor Dysfunction,* v. 8, n. 5, p. 314-317, set. 1997.

Kegel, A. H. Progressive resistance exercise in the functional restoration of the perineal muscles. *American journal of obstetrics and gynecology,* v. 56, n. 2, p. 238-248, ago. 1948.

Kegel, A. H. Physiologic therapy for urinary stress incontinence. *Journal of the American Medical Association,* v. 146, n. 10, p. 915-917, jul. 1951.

Moreno, A. L. Fisioterapia em Uroginecologia. 1. ed. [S.l.] Ed. *Manole,* 2004. p. 1-22, 51-59, 99-112, 133-136

Payne, C. K. Behavioral therapy for overactive bladder. *Urology,* v. 55, n. 5A Suppl, p. 3-6; discussion 14-6, maio. 2000.

Peattie, A.B., Plevnik, S., Station, S. L. Vaginal cones: a conservative method of treating genuine stress incontinence. *Br. J. Obstet. Gynecol.*, v. 95, p. 1049-1053, 1988.

Plevnik, S. New methods for testing and strengthening the pelvic floor muscles. In: *Annual Meeting of The International Continence Society. International Continence Society-ICS,* p. 267-268, 1985.

Schubler, B. Pelvic floor reeducation: principles and practise. *Int. Urogynecol. J.,* v. 10, p. 93-98, 1994.

Shamliyan, T. A et al. Systematic review: randomized, controlled trials of nonsurgical treatments for urinary incontinence in women. *Annals of internal medicine,* v. 148, n. 6, p. 459-73, 18 mar. 2008.

Spence, A. P. Anatomia Humana Básica. 2. ed. [S.l.] Ed. *Manole*, 1991. p. 215-219

Wagner, T. H.; Hu, T. W. Economic costs of urinary incontinence in 1995. *Urology,* v. 51, n. 3, p. 355-61, mar. 1998.

In: Urinary Incontinence
Editor: Eric Chung

ISBN: 978-1-62618-482-4

Chapter 8

Medical Treatments of Overactive Bladder: Current and Future Therapeutic Applications

Eric Chung*
Department of Urology, Princess Alexandra Hospital, Brisbane QLD, Australia

Abstract

Overactive bladder (OAB) is a clinical syndrome of lower urinary tract dysfunction and there is a strong correlation between OAB and detrusor overactivity (DO). At present, the exact pathogenesis of OAB remains unclear and it is likely that there are multiple factors involved in the disease complex. OAB remains under-diagnosed and under-treated due to the lack of awareness, embarrassment and/or misconception that OAB is a natural consequence of ageing, as well as lack of ideal medical therapeutic options. The available medical treatment is associated with poor compliance and high discontinuation rates secondary to high incidence of adverse events. In recent years, considerable effort has been made to identify an ideal drug for the treatment of OAB that is uro-selective i.e. able to discriminate between normal and abnormal bladder contractions. Several promising pharmacological targets include β3-agonist, NK1 receptor antagonists, Rho kinase inhibitors, K^+ channels blockers and purinergic receptor antagonist. The following chapter reviews the current and novel medical therapeutic agents for the treatment of OAB.

Introduction

Overactive bladder (OAB) is a clinical syndrome of lower urinary tract dysfunction characterised by the symptoms of urgency, with or without urge incontinence, usually with frequency and nocturia [1]. The prevalence of OAB increases with age and it is estimated that

* Corresponding author: Dr Eric Chung, Department of Urology, Princess Alexandra Hospital, Ipswich Rd, Brisbane, QLD 4103, Australia, (T): +617-33242468, (F):+617-33242546, ericchg@hotmail.com.

42% of men and 31% of women aged greater than 75 years old have OAB [2]. This highly prevalent condition places considerable impact on the overall quality of life, impairing several areas with physical, social, emotional and sexual limitations [3].

There is a strong correlation between OAB and detrusor overactivity (DO). In contrast to the clinical description of OAB, DO is a urodynamic observation of involuntary contractions during bladder filling that commonly associated with a corresponding sensation of urgency [1]. It is important to be aware that heightened or altered sensation of the bladder may manifest as urgency in the absence of DO, impaired bladder compliance, or urinary leak. In the past, terminology such as OAB wet and OAB dry have been used to describe the symptoms of urgency with or without incontinent episodes [4]. While it is justifiable to assume that DO contributes to OAB, OAB is a constellation of clinical symptoms and therefore is likely a consequence of multiple aetiologies.

Pathophysiology of DO: (Figure 1)

Despite the presence of an intrinsic myocyte activity within the detrusor for spontaneous bladder contraction, normal contraction of the bladder during voiding is mainly mediated through the activation of the muscarinic receptors on the detrusor muscle by acetylcholine (ACh) [5]. There are at least 5 known muscarinic receptor subtypes, M1 to M5 and it appears that the majority of the muscarinic receptors in human smooth muscle are of the M2 subtype although M3 receptor subtype has been shown to be more active. These muscarinic receptors are found not only on smooth muscle cells of the bladder, but also on presynaptic nerve terminals to the bladder, urothelial cells, suburothelial nerves, and on suburothelial structures such as interstitial cells, and potentially contribute to the pathophysiology of OAB [6]. In addition to muscarinic receptors, nicotinic receptors are also found in the human urothelium [7]. At present the exact role of ACh in the pathogenesis of DO remains uncertain but evidence is pointing to both a dys-regulation in both the afferent and efferent control of detrusor contractions [5]. In recent times, atropine resistance (non-adrenergic, non cholinergic, NANC) contractions have been reported in normal human detrusor and, in particular, observed in bladder dysfunction associated with lower urinary tract symptoms such as in DO. There is now strong evidence to suggest that ACh is responsible for the NANC component of ATP acting on purinergic receptors within the detrusor muscle [8].

1. **Muscarinic, nicotinic and beta-adrenergic receptors abnormality**
2. **NANC receptors abnormality**
3. **Afferent nerve activity**
4. **Prostanoids**
5. **Efferent activity**
6. **Calcium and Potassium channels hypersensitivity**
7. **Rhoa/Rho kinase pathway**

Figure 1. Proposed pathophysiology of DO.

The importance of afferent nerve activity in the pathogenesis of DO is undisputed and the roles of the urothelium and suburothelial myofibroblasts in afferent activation have became the focus of intense interest [9]. Local release of tachykinins and other peptides from the sensory nerves in the bladder wall has been shown to produce bladder contraction [10]. Prostanoids such as prostaglandin (PG) F2α, PG-E1 α and thromboxane A2 are synthesized locally in both detrusor and bladder mucosa. These prostanoids may affect bladder activity directly by effects on smooth muscles or indirectly via effects on neurotransmission. However the exact role of prostanoids in the pathogenesis of OAB remains unclear. Muscarinic receptors are also known to be expressed on sympathetic nerve endings and play an important role in the regulation of norepinephrine release [11]. In fact it has been postulated that there is an activation of the C-fibers leading to the heightened sensation of bladder filling. The non-neuronal release of neurotransmitters may also represent another mechanism of a direct stimulatory effect on the C-fibers [12].

Activation of detrusor muscle requires an influx of extracellular calcium (Ca^{2+}) through Ca^{2+} channels as well as mobilisation of intracellular Ca^{2+}. The influx of intracellular Ca^{2+} can be blocked by Ca^{2+} antagonists or by opening the K^+ channels. The opening K^+ channels hyperpolarises not only the smooth muscle cells, but also the afferent nerves and decreases the opening probability of Ca^{2+} channels. Therefore it is possible that DO is a result of increased sensitivity to the depolarising stimuli [13]. Human detrusor muscle consists of 2 main types, the K^+ channels (K_{ATP}) and the large conductance Ca^{2+} -activated big K^+ channels (BK_{Ca}). There is also an abundance of β-adrenoceptor within the detrusor layer that is responsible for bladder relaxation in response to noradrenaline. Animal studies have shown that β_3 agonists may have the potential to inhibit spontaneous bladder contraction and increase the bladder capacity [14]. More recently, RhoA/Rho kinase pathway, a Ca^{2+} sensitising pathway has been identified to play a key role in abnormal bladder contractions [15].

Current Medical Therapies of OAB

Given that the pathophysiology of OAB is multifactorial and not fully elucidated the available treatment options for this distressing and debilitating condition remains far from ideal. Conservative treatment is the mainstay of therapy for OAB. The available treatment options include diet and behavioural modifications, bladder retraining, biofeedback, electrical stimulation, pharmacotherapy or a combination of these options. Presently, pharmacotherapy of OAB remains the treatment of choice and is directed towards the detrusor and also both the central and peripheral neural control pathways. The current pharmacological treatment for OAB is aimed at increasing the bladder capacity, decreasing bladder activity and contractility, and/or decreasing sensory (afferent input).

1. Antimuscarinic Agents (Table 1)

Since the physiologic bladder contractions are thought to be primarily triggered by ACh-induced stimulation of the post-ganglionic muscarinic receptor sites on the bladder smooth muscle, antagonists of ACh will depress normal bladder contractions and involuntary bladder contractions. Furthermore, these agents will increase the volume to first involuntary bladder contraction and the total bladder capacity, and decrease the amplitude of the bladder contraction [16]. There is direct experimental evidence that anti-muscarinics decreased activity in both C and A-delta afferent fibres from the bladder during filling and altered the underlying detrusor tone [17].

Table 1. Current pharmacological treatment of OAB

Name	Mechanism of action	Active metabolite	Doses	Specific features
Oxybutynin	Anti(m) Musculotropic relaxant LA	N-DEO	IR-5mg tds/qid ER-5,10 or 15mg TDS-3.9mg twice weekly	Many delivery systems- oral, transdermal, gel and intravesical
Tolterodine	Anti(m)	5-HMT	IR-2mg bd ER-2 or 4mg	Less cognitive side effect
Trospium	Anti(m)	-	IR-20mg bd/tds ER-60mg	Quartenary amines; Tubular excretion
Solifenacin	Anti(m); m3>m2 receptors	-	5 or 10mg	Less cognitive side effect
Darifenacin	Anti(m); m3 receptor selective	-	7.5 or 15 mg	Less cognitive side effect
Fesoterodine	Anti(m)	5-HMT	4 or 8 mg	Less cognitive side effect
Duloxetine	SNRI	-	80 or 120mg	Suicidal tendency among psychiatric patients
Imipramine	Anti(m) Noradrenaline uptake inhibitor	-	25mg incremental increase to 150mg	Ventricular arrhythmias and prolongation of QT interval

(m=muscarinic; LA=local anaesthetic; N-DEO= N-desethyl-oxybutynin; 5-HMT= 5-hydroxymethyl tolterodine; IR=immediate formulation; ER=extended formulation; TDS=transdermal delivery system; SNRI=serotonin noradrenaline reuptake inhibitor)

Antimuscarinic drugs are proven efficacious and safe and are the mainstay of treatment for OAB. They can be divided into tertiary and quaternary amines which differ in molecular size, charge and lipophilicity [5]. The advantage of quaternary compounds is theorectically lower risk of central nervous system (CNS) side effects as they have larger molecular charge and less lipophilicity resulting in limited passage into the CNS [18]. A recent meta-analysis on antimuscarinic agents found that these agents are more effective and significantly reduce urge incontinence episodes, severity of urgency, micturition frequency and provide significant improvements in quality of life [19]. Head-to-head studies comparing these agents are not available and therefore no "best-in-class" recommendation can be given. The vast majority of agents studied have comparable efficacy and provided improvement in health-related quality of life. However the drug profiles, dosing schedules, drug interactions and tolerability differ and therefore should be individualised when given to certain patients. "Salvaging" non-responders to one drug with another has been shown in several studies and that switching between drugs is a reasonable approach in patients failing initial treatment [20].

As the currently available antimuscarinic agents lack super-selectivity for the M2 and M3 receptors in the bladder, they can produce widespread side-effects on various organ systems. The slight differences in the safety profiles of these antimuscarinic agents are related to their selectivity for specific muscarinic receptor subtypes, selectivity for the bladder compared to salivary glands, their lipophilicity and the ability to cross the blood-brain barriers, as well as their pharmacokinetics. The most common adverse effects include dry mouth, blurred vision, tachycardia, constipation, somnolence, impaired cognition and headache. In general the extended release (ER) formulations are better tolerated that the immediate release (IR) formulations. Antimuscarinic drug is contraindicated in patients with urinary retention, impaired gastric or gastrointestinal motility disorders and uncontrolled narrow-angle glaucoma. The current prescribed doses of antimuscarinic agents are not commonly associated with urinary retention but monitoring of post void residual urine volumes in patients with prostatic enlargement or incomplete bladder emptying is still recommended; however, these diagnoses should not be considered as absolute contraindications to the use of antimuscarinics in such patients with OAB [21]. The risk of blindness in narrow-angle glaucoma is high only if iridotomy had not been performed or that the glaucoma disease is not well- controlled [22]. While newer antimuscarinic agents have improved drug profiles, compliance remains an issue and many patients discontinue the drug therapy after 1 year due to dissatisfaction with the balance between drug efficacy and tolerability [23]. Nonetheless, most physicians prescribe a trial of antimuscarinic therapy in addition to behavioural modification in patients with OAB and recommend a second trial using a different drug or formulation if the former was unsuccessful.

1.1. Oxybutynin

Oxybutynin was first introduced into the market in 1982 and in addition to the antimuscarinic effect it has a strong independent musculo-tropic relaxant activity and local anaesthetic activity. It is a tertiary amine that is metabolized primarily by cytochrome P (CYP) system into its primary metabolite, N-desethyl-oxybutynin (DEO) [24]. The recommended oral adult dose for IR formulation is 5 mg three or four times daily. An ER oxybutynin in 5, 10 or 15 mg once daily oral formulation and transdermal delivery system (TDS) prescribed as 3.9 mg twice weekly dosing, and a transdermal gel with once daily dosing in 100 mg/1 g application are also available. Studies confirmed that ER is associated with lower side effects than IR form due to less absorption in the gut and first pass metabolism [25]. Transdermal administration of oxybutynin alters the metabolism of the drug, further reducing the production of DEO compared to oxybutynin ER [26] but is associated with moderate rate of local skin reaction [27]. In contrast, oxybutynin topical gel has improved skin tolerability over the TDS delivery system and this is likely related to the lack of adhesive and skin occlusion [28]. Lastly, intravesical administration of oxybutynin is a conceptually attractive form of drug delivery but at present no specific intravesical formulation is available and patients would need to dissolve the oral formulation in solution and deliver periodically into the bladder by a urinary catheter, and has been shown to be as effective as oral oxybutynin [29].

1.2. Tolterodine

Tolterodine was introduced in 1998 and is a tertiary amine with a major active metabolite, 5-hydroxymethyl tolterodine. The effects of tolteroedine and its metabolite on the bladder seemed to be more long-lasting [30]. Tolterodine is available in two formulations: an IR form prescribed as 2 mg twice daily, and an ER form prescribed 2 or 4 mg once daily. There appears to be very low incidence of cognitive side-effects with tolterodine which is likely due to the low lipophilicity of the drug and its metabolite, minimizing penetration into the CNS [31]. However a subset of patients who lack the specific CYP enzyme, 2D6, that metaboliszes tolterodine to its metabolite will experience a higher side-effect profile.

1.3. Trospium

Trospium was brought into the market in 2004 as a hydrophilic, quaternary amine with limited ability to cross the blood-brain barrier and therefore is associated with minimal risk of cognitive impairment [32]. In contrast to other antimuscarinics, trospium is not metabolized by the CYP enzyme system and is mainly excreted by the renal tubular secretion. In comparison with oxybutynin, trospium has been shown to be comparable in improving the urinary symptoms but with a better benefit-risk ratio due to better tolerability [33]. The ER formulation of 60 mg once daily has been shown in studies to have similar efficacy and side-effects as the IR formulation which is 20 mg twice daily preparation [34].

1.4. Soifenacin

Solifenacin was introduced in 2005 as a tertiary amine with modest selectivity for M3 receptor over the M2 receptor [5]. The formulation for solifenacin is either 5 or 10 mg once a day and is predominantly metabolized by the liver by CYP3A4 enzyme. The STAR (Solifenacin and Tolterodine as Active comparator in a Randomized) trial showed non-inferiority of solifenacin flexible dosing and that solifenacin was associated with better efficacy but higher adverse events especially constipation [35].

1.5. Darifenacin

Similarly to solifenacin, darifenacin was also introduced into the market around 2005 and is a relatively selective M3 receptor antagonist. The M3 receptor selectivity has been postulated to be associated with minimal cognitive impairment in the elderly population [36]. Review of available literature concluded that darifenacin did not cause an impairment of memory among other cognitive functions [37]. Darifenacin is available as a controlled release formulation of 7.5 and 15 mg once daily dosing.

1.6. Fesoterodine

Fesoterodine was introduced later in 2007 and is metabolized rapidly to 5-hydroxymethyl tolterodine, the same active metabolite of tolterodine. However, unlike tolterodine, fesoterodine is not affected by CYP2D6 enzyme and is considerably less lipophilic and therefore has minimal or no cognitive effects. While fesoterodine is available at doses of 4 and 8 mg daily, the higher dose has been shown to have greater efficacy but at the expense of higher rate of dry mouth [38].

2. Antidepressant (Table 1)

Several antidepressants have been shown to decrease bladder contraction and increase outlet resistance resulting in better bladder storage symptoms. In general, they have anticholinergic effects both centrally and peripherally, and they block the re-uptake of serotonin and noradrenaline [39]. In addition to the common antimuscarinics side effects, tricyclic antidepressants can have cardiotoxic and CNS effects such as parkinsonian effects, insomnia and sedation [39].

2.1. Duloxetine

Duloxetine is a combined serotonin-norepinephrine re-uptake inhibitor (SNRI) and has been shown to be effective in treating both urge and stress urinary incontinence. It can be taken either as 80 or 120 mg daily. The product information for this drug contains a black box warning due to increased suicidal thinking and behaviour in those taking the drug for psychiatric disorders.

2.2. Imipramine

Imipramine is a tricyclic antidepressant with prominent systemic anticholinergic effects but only weak antimuscarinic effect on bladder smooth muscle [40]. The effect of imipramine on noradrenaline re-uptake is non-selective, and can affect both the lower urinary tract system and the brain [41]. Imipramine is prescribed as 25 mg nightly and can be increased by 25 mg every 3 days until either the patient was continent, had side-effects, or dose of 150 mg was reached [42]. Serious toxic side-effects can occur with therapeutic doses of imipramine such as orthostatic hypotension, ventricular arrhythmias and prolongation of QT interval.

Newer Medical Therapies for OAB (Figure 2)

1. Phosphodisterase Type 5 (PDE5) Inhibitor

Recent understanding in the specific modulation of intracellular second messenger pathways such as the cAMP and Rho-kinase pathways as well as the identification of phosphodiesterase (PDE) receptors in detrusor muscle have highlighted the role of nitric oxide (NO) in detrusor smooth muscle relaxation [43, 44]. PDE5 inhibitors act by increasing the concentration of NO in smooth muscle, which relaxes the prostate as well as acting on the bladder neck [45]. It is also postulated that PDE5 inhibitors may also prevent deleterious alterations of the histological structure of the urinary bladder such as muscle hypertrophy and collagen deposition that may lead to disturbances in urine storage and voiding [46]. More recently, it was found that PDE5 inhibitor reduces the input of the afferent nerve activity and bladder sensory input [47]. While several well designed randomised controlled trial have demonstrated the efficacy of PDE5 inhibitors on the treatment of lower urinary tract dysfunction in the setting of benign prostatic hyperplasia [48, 49], it remains unclear around the actual role of PDE5 inhibitors on OAB. Recently, PDE5 inhibitor, vardenafil has been shown to improve the urodynamic parameters and bladder urgency symptoms in patients with neurogenic bladder who were on oxybutynin treatment [50]. In the future it is likely that combination of an antimuscarinic and PDE5 inhibitor may be considered.

1. **Phosphodiesterase type 5 inhibitors**
2. **Adrenergic receptor antagonist**
3. **Neurokinin receptor antagonist**
4. **Potassium channels blockers**
5. **Transient receptor vanilloid type 1 blocker**
6. **Prostanoids**
7. **RhoA/Rho kinase inhibitor**
8. **Purinergic receptor antagonist**
9. **$5HT_{1A}$ antagonist**

Figure 2. Novel therapeutic agents for OAB.

2. Adrenergic Receptor Agonists

Both alpha (α)- and beta (β)-adrenergic receptors (AR) have been identified in the human urinary bladder. Within the detrusor muscle layer, the predominant β-AR population mediates smooth muscle relaxation in response to noradrenaline. Therefore drugs with β-AR agonist activity are likely to inhibit nerve-induced contractions of the detrusor muscle and that the administration of such drugs in humans can increase bladder capacity. Of the 3 β subtypes, β3 AR is the most prevalent in human detrusor muscle [51]. Early clinical trial with YM-178 (mirabegron), a β3 AR agonist showed proof-of-concept results with improvement in OAB symptoms such as urge incontinence, urinary frequency and urgency [52]. While the drug appeared to be well tolerated, larger studies are necessary to establish the exact role of this drug in the myriad of antimuscarinic treatments.

3. Neurokinin Receptor Antagonists

The importance of afferent nerve activity in the pathogenesis of DO has been proven in many studies and the local release of tachykinins and other peptides from sensory nerves in the bladder wall has been shown to produce DO. The neurokinins (NK) are a family of neuropeptides that include substance P and NK A and B, all of which are widely distributed in the human bladder. Antagonists of NK receptor NK1 and NK 2 were shown to increase bladder capacity in animal models of DO [53]. Aprepitant is a selective NK1 receptor antagonist that has been shown to decrease the urgency, urge incontinence and frequency in OAB patients [54]. More recently, serlopitant, another NK 1 antagonist was reported to show no dose response and an inferior efficacy to tolterodine [55]. Two other NK1 antagonists, SSR-240600 and TA-5538, are being investigated for the treatment of OAB [10].

4. Potassium Channel Blockers

Given that K^+ channels are expressed not only in detrusor smooth muscle but vascular smooth muscle, K^+ channels openers may affect cardiovascular function [56]. Therefore newer K^+ channels openers are designed with minimal cardiac adverse effects and ZD0947 is a type of K^+ channels opener that is devoid of cardiovascular side effects. While the preclinical studies have shown that ZD-0947 was associated with dose-dependent decreased in bladder contractions, the results from the clinical trial have been disappointing and did not show any superiority of the drug on the OAB symptoms [57]. On the other hand, NS-8 is a Ca^{2+} sensitive K^+ channel activator that is being investigated for the potential treatment of pollakiuria and incontinence. The animal model demonstrated that systemic administration of NS-8 suppresses the micturition reflex by inhibiting afferent pelvic nerve activity [58]. Unfortunately, phase II clinical trial was discontinued due to the lack of sufficient efficacy at the expected therapeutic dose in the proof-of-concept study [59].

Novel Treatment of OAB (Figure 2)

1. Transient Receptor Potential Vanilloid Type 1

The transient receptor potential vanilloid type 1 (TRPV1) or previously known as vanilloid receptor is known to be closely involved in DO in animal models of OAB [60]. A proof-of-concept study demonstrated that intravesical resiniferatoxin desensitized TRPV1 and improved the OAB symptoms among a selected group of patients with idiopathic DO [61].

2. Prostanoids

The human detrusor muscle is able to synthesize prostaglandins and cyclo-oxygenases. Nitroflurbiprofen (NicOx) is a NO-donating derivative of flurbiprofen, a well known non-steroidal anti-inflammatory drug designed to minimise the local negative effects of prostacyclin deficiency mainly by local NO release, and retains all the therapeutic effects of a parent compound such as analgesic, anti-inflammatory and antithrombotic effects [62]. Administration of nitroflurbiprofen demonstrated good overall safety and no differences in adverse events compared to placebo, and resulted in some improvements in urinary urgency, pain intensity and the sensation of complete bladder emptying. Interestingly, flurbiprofen did not abolish DO [63]. Another compound, ONO-8539, a PGE2 receptor subtype EP1 antagonist have recently completed a Phase I study with encouraging safety profile [64].

3. RhoA/Rho-Kinase Pathway

The Rho-kinase pathway has been shown to be involved in detrusor contraction following noradrenaline stimulation [65]. Rho-kinases inhibitor, Y-27632 was shown to induce a significant concentration-dependent inhibition of carbachol-induced contraction of human detrusor strips [66]. Elocalcitrol (BXL-628), a vitamin D2 analogue, is responsible for mediating the activation of vitamin D-responsive pathways resulting in modulation of smooth muscle cells gene expression of contractile and cytoskeleton proteins that regulate bladder contractions [67]. This drug has recently been shown to inhibit the RhoA/Rho kinase pathway, a Ca^{2+} sensitising pathway that is strictly involved in abnormal bladder contraction [68]. The administration of elocalcitol has been shown to be effective in increasing the mean volume voided in OAB patients after 4 weeks of treatment and appears to be extremely well tolerated.

4. Purinergic Receptor Antagonist

While normal human detrusor contraction is mediated primarily through the activation of muscarinic receptors, NANC contractions can occur in the diseased bladder states. There is now good evidence that the transmitter responsible for the NANC component is ATP acting on P2X receptors found in human detrusor muscle membrane [69]. Pre-clinical data suggests that P2X1 antagonist reduced the bladder smooth muscle contraction force while P2X3 antagonist acted on the afferent signalling from the bladder [70]. Studies using P2X3 knock-out mice have provided support that purinergic receptors are involved in the mechanoafferent transduction in the bladder [71] and P2X3 receptor-deficient mice exhibited detrusor hyporeflexia and fewer bladder contractions in response to saline distension [72].

5. 5-HT_{1a} Antagonist

Many central nervous system (CNS) regions are known to be involved in the control of micturition. Several animal studies in the CNS have suggested that the 5-HT_{1a} receptors and 5-HT-re-uptake mechanisms may represent therapeutic target for OAB treatment [10]. Recordati or REC-0545 is a 5-HT_{1a} antagonist and has been shown to increase the bladder volume capacity and/or time between micturitions without blunting the bladder contractility in a Phase II proof-of-concept study [73]. Besipirdine is a potent blocker of voltage gated Na^+ channels and increases adrenaline and 5-HT mediated transmission, mainly through inhibition of noradrenaline and 5-HT re-uptake. This drug is currently in a Phase III clinical trial and the result is yet to be communicated [10].

Conclusion

At present, the exact pathogenesis of OAB remains unclear and it is likely that there are multiple factors involved in the disease complex. Despite its high prevalence especially among the elderly, OAB remains an under-diagnosed and under-treated [74]. This could be related to the lack of awareness, embarrassment and/or misconception that OAB is a natural consequence of ageing. The available medical treatment remains far from ideal due to poor compliance and high discontinuation rates from the high incidence of adverse events. Therefore considerable effort has been made to identify an ideal drug for the treatment of

OAB that is uro-selective, to discriminate between normal and abnormal bladder contractions. Several promising pharmacological targets include β3-agonist, NK1 receptor antagonists, Rho kinase inhibitors, K^+ channels blockers and purinergic receptor antagonist. It is also likely that perhaps combination therapy and not monotherapy will play a major role in the treatment of OAB. Intravesical botulinum toxin has resulted in significant improvement in OAB symptoms, been established as an effective therapy in the treatment of medication-refractory OAB, and provides an alternative minimally invasive therapeutic options instead of neuromodulation and augmentation cystoplasty [75.76].

References

[1] Haylen BT, de Ridder D, Freeman RM et al. An International Urogynaecological Association (IUGA)/International Continence Society (ICS) joint report on the terminology for female pelvic floor dysfunction. *Neurourol Urodyn* 2010;19(1)::4-20

[2] Milson I, Abrams P, Cardozo L et al. How widespread are the symptoms of an overactive bladder and how are they managed? A population-based prevalence study. *Br J Urol Int* 2001;81(9):760-6

[3] Coyne KS, Sexton CC, Irwin DE et al. The impact of overactive bladder, incontinence and other lower urinary tract symptoms on quality of life, work productivity, sexuality and emotional wellbeing in men and women: results from the EPIC study. *BJU Int* 2008;101(11):1388-95

[4] Milson I. Epidemiology of stress, urgency, and mixed incontinence: where do the boundaries cross? *Eur Urol* 2006;16(Suppl 5):842-8

[5] Abrams P, Andersson KE. Muscarinic receptor antagonists for overactive bladder. *BJU Int* 2007;100:987-1006

[6] Chess-Williams R. Muscarinic receptors of the urinary bladder: Detrusor, urothelial and prejunctional. *Auton Autacoid Pharmacol.* 2002;22:133-45

[7] Bschleipfer T, Schukowski K, Weidner W et al. Expression and distribution of cholinergic receptors in the human urothelium. *Life Sci* 2007;80:2303-7

[8] Chen CC, Akopian AN, Sivilotti L et al. A P2X purinoceptor expressed by subset of sensory neurons. *Nature* 1995;377:428-31

[9] Andersson KE. Bladder activation: afferent mechanisms. *Urology* 2002;59:43-50

[10] Colli E, Digesu GA, Olivieri L. Overactive bladder treatments in early phase clinical trials. *Expert Opin. Investig. Drugs* 2007;16(7):999-1007

[11] Tredelenburg AU, Meyer A, Wess A et al. Distinct mixtures of muscarinic receptor subtypes mediate inhibition of noradrenalin release in different mouse peripheral tissues, as studied with receptor knockout mouse. *Br J Pharmacol* 2005;145:1153-9

[12] Yoshida M, Masunaga K, Satoji Y et al. Basic and clinical aspects of non-neuronal acetylcholine: expression of non-neuronal acetylcholine in urothelium and its clinical significance. *J Pharmacol Sci* 2008;106:193-8

[13] Barras M, Van der Graf PH, Chritoph P, Itzchak A. Relaxant efficacy of potassium channel openers in rabbit isolated bladder and mesenteric artery. *Eur J Urol* 1996;30(Suppl 2):240

[14] Yamazaki Y, Tatemichi S, Maruyama I et al. Characterisation of KUC-7483 and its active metabolite, KUC-7322, a selective β_3 –adrenoceptor agonist, on bladder function in rats. *Neururol Urodyn* 2002;21(4):405-6
[15] Morelli A, Vignozzi L, Filippi S et al. BXL-628, a vitamin D receptor antagonist effective in benign prostatic hyperplasia treatment, prevents RhoA activation and inhibits RhoA//Rho kinase signalling in rat and human bladder. *Prostate* 2006;X:XX-XX
[16] Anderson KE, Yoshida M. Antimuscarinics and the overactive detrusor-which is the main mechanism of action? *Eur Urol* 2003;43:1-5
[17] Andersson KE, Chapple CR, Cardozo L et al. Pharmacological treatment of urinary incontinence. In: Abrams P, Cardozo L, Khoury S, Wein AJ, editors. *Incontinence. 4th ed. Paris: Health Publication Ltd*; 2009. P. 631-700
[18] Guay DR. Clinical pharmacokinetics of drugs used to treat urge incontinence. *Clin Pharmacokinet.* 2003;42:1243-85
[19] Chapple CR, Khullar V, Gabriel Z et al. The effects of antimuscarinic treatments in overactive bladder: an update of a systemic review and meta-analysis. *Eur Urol* 2008;54:543-62
[20] Chapple CR, Rosenberg MT, Brenes FL. Listening to the patient: A flexible approach to the use of antimuscarinic agents in overactive bladder syndrome. *BJU Int* 2009;104(7):960-7
[21] Smith AL, Wein AJ. Urinary incontinence-pharmacotherapy options. *Ann of Med.* 2011;43:461-76
[22] Kato K, Furuhashi K, Suzuki K et al. Overactive bladder and glaucoma: a survey at outpatient clinics in Japan. *Int J Urol* 2007;14:595-7
[23] Chapple CR. Muscarinic receptor antagonists in the treatment of overactive bladder. *Urology*. 2000;55(5A Suppl):47-9, discussion 50
[24] Waldeck K, Larsson B, Andersson KE. Comparison of oxybutynin and its active metabolite, N-desethyl-oxybutynin, in the human detrusor and parotid gland. *J Urol* 1997;157:1093-7
[25] Gupta SK, Sathyan G. Pharmacokinetics of an oral once-a-day controlled-release oxybutynin formulation compared with immediate-release oxybutynin. *J Clin Pharmacol.* 1999;39:289-96
[26] Dmochowski RR, Davila GW, Sinner NR et al. Efficacy and safety of transdermal oxybutynin in patients with urge and mixed urinary incontinence. *J Urol* 2002;168: 580-6
[27] Cartwright R, Cardozo L. Transdermal oxybutynin: sticking to the facts. *Eur Urol* 2007;51:907-14
[28] Staskin DR, Dmochowski RR, Sand PK et al. Efficacy and safety of oxybutynin chloride topical gel for overactive bladder: a randomized, double-blind, placebo controlled, multicenter study. *J Urol* 2009;181:1764-72
[29] Szollar SM, Lee SM. Intravesical oxybutynin for spinal cord injury patients. *Spinal Cord.* 1996;34:284-7
[30] Brynne N, Stahl MMS, Hallen B et al. Pharmacokinetics and pharmacodynamics of tolterodine in man: a new drug for the treatment of urinary bladder overactivity. *Int J Clin Pharmacol Ther.* 1997;35:287
[31] Hills CJ, Winter SA, Balfour JA. *Tolterodine. Drugs* 1998;55:813

[32] Todorova A, Vonderheid-Guth B, Dimpfel W. Effects of tolterodine, trospium chloride, and oxybutynin on the central nervous system. *J Clin Pharmacol.* 2001;41:636-44
[33] Halaska M, Ralph G, Wiedemann A et al. Controlled, double-blind, multicenter clinical trial to investigate long-term tolerability and efficacy of trospium chloride in patients with detrusor instability. *World J Urol.* 2003;20:392-9
[34] Dmochowski RR, Sand PK, Zinner NR, Staskin DR. Trospium 60 mg once daily (QD) for overactive bladder syndrome: results from a placebo-controlled interventional study. *Urology* 2008;71:449-54
[35] Chapple CR, Martinez-Garcia R, Selvaggi L et al. STAR study group. A comparison of the efficacy and tolerability of solifenacin succinate and extended release tolterodine at treating overactive bladder syndrome: Results of the STAR Trial. *Eur Urol* 2005;48:464-70
[36] Lipton RB, Kolodner K, Wesnes K. Assessment of cognitive function of the elderly population: effects of darifenacin. *J Urol* 2005;173:493-8
[37] Kay GG, Ebinger U. Preserving cognitive function for patients with overactive bladder: evidence for a differential effect with darifenacin. *Int J Clin Pract.* 2008;62(11):1792-1800
[38] Khullar V, Rovner ES, Dmochowski R et al. Fesoterodine dose response in subjects with overactive bladder syndrome. *Urology* 2008;71:839-43
[39] Hollister LE. Current antidepressants. *Annu Rev Pharmacol Toxicol.* 1986;26:23-37
[40] Olubadewo J. The effect of imipramine on rate detrusor muscle contractility. *Arch Int Pharmacodn Ther.* 1980;145:84-94
[41] Freeman MM, McNulty AM. Alterations in K (+)-evoked release of 3H-norepineprhione and contractile responses in urethral and bladder tissues induced by norepinephrine reuptake inhibition. *Life Sci* 1993;53:193-200
[42] Castleden CM, George CF, Renwick AG et al. Imipramine-possible alternative to current therapy for urinary incontinence in elderly. *J Urol* 1981;125:318-20
[43] Truss MC, Uckert S, Stief CG, Kuczyk MA, Jonas U. Cyclic nucleotide phosphodiesterase (PDE) isoenzymes in the human detrusor smooth muscle: I. Identification and characterization. *Urol Res* 1996;24:123-8
[44] Gomelsky A, Dmochowski RR. Urodynamic effects of once-daily tadalafil in men with LUTS secondary to clinical BPH. *Curr Urol Rep.* 2010;11(4)::254-60
[45] Wang C. Phosphodiesterase -5 inhibitors and benign prostatic hyperplasia. *Curr Opin Urol* 2010;20:49-54
[46] Beamon CR, Mazar C, Salkini MW, Phull HS, Comiter CV. The effect of sildenafil citrate on bladder outlet obstruction: a mouse model. *BJU Int* 2009;104:252-6
[47] Behr-Roussel D, Oger S, Caisey S et al. Vardenafil decreases bladder afferent nerve activity in unanesthetized, decerebrate, spinal-cord-injured rats. *Eur Urol* 2010;X: XX-XX
[48] McVary KT, Monnig W, Camps JL Jr et al. Sildenafil citrate improves erectile function and urinary symptoms in men with erectile dysfunction and lower urinary tract symptoms associated with benign prostatic hyperplasia: a randomized, double-blind trial. *J Urol* 2007;177(3):1071-7
[49] Andersson KE, de Groat WC, McVary KT et al. Tadalafil for the treatment of lower urinary tract symptoms secondary to benign prostatic hyperplasia: Pathophysiology and mechanism(s) of action. *Neurourol Urodyn* 2011;30:292-301

[50] Gacci M, del Popolo G, Macchiarella A et al. Vardenafil improves urodynamic parameters in men with spinal cord injury: results from a single dose, pilot study. *J Urol* 2007;178:2040-3
[51] Levin RM, Ruggieri MR, Wein AJ. Identificatin of receptor subtypes in the rabbit and human urinary bladder by selective radio-ligand binding. *J Urol* 1988;139(4):844-8
[52] Chapple CR, Yamaguchi O, Ridder A et al. Clinical proof of concept study (BLOSOM) shows novel beta3 adrenoceptor agonist YM178 is effective and well tolerated in the treatment of symptoms of overactive bladder. *Eur Urol Suppl* 2008;3:239
[53] Smet PJ, Moore KH, Jonavicius J. Distributino and colocalization of calcitonin gene-related peptide, tachykinis, and vasoactive intestinal peptide in normal and idiopathic unstable human urinary bladder. *Lab Invest* 1997;77(1):37-49
[54] Green SA, Alon A, Ianus J et al. Efficacy and safety of a neurokini-1 receptor antagonist in postmenopausal women with overactive bladder with urge urinary incontinence. *J Urol* 2006;176(6 Pt 1):2535-40
[55] Frenkl TL, Zhu H, Reiss T et al. A multicenter, double-blind, randomized, placebo controlled trial of a neurokinin-1 receptor antagonist for overactive bladder. *J Urol* 2010;184(2):616-22
[56] Connolly MJ, Astridge PS, White EG. Et al. Torsades de pointes ventricular tachycardia and terodiline. *Lancet* 1991;338(8763):344-5
[57] Chapple CR, Patroneva A, Raines SR. Effect of an ATP-sensitive potassium channel opener in subjects with overactive bladder: a randomized, double-blind, placebo-controlled study (ZD0947IL/0004). *Eur Urol* 2006;49:879-86
[58] Tanaka M, Sasaki Y, Kimura Y et al. A novel pyrrole derivative, NS-8, suppresses the rate micturition reflex by inhibiting afferent pelvic nerve activity. *BJU Int* 2003;92(9):1031-36
[59] *http://www.apogepha.de/en/* Apogepha website 2007
[60] Charrua A, Cruz CD, Cruz F, Avelino A. Transient receptor potential vanilloid subfamily 1 is essential for the generatin of noxious bladder input and bladder overactivity in cystitis. *J Urol* 2007;177(4):1537-41
[61] Silva C, Ribeiro MJ, Cruz F The effect of intravesical resiniferatoxin in patients with idiopathic detrusor instability suggests that involuntary detrusor contraction are triggered by C-fiber input. *J Urol* 2002;168(2):575-9
[62] Palmer J. Report of a double-blind crossover study of flurbiprofen and placebo in detrusor instability. *J Int Med Res* 1983;11 Suppl 2):11
[63] Athanasopoulos A, Cruz F. The medical treatment of overactive bladder, including current and future treatments. *Expert Opin. Pharmacother.* 2011;12(7):1041-55
[64] Wilbraham D, Masuda T, Deacon S et al. Safety, tolerability, and pharmacokinetic of multiple ascending doses of the EP-1 receptor antagonist ONO-8539, a potential new and novel therapy to overactive bladder in healthy young and elderly subjects. *Eur Urol Suppl* 2010;2:250
[65] Rajasekaran M, Wilkes N, Kuntz S, Albo EM. Rho-kinase inhibition suppresses bladder hyperactivity in spontaneously hypertensive rats. *Neurourol Urodyn* 2005;24(3): 295-300
[66] Broqueres-You, Behr-Roussel D, Oger S et al. Rho-kinase inhibition impacts neurogenic detrusor overactivity in chronic spinalized rats. *Eur Urol Suppl* 2010;2:112

[67] Crescioli C, Morelli A, Adorini L et al. Human bladder as a novel target for vitamin D receptor ligands. *J Endocrinol Metab*. 2004;90(2):962-72

[68] Morelli A, Vignozzi L, Fillippi S et al. BXL-628, a vitamin D receptor antagonist effective in benign prostatic hyperplasia treatment, prevents RhoA activation and inhibits RhoA/Rho kinase signalling in rat and human bladder. *Prostate* 2006;x:XXX

[69] O'Reilly BA, Kosaka AH, Knight GF et al. P2X receptors and their role in female idiopathic detrusor instability. *J Urol* 2002;167:157-64

[70] Vlaskovska M, Kasakov L, Rong W et al. P2X3 knock-out mice reveal a major sensory role for urothelially released ATP. *J Neurosci*. 2001;21:5670-77

[71] Cockayne DA, Hamilton SG, Zhu QM et al. Urinary bladder hyporeflexia and reduced pain-related behaviour in P2X3-deficient mice. *Nature* 2000;407:1011-5

[72] Kibble A. Division of medicinal chemistry-P2 nucleotide receptors. *IDrugs* 2000;3(11):1270-71

[73] *http://www.recordati.it*, Recordati website 2007

[74] Brubaker L, Chapple C, Coyne KS, KoppZ. Patient-reported outcomes in overactive bladder: importance for determining clinical effectiveness of treatment. *Urology* 2006;68(Suppl 2):3-8

[75] Anger JT, Weinberg A, Suttorp MJ et al. Outcomes of intravesical botulinum toxin for idiopathic overactive bladder symptoms: A systematic review of the literature. *J Urol* 2010;183(6):2258-64

[76] Duthie J, Wilson DI, Herbison GP et al. Botulinum toxin injections for adults with overactive bladder syndrome. *Cochrane Database Syst Rev*. 2007 CD005493

In: Urinary Incontinence
Editor: Eric Chung
ISBN: 978-1-62618-482-4

Chapter 9

Non-medical Management of Overactive Bladder/Urge Urinary Incontinence

Dominic Lee and O. Lenaine Westney
University of Texas, M.D. Anderson Cancer Center, Houston, Texas, US

Abstract

Overactive bladder (OAB) syndrome with or without urinary incontinence is a prevalent condition with considerable cost to the individual and to the community. With our aging population the incidence is set to rise.

However the current medical management has not really progressed with time as we are still using the derivatives of anticholinergic compounds for first line therapy. Clearly this is fertile soil for basic science research and to some extent, novel drug therapies are emerging targeting different symptom pathways. However patients failing conservative therapy are still considerable. Our understanding of the neural pathways is slowly paving the way for more effective strategies and minimally invasive techniques with nerve modulation are clearly an emerging modality. As our knowledge grows so will the options for wider therapeutics, which will enhance the quality of life of our patients. This chapter is by no means comprehensive but it aims to review the current data and gives a general overview to the current surgical management options available for our patients.

Introduction

Overactive Bladder Syndrome is a common presenting problem to any Urologists. It is defined by the International Continence Society (ICS) as '*urgency with or without urge urinary incontinence but usually with urinary frequency and nocturia in the absence of urinary tract infection or other obvious pathology*' [1]. Its estimated prevalence in the US from the National Overactive BLadder Evaluation (NOBLE) Program study is estimated at

17% and the incidence rises with age [2]. The estimated direct and indirect cost of OAB to the US healthcare system has been estimated at $65.9 billion per annum [3].

There are numerous pharmaceutical agents approved by the US Food and Drug Administration (FDA) for treatment. The side-effects are not inconsiderable with significant anti-cholinergic effects on salivary and lacrimal production, visual changes as well as constipation and worsening cognition amongst the elderly [4]. Withdrawal of treatment within the first month of therapy can be as high as 40% [5]. The general response with non-surgical management (first line therapy) is estimated at 50% to 70% [6]. The matter in question is what happens if these OAB patients become refractory to these conservative measures and/ or are intolerant of the adverse effects of the medications. Before considering more invasive measures it is prudent to quantify the degree of bother with validated questionnaires and re-evaluate these patients with urinalysis, pad testing, flexible cystoscopy and/or Urodynamic evaluation as is necessary especially if the clinical history is incongruent. The International Consultation on Incontinence (ICS) 2010 has established guidelines on OAB management [1]. With therapeutic advances the following options are established secondary treatments for refractory patients and will discussed in this chapter. They include intravesical botulinum toxin A (BTX-A), electrical stimulation (ES) with sacral neuro-modulation (SNM) or posterior tibial nerve stimulation (PTNS), bladder reconstruction surgery with augmentation cystoplasty, detrusor myomectomy and urinary diversion. The penultimate aim of all these modalities is to decrease feeling of urge and resolve incontinence episodes by way of inducing stability to overactive bladder contraction, decrease the cystometric filling pressure and increase cystometric capacity.

Electro-Stimulation (ES)

The use of electrical stimulation to elicit bladder contraction was first demonstrated in the late 50s and early 60s. Early work by Boyce et al. demonstrated objective bladder contractions with direct electrode stimulation [7]. Subsequent animal research on spinal cord stimulation by Nashold at S2 level elicited bladder contractions [8]. This paved the way for Tanagho and Schmidt to further capitalize on the concept via trans-foraminal stimulation which led to the development of modern day sacral neuro-modulation (SNM)[9]. Concurrently, peripheral neuro-modulative techniques were also being evaluated at the time, inspired to an extent by Chinese acupuncture.

McGuire et al. in 1983 was able to show significant improvement in his heterogenous group of neurogenic and non-neurogenic OAB patients treated with trans-cutaneous peroneal and tibial nerve stimulation [10]. Stoller carried this further with his experiments on pig-tailed monkeys and devised the Stoller afferent nerve stimulator (SANS) using steel acupuncture needles targeting the tibial nerve in humans (SP 6 in acupuncture) [11].

I. Sacral Neuro-Modulation (SNM)

Mechanism of Action

The exact mechanism of action for sacral neuro-modulation has yet to be determined. Early work was performed by Nashold who demonstrated raised intravesical pressures on stimulation of S2 spinal cord and; with the use of bipolar leads was able to induce bladder emptying upon stimulation of S1-S2 grey matter. Tanagho and Schmidt were further luminaries in the field where their pioneering research on canine and eventually human subjects enhanced our understanding of motor and sensory responses upon sacral root stimulation. They discovered that activation of the rhabdosphincter mitigated by the Pudendal nerve branches caused suppression of bladder contractions as part of the arc of the primitive voiding reflex [9]. Indeed it is postulated that from a neurogenic standpoint, there is dysregulation of the excitatory and inhibitory signals on the voiding reflexes and modulating of the sacral nerve plexus corrects this and restores the coordination. SMN generates afferent impulses to the central nervous system (CNS) that resets the somatic impulses input by modulating sensory processing and the micturition reflex pathway [12]. In 1997 the US Food and Drug Administration (FDA) approved SNM with the Interstim™ therapy device (Medtronic Minneapolis, MN, USA) for use in Urge Incontinence. The indication was expanded to include urgency/frequency syndrome and non-obstructive urinary retention in 1999.

Patient Selection

As the clinical symptoms have such a broad etiology with neurogenic and non-neurogenic causes, factors predicting success is difficult to assess. Amundsen et al. explored this in a prospective trial with mean duration of 29 months follow up and reported that age less than 55 years has a statistically greater cure rate (65% vs. 37% for older individuals; $P < 0.05$). 3 or more chronic co-morbidities as well as patients with neurological conditions were however associated with lower success outcomes across the board [13]. Sherman et al. looking at refractory urge incontinence in women status post stress urinary incontinence surgery found that predictive factors for success included: age < 55 years ($P = 0.01$), test stimulation performed within 4 years of the stress incontinence procedure ($P = 0.01$), and evidence of pelvic floor muscle activity ($P = 0.03$) [14].

Peripheral Nerve Evaluation (PNE) versus Permanent Lead Test Procedure

In order for patients to undergo definitive implantation of the implantable pulse generator (IPG) they must under pre-implantation response testing with the electrode lead. This can be done in 2 ways. The first is (PNE) – outpatient procedure with non-permanent lead and 3-7 days testing period. This can be done with or without fluoroscopic control. The other is to undergo a first stage permanent tined-lead implant with fluoroscopy under sedation in an ambulatory care setting or operating room with longer testing period. All patients in the screening phase are fitted with an external stimulator device that can be adjusted for optimal effect at a comfortable level and completes a strict voiding diary as an objective measure of response before progression to stage 2 IPG implant. A positive clinical response is defined as subjective improvement with *a 50% or greater reduction in voiding parameters of urgency, frequency or incontinence episodes.*

Prior to the introduction of the quadripolar tined-lead in 2002, PNE was the only method for screening patients. An insulated unipolar test lead was placed blindly bilaterally under local anesthesia and a motor and/or sensory response was evoked and the wire subsequently taped and the wires connected to the external stimulator for neuromodulation over a 3 to 7 day period. Lead migration was not an uncommon problem which occurred in about 10% to 15% of patients. Short-term failure rates were as high as 27% in some studies [15]. There was still a potential false-negative response due to limited testing time as Kessler et al. reported a 30% increase in IPG implantation when the testing time was doubled [16]. There has been resurgence in the technique using fluoroscopy to optimize lead placement in addition to being office based for insertion and removal of lead and a greater simplification to a one stage procedure with a positive response.

To overcome the questionable response rate in PNE subjects, the utilization of the permanent electrode as a testing measure in what is known as the 2 stage implant was adopted. The advantage of the permanent lead test was an availability of extended testing, stable nerve-lead interface and low risk of lead migration. A randomized control trial by Everaert et al. on PNE vs. tined lead showed a greater success in the permanent lead group (14% vs. 33%) at 24 months follow-up. All of the patients randomized to the permanent group had successful implantation [17]. In addition, patients with permanent lead re-testing following equivocal PNE studies had an 80% success [18]. Leong et al. reported on their 2 year prospective case series comparing PNE versus first stage tined-lead testing in 100 patients (69 with OAB) and found a positive response rate of 47% (PNE) versus 69% (Tined-lead) suggesting a higher sensitivity in screening for SMN therapy [19].

Sensory versus Motor Responses

Evoked intra-operative neural responses are what guide us to our lead positioning during the testing phase. The anticipated S3 motor and sensory responses include anal bellows, dorsiflexion of great toe and sometimes plantar flexion of the foot and perineal, genital or anal tingling or pulling sensation respectively. S4 response is limited to anal bellows for motor response and perianal sensation for sensory response. At times S4 maybe the preferred nerve target as some patients with excessive S3 motor responses find this bothersome. Cohen et al. found that the motor response was superior in predicting successful implantation with 95% versus 21.4% with and without motor response respectively. Only 4.7% of patients with sensory response only progressed to successful implantation [20]. A recent abstract presented at the AUA by Guralnick et al. was less confirmatory, reporting on 51% successful implantation in 81% of patients with both motor and sensory responses. However with isolated sensory (6%) and motor response (8%) success rates were 40% and 38% respectively. 6% of patients with no S3 response at all had no success indicating that optimal stimulation will require both responses [21].

Surgical Technique

The patient is prepped in a prone position with pillows to flatten the sacrum and the feet free for access under non-paralytic anesthesia with sedation to gauge patient response. The buttocks are parted gently to observe for anal bellows. Fluoroscopy is used to establish landmark and for placement of quadripolar tined-lead. Biplanar (AP and lateral views) are utilized. The S3 foramen is located 1.5 to 2cm lateral to midline at the level of the sacral notches or 9 cm above the coccygeal drop –off. Local anesthesia is used to anesthetize the skin to the level of bone but not into foramina. A beveled 3.5-inch needle is used to access foramina till desired level. Testing is confirmed at the lowest voltage for sensory and motor response. A small incision is made at skin level. The needle stylet is removed and a directional guide-wire is placed and confirmed fluoroscopically. The dilator with introducer sheath is placed over the wire and directed into foramen until the marker of the dilator is seen at the anterior rim of the sacrum. The tined lead is inserted through sheath to the first white line and deployed when the 3 electrodes are visible below sacrum.

Lead is retested and the sheath is retracted. A subcutaneous pocket is made posterior to iliac crest for the IPG. A tunneling tool is used to route the lead through subcutaneously from the lead site to the subcutaneous pocket. The IPG is connected and the subcutaneous pocket closed after antibiotic irrigation. Impedance is verified and programming performed.

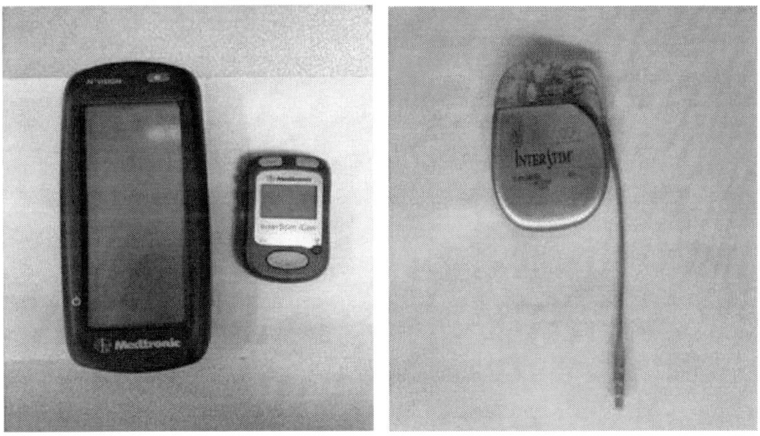

Figure 1. Interstim ™ therapy with programmer and implantable pulse generator (IPG).

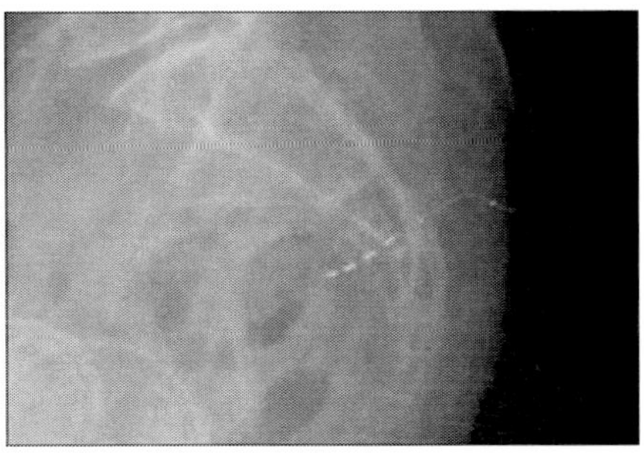

Figure 2. Deployment of tined lead on lateral X-ray. Note the 3 radio-opaque electrodes anterior to the inner table of the sacrum.

Outcomes

There is much published evidence on the efficacy of SNM to treat Urgency/Urge incontinence in both short and long term follow up. The fourth ICI has recommended SNM as a 2nd line treatment in both men and women for refractory OAB[1].

In the first multi-center RCT trial with SNM versus medical therapy, the Sacral Nerve Stimulation Study Group reported a 47% cure for UI and an additional 29% with greater than 50% improvement with an overall clinical success of 76 % at 6 months follow up which was sustained at 18 months. However the surgical revision rates of 32.5% were high [22]. Van Kerrebeoeck et al. published their multi-center trial data at 5 years and reported an impressive 56% and 68% sustained improvement for urgency-frequency and urge incontinence respectively [23].

Brazelli et al. systematically reviewed the evidence on sacral nerve stimulation (SNS) for severe urge incontinence. From 4 RCTS and 30 case series with a total of 1827 patients, 80% of the RCT and 67% of the case series patients achieved continence or >50% improvement in symptom control.

Benefits were sustained over 3 to 5 years after implantation. The overall reoperation rate was 33% [24]. [Table 2] summarizes the published literature on SNM [23-33].

Table 1. Published literature on the use of SNM for refractory OAB

Study	Year	Technique	N	Follow up	Efficacy (%)
Weil [25]	2000	PNE	21	6	56
Schmidt [26]	1999	PNE	34	6	75
Bosch [27]	2000	PNE	40	47	60
Hassouna [28]	2000	PNE	25	6	56
van Kerrebroeck [23]	2007	PNE	121	60	56-68
van Voskuilen [29]	2007	1/2 stage	39	15.5	90
Greonendijk [30]	2008	PNE	111	6	61-73
Brazelli [24]	2006	PNE	120	NA	80
Siegel [31]	2000	PNE	29	18-36	46-56
Spinelli [32]	2001	2 stage	196	12	60
Latini [33]	2006	1/2 stage	41	12	90

Surgery revision rates are estimated around 32% and include pulse generator site or implant site pain in 15.9% to 25%, lead migration in 7.0% to 16%. Infection and generator problems are about 5% [24, 31].

In an 11 year series, tined-leads had lower complication rates compared to non-tined leads: 28% and 73%, respectively [34].

II. Posterior Tibial Nerve Stimulation

Mechanism of Action

As with SNS, the exact mechanism of PTNS is not established but afferent inhibition plays a major role. Posterior tibial nerve is a mixed nerve with somatic and autonomic fibers extending from L3 to S4. It shares the same spinal segments as the micturition center S2-S4 with S3 predominantly innervating the detrusor muscle and levator musculature. It is proposed that retrograde stimulation of the nerve recruits the spinal inhibitory neurons to suppress detrusor contractions [35]. In addition, Fall et al. proposed the concept of 'neuronal reorganization' where prolonged afferent nerve stimulation remodels and reprograms the micturition reflex [36].

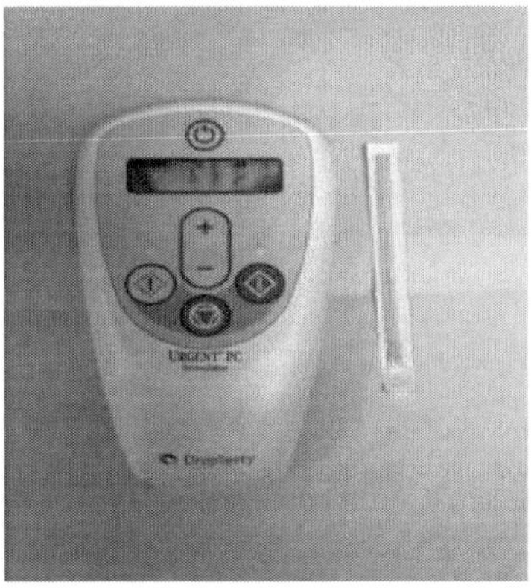

Figure 3. Urgent PC ™ by Uroplasty Inc.

Technique

The patient is positioned supine. Surface landmark for the posterior nerve is 3 finger-breaths above the medial malleolus between the posterior edge of the tibial bone and soleus muscle. 34-gauge steel acupuncture needle is inserted 3 to 4 cm into this point. Grounding electrode is attached to the sole of the feet. Both the electrode and needle are connected to the stimulator box (Urgent PC ™, Uroplasty Inc.). Motor response is big toe flexion or fanning of the toes. Sensory response is a tingling sensation in the sole of the feet. Stimulation at a comfortable level is maintained for 30 minutes.

Outcomes

Stoller devised the Stoller afferent nerve stimulator (SANS) - the prototype of the PTNS. He was able to demonstrate a sustained 80% clinical response in 90 patients with lower urinary tract symptoms (LUTS) and voiding dysfunction with a mean duration follow-up of 5.1 years [11]. Since the introduction of PTNS, there have been more than 30 published studies in peer-reviewed journals.

Table 2. Published series on PTNS

Study	Year	Indication	N	Duration (weeks)	Follow -up (months)	Efficacy (%)
Stoller #[11]	1999	LUTS	90	10	5.1	81
Klinger [41]	2000	Frequency/Urgency	15	12	10.9	67
Van Ballen [42]	2001	OAB	37	12	NA	60
Govier [37]	2001	OAB	53	12	3	71
Vandoninck [43]	2003	UI	35	12	3	70
Vandoninck [44]	2003	OAB	90	12	3	56
Congregado-Ruiz [45]	2004	OAB/UI	51	10	21	86
De Gennaro[46]	2004	OAB	17	12	3	80
Karademir #[38]	2005	OAB	43	8	2	61.6/83.2
Peters **[40]	2009	OAB	50	12	3	80
Peters +[39]	2010	OAB	220	12	3.2	58

# denotes using SANS, + SUmit trial, ** OrBiT trial.

These have similar results, with 70-80% of patients showing an improvement in their OAB symptoms. Govier et al. reported on the first national multi-center trial in 51 patients with refractory OAB with 71% success based on objective and questionnaire led outcomes. There was statistically significant reduction in frequency, nocturia and urge incontinence [37]. Karademir et al. looked at a series of 43 patients randomized to SANS alone and SANS with 5mg Oxybutynin and found that treatment response rate was 61.6% and 83.2% respectively [38]. Peters et al. recently published his multi-center SUmit trial- a RCT between PTNS versus sham surgery evaluated at 6 weeks and 12 weeks. His outcomes corroborates with previous studies and provides vital level 1 evidence with a 55% response to treatment in the 'real' PTNS group compared to 21% of sham subjects at 12 weeks [39]. The multi-center, randomized controlled OrBIT trial with 100 OAB patients was also pivotal comparing the effectiveness of PTNS to 4 mg daily extended-release tolterodine where 80% of PTNS group reported improvement compared to 55% of those on medication. Of those that responded to PTNS, 73% continued treatment for 1 year and were able to sustain improvement with maintenance treatment every 21 days [40]. [Table 2] summarizes the major case series in PTNS efficacy [11, 39-46].

Intravesical Botulinum Toxin A

The paralyzing effect of botulinum toxin is well known since 1871 when it was first described by van Ermenegem [47]. The toxin is derived from the fastidious Gram-positive bacteria Clostridium Botulinum. There are several characteristic serotypes (A,B,C,D,E,F and G) [48]. Serotype A is utilized therapeutically in Urology- BTX A. Normally, transmission of action potential impulses from pre-synaptic to postsynaptic membrane is actioned via neurotransmitters such as acetylcholine, which are contained within vesicles and are released by exocytosis from the pre-synaptic membrane via SNARE (soluble N-ethylmaleimide-sensitive factor attachment protein receptor) protein complex coupling. Botox A cleaves the SNAP-25 (synaptosome-associated protein 25 kd) protein which is vital for the formation of the SNARE protein complex and inhibits the process of exocytosis altogether and thus produces a chemical denervation effect. In the detrusor muscle complex of the urinary bladder this results in smooth muscle relaxation[49].

Its action is primarily on the inhibition of neurotransmitter release from the pre-synaptic membrane into the synaptic cleft and prevents post-synaptic receptor activation and generation of action potential by ionic channel activation.

Upon intra-detrusor injection, the toxin is endocytosed by the pre-synaptic membrane and disrupts the formation of SNARE proteins and halts the exocytosis process leading to muscle cell relaxation. In addition recent studies suggest it has a role in afferent desensitization by inhibiting other interactive neurotransmitters (substance P, adenosine triphophate –ATP) and down-regulation of axonal purinergic -P2CX3 and capsaicin TPRV-1 receptors in the urothelium [50]. The use of BTX-A came into effect with Stohrer's landmark paper in 2000 where he showed significant reduction in urge incontinence in neurogenic patients treated with intravesical BTX-A [51]. There has been numerous case series published since evaluating its efficacy in the neurogenic population, which recently obtained FDA approval. Comparatively for non-neurogenic refractory OAB, its use remains 'off-label'. There is no current consensus on treatment protocols with BTX-A for idiopathic OAB although several multi-center trials are currently underway to explore this [52].

Most published literature are clinical case series with significant heterogeneity in application (dose, number of injections) and outcome measures (efficacy, side effects) making objective assessment difficult. Most series demonstrate efficacy at 3 to 6 months intervals with 100-300 U (Botox®) or 500 U (Dysport®) use.

There has been a trend to use smaller doses in order to avoid some of the adverse effects. Most authors execute 20-30 injections with 1 ml per injections and spared the trigone to avoid potential vesico-ureteric reflux although these concerns have been negated in recent publications [53]. Schmid et al. has one of the largest prospective series with a 100 non-NGB patients and a mean follow up of 36 weeks.

All were treated at a dose of 100 U with 30 injections with 88% reporting significant improvement in subjective symptoms, quality of life and urodynamic parameters. 86% were cured of their urge incontinence, mean cystometric capacity increased by 56% and compliance increased from 24 to 41 ml/cm H2O [54]. There have been 3 randomized placebo control trials with demonstrable efficacy ranging between 50-60 % with up to 12 months follow up [55-57].

The major adverse events are mild hematuria, UTI and voiding difficulties requiring CIC as high as 45% in some of the published series[61]. In view of this all patients are counseled with regards to potential need for CIC pre-operatively.

Currently multi-center trials are underway to establish optimal dosage and to evaluate outcomes and adverse events with the varying doses. [Table 3] provides a summary of current published data on BTX-A in non-neurogenic OAB population [54-66].

Bladder Reconstructive Surgery

Historically surgery has been in the arsenal to treat small capacity bladders since the 19th century using various tissues ranging from bowel segments to fascia grafts. It became a widely adopted technique when clean intermittent catheterization (CIC) became available in the mid-1950s. With the advent of oral medications and effective minimally invasive techniques such as botulinum toxin A, SNM and PTNS being made available, the role of major surgery has lessened.

However, it remains a viable option for patients who have exhausted all these treatment modalities or are intolerant of its adverse effects. The main objective is to increase bladder capacity, decrease intra-vesical pressure as well as short-circuiting the neuronal stimulus for over-activity while protecting the upper urinary tract.

Augmentation Cystoplasty (AC)

Patients with poor bladder compliance or high-pressure detrusor overactivity are good candidates for augmentation. Intestinal segments mainly ileum are utilized in most circumstances.

The risk of urinary retention is high and in addition to mucus production, CIC is a prerequisite in most cases either per urethra or through a continent catheterizable stoma. Awad et al. reported a CIC rate of 39% in their cohort of 51 women [68]. Most published literature evaluating outcomes with augments have been in the neurogenic population. Venn et al. characterized a 78% continence rate in their series of neurogenic bladder AC. The success with non-neurogenic bladder AC is more impressive with 93% continence rate [69]. Daher et al. reported a 95% success rate on their 10 year follow-up in a series of 21 pediatric patients [70].

Blaivas et al. reported his series of long-term follow up (mean 8.9 years) on 49 out of 71 patients with AC and reported an overall 89% success rate [71]. To minimize morbidity, Reyblat et al. reported on an extra-peritoneal versus conventional approach for AC with mean follow up of 2.5 years with statistically significant difference in operative time, length of hospital stay and return of bowel function with no difference in complication rate [72]. Laparoscopic and robotic techniques have been described but longer term follow-up is required [73-74].

Conduit diversion is a last resort option reserved for severe intractable cases unresponsive to other therapies but recent systematic review was inconclusive (small sample size) regarding its therapeutic value in comparison to bladder reconstruction [75]. Detrusor myomectomy along with trans-trigonal phenol ablation has lost favor in most contemporary adult management and is no longer a choice option.

Long term follow up of AC patients on cystoscopy has not yielded significant rates of secondary cancers and recommendation for close cystoscopic surveillance seems unnecessary in this patient cohort [76].

Table 3. Published studies on BTX-A for non-neurogenic OAB

Study	Year	N	Dose (U)	Efficacy	Follow-up (months)	CISC (%)
Rapp [58]	2004	35	300	60	6	NA
Flynn[59]	2004	10	150	50	3	NA
Kuo [60]	2004	20	200	45	3	30
Kessler [61]	2005	11	300	91	3	45
Werner[62]	2005	26	100	65	9	7
Schulte-Baukloh [63]	2005	44	200-300	86	9	NA
Schulte-Baukloh [64]	2005	7	300	71	3	NA
Popat [65]	2005	31	200	50.7	4	19.3
Rajkumar [66]	2005	15	300	46	3	NA
Schmid [54]	2006	100	100	88	3	NA
Sahai +(RCT)[57]	2007	16	200	50	6	37.5
Brubaker +(RCT)[55]	2008	28	200	60	12.4	43
Flynn +(RCT)[56]	2009	22	200	57.5	1.5	6.7
Khan [67]	2009	81	200	43	33.6	43

+ denotes randomized control trial.

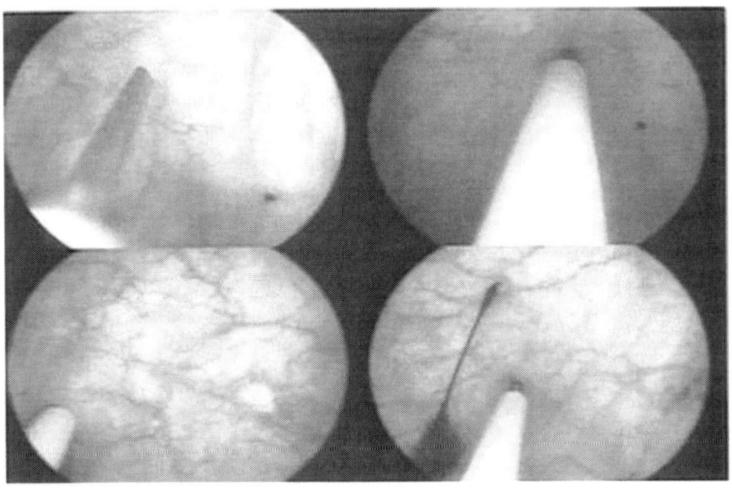

Figure 5. Cystoscopic view of intravesical BTX-A injections.

Conclusion

OAB syndrome is a non-terminal event that can be life-long and greatly impact on quality of life. Despite an explosion of available pharmacotherapy, the efficacy, non-compliance rate and side effect profile is considerable. Modern therapeutics has now arrived at a threshold that offers more effective minimally invasive surgical options to restore health and quality of life in these patients. The efficacy is by no means exceptional given our incomplete understanding of the underlying patho-physiology and many challenges lie ahead. With ongoing basic scientific research, innovative therapeutics and clinical trials the future looks promising.

References

[1] Abrams P, Andersson KE, Birder L, Brubaker L, Cardozo L, Chapple C, Cottenden A, Davila W, de Ridder D, Dmochowski R, Drake M, Dubeau C, Fry C, Hanno P, Smith JH, Herschorn S, Hosker G, Kelleher C, Koelbl H, Khoury S, Madoff R, Milsom I, Moore K, Newman D, Nitti V, Norton C, Nygaard I, Payne C, Smith A, Staskin D, Tekgul S, Thuroff J, Tubaro A, Vodusek D, Wein A, Wyndaele JJ. Fourth International Consultation on Incontinence Recommendations of the International Scientific Committee: Evaluation and treatment *Neurourol Urodyn.* 2010;29(1):213-40.

[2] Stewart WF, Van Rooyen JB, Cundiff GW, Abrams P, Herzog AR, Corey R, Hunt TL, Wein AJ. Prevalence and burden of overactive bladder in the United States. *World J Urol.* 2003 May;20(6):327-36.

[3] Ganz ML, Smalarz AM, Krupski TL, Anger JT, Hu JC, Wittrup-Jensen KU, Pashos CL.Economic costs of overactive bladder in the United States. *Urology.* 2010 Mar;75(3):526-32, 532.e1-18.

[4] Tune LE. Anticholinergic effects of medication *J Clin Psychiatry.* 2001;62 Suppl 21:11-4. Review.

[5] Chapple CR, Khullar V, Gabriel Z, Muston D, Bitoun CE, Weinstein D. The effects of antimuscarinic treatments in overactive bladder: An update of a systematic review and meta-analysis. *Eur Urol* 2008;54:543-62.

[6] MacDiarmid SA. Maximizing anticholinergic *BJU Int.* 2007 Jun;99 Suppl 3:8-12. Review.

[7] Boyce W, Lathem J, Hunt L. Research related to the development of an artificial electrical stimulator for the paralyzed human *J Urol.* 1964 Jan;91:41-51

[8] Nashold BS Jr, Friedman H, Boyarsky S. Electrical activation of micturition by spinal cord stimulation. *J Surg Res* 1971;11:144-7

[9] Schmidt RA, Bruschini H, Van Gool J, Tanagho EA. Micturition and the male genitourinary response *Invest Urol.* 1979 Sep;17(2):125-9.

[10] McGuire EJ, Zhang SC, Horwinski ER, Lytton B. Treatment of motor and sensory detrusor instability by electrical stimulation *J Urol.* 1983 Jan;129(1):78-9.

[11] Stoller M. Afferent nerve stimulation for pelvic floor dysfunction. *European Urology* 1999 35 (Supp.2); 16. 1999

[12] De Groat WC. A neurologic basis for the overactive bladder. *Urology* 1997;50:36-52.

[13] Amundsen CL, Romero AA, Jamison MG, Webster GD. Sacral neuromodulation for intractable urge incontinence: are there factors associated with cure *Urology.* 2005 Oct;66(4):746-50.

[14] Sherman ND, Jamison MG, Webster GD, Amundsen CL. Sacral neuromodulation for the treatment *Am J Obstet Gynecol.* 2005 Dec;193(6):2083-7

[15] Koldewijn EL, Rosier PF, Meuleman EJ, Koster AM, Debruyne FM, van Kerrebroeck PE. Predictors of success with neuromodulation in lower urinary tract *J Urol.* 1994 Dec;152(6 Pt 1):2071-5.

[16] Kessler TM, Madersbacher H, Kiss G. Prolonged sacral neuromodulation testing *Eur Urol.* 2005 May;47(5):660-5.

[17] Everaert K, Kerckhaert W, Caluwaerts H, Audenaert M, Vereecke H, De Cuypere G, Boelaert A, Van den Hombergh U, Oosterlinck W. A prospective randomized trial *Eur Urol.* 2004 May;45(5):649-54.

[18] Van Voskuilen AC, Oerlemans DJ, Weil EH, van den Hombergh U, van Kerrebroeck PE. Medium-term experience of sacral neuromodulation by tined lead implantation. *BJU Int.* 2007 Jan;99(1):107-10.

[19] Leong RK, De Wachter SG, Nieman FH, de Bie RA, van Kerrebroeck PE. PNE versus 1st stage tined lead procedure: a direct comparison to select the most sensitive test method to identify patients suitable for sacral neuromodulation therapy. *Neurourol Urodyn.* 2011 Sep;30(7):1249-52.

[20] Cohen BL, Tunuguntla HS, Gousse A. Predictors of success for first stage neuromodulation: motor versus sensory response *J Urol.* 2006 Jun;175(6):2178-80; discussion 2180-1.

[21] Guralnick M, Rasmussen N, Szabo A, O'Connor R. Milwaukee, WI. Sensory or motor responses: which are more important for sacral neuromodulation for voidingAbstract 1344, *AUA* 2011. Washington DC

[22] Schmidt RA, Jonas U, Oleson KA, Janknegt RA, Hassouna MM, Siegel SW, et al. Sacral nerve stimulation for treatment of refractory urinary urge incontinence: Sacral Nerve Stimulation Study Group. *J Urol* 1999;162:352-7.

[23] van Kerrebroeck PE, van Voskuilen AC, Heesakkers JP, Lycklama á Nijholt AA, Siegel S, Jonas U, Fowler CJ, Fall M, Gajewski JB, Hassouna MM, Cappellano F, Elhilali MM, Milam DF, Das AK, Dijkema HE, van den Hombergh U. Results of sacral neuromodulation therapy *J Urol.* 2007 Nov;178(5):2029-34.

[24] Brazzelli M, Murray A, Fraser C. Efficacy and safety of sacral nerve stimulation for urinary urge incontinence: A systematic review. *J Urol* 2006;175:835-41.

[25] Weil EH, Ruiz-Cerdα JL, Eerdmans PH, Janknegt RA, Bemelmans BL, van Kerrebroeck PE. Sacral root neuromodulation in the treatment of refractory urinary urge incontinence: A prospective randomized clinical trial. *Eur Urol* 2000;37:161-71

[26] Schmidt RA, Jonas U, Oleson KA, Janknegt RA, Hassouna MM, Siegel SW, et al. Sacral nerve stimulation for treatment of refractory urinary urge incontinence: Sacral Nerve Stimulation Study Group. *J Urol* 1999;162:352-7

[27] Bosch JL, Groen J.Sacral nerve *J Urol.* 2000 Apr;163(4):1219-22.

[28] Hassouna MM, Siegel SW, Neholt AA, Elhilali MM, van Kerrebroeck PE, Das AK, et al. Sacral neuromodulation in the treatment of urgency-frequency symptoms: A multicenter study on efficacy and safety. *J Urol* 2000;163:1849-54.

[29] Van Voskuilen AC, Oerlemans DJ, Weil EH, van den Hombergh U, van Kerrebroeck PE. Medium-term experience of sacral neuromodulation by tined lead *BJU Int.* 2007 Jan;99(1):107-10.

[30] Groenendijk PM, Lycklama à Nyeholt AA, Heesakkers JP, van Kerrebroeck PE, Hassouna MM, Gajewski JB, Cappellano F, Siegel SW, Fall M, Dijkema HE, Jonas U, van den Hombergh U; Sacral Nerve Stimulation Study Group. Urodynamic evaluation of sacral neuromodulation for urge urinary incontinence. *BJU Int.* 2008 Feb;101(3):325-9.

[31] Siegel SW, Catanzaro F, Dijkema HE, Elhilali MM, Fowler CJ, Gajewski JB, et al. Long-term results of a multicenter study on sacral nerve stimulation for treatment of urinary urge incontinence, urgency-frequency, and retention. *Urology* 2000;56:87-91

[32] Spinelli M, Bertapelle P, Cappellano F, Zanollo A, Carone R, Catanzaro F, et al. Chronic sacral neuromodulation in patients with lower urinary tract symptoms: Results from a national register. *J Urol* 2001;166:541-5

[33] Latini JM, Alipour M, Kreder KJ Jr. ficacy of sacral neuromodulation for symptomatic treatment of refractory urinary urge incontinence. *Urology* 2006;67:550-3.

[34] Sutherland SE, Lavers A, Carlson A, Holtz C, Kesha J, Siegel SW. Sacral nerve *Neurourol Urodyn.* 2007;26(1):19-28

[35] Hasan ST, Robson WA, Pridie AK, Neal DE. Transcutaneous electrical nerve *J Urol.* 1996 Jun;155(6):2005-11.

[36] Fall M, Lindstrom S. Electrical Stimulation: A physiologicl approcach to the treatment of urinary incontinence. *Urology Clinics of North America* 18:393-407.

[37] Govier FE, Litwiller S, Nitti V, Kreder KJ Jr, Rosenblatt P. Percutaneous afferent neuromodulation for the refractory overactive bladder: results of a multicenter study. *J Urol.* 2001 Apr;165(4):1193-8.

[38] Karademir K, Baykal K, Sen B, Senkul T, Iseri C, Erden D. A peripheric neuromodulation technique for curing detrusor overactivity: Stoller afferent neurostimulation. *Scand J Urol Nephrol.* 2005;39(3):230-3.

[39] Peters KM, Carrico DJ, Perez-Marrero RA, Khan AU, Wooldridge LS, Davis GL, Macdiarmid SA. Randomized trial *J Urol.* 2010 Apr;183(4):1438-43.

[40] Peters KM, Macdiarmid SA, Wooldridge LS, Leong FC, Shobeiri SA, Rovner ES, Siegel SW, Tate SB, Jarnagin BK, Rosenblatt PL, Feagins BA. Randomized trial of percutaneous tibial nerve stimulation versus extended-release tolterodine: results from the overactive bladder innovative therapy trial. *J Urol.* 2009 Sep;182(3):1055-61.

[41] Klingler HC, Pycha A, Schmidbauer J, Marberger M. Use of peripheral neuromodulation of the S3 region for treatment *Urology.* 2000 Nov 1;56(5):766-71.

[42] van Balken MR, Vandoninck V, Gisolf KW, Vergunst H, Kiemeney LA, Debruyne FM, Bemelmans BL. Posterior tibial nerve stimulation as neuromodulative treatment of lower urinary tract dysfunction. *J Urol.* 2001 Sep;166(3):914-8.

[43] Vandoninck V, Van Balken MR, Finazzi Agró E, Petta F, Caltagirone C, Heesakkers JP, Kiemeney LA, Debruyne FM, Bemelmans BL. Posterior tibial nerve *Neurourol Urodyn.* 2003;22(1):17-23.

[44] Vandoninck V, van Balken MR, Finazzi Agrò E, Petta F, Micali F, Heesakkers JP, Debruyne FM, Kiemeney LA, Bemelmans BL. Percutaneous tibial nerve stimulation in the treatment of overactive bladder: urodynamic data. *Neurourol Urodyn.* 2003;22(3):227-32.

[45] Congregado Ruiz B, Pena Outeiriño XM, Campoy Martínez P, León Dueñas E, Leal López A. Peripheral afferent nerve *Eur Urol.* 2004 Jan;45(1):

[46] De Gennaro M, Capitanucci ML, Mastracci P, Silveri M, Gatti C, Mosiello G. Percutaneous tibial nerve neuromodulation is well tolerated in children and effective for treating refractory vesical dysfunction. *J Urol.* 2004 May;171(5):1911-3.
[47] Erbguth FJ. Historical notes on botulism, Clostridium botulinum, botulinum toxin, and the idea of the therapeutic use of the toxin. *Mov Disord* 2004;19:S2-6.
[48] Oguma K, Fujinaga Y, Inoue K. Structure and function of Clostridium botulinum toxins. *Microbiol Immunol.* 1995;39(3):161-8. Review
[49] Nitti VW. Botulinum toxin for the treatment of idiopathic and neurogenic overactive bladder: State of the art. *Rev Urol* 2006;8:198-208
[50] Apostolidis A, Dasgupta P, Fowler CJ. Proposed mechanism for the efficacy of injected botulinum toxin *Eur Urol.* 2006 Apr;49(4):644-50. Epub 2006 Jan 4. Review
[51] Stohrer M, Schurch B, Kramer G. Botulinum A-toxin in the treatment of detrusor hyperreflexia in spinal cord patients: A new alternative to medical and surgical managements procedures? *Neurol Urodyn* 2000;18:401
[52] Dmochowski R, Sand PK. Botulinum toxin *BJU Int.* 2007 Feb;99(2):247-62. Review
[53] Kuo HC. Bladder base *Neurourol Urodyn.* 2011 Sep;30(7):1242-8.
[54] Schmid DM, Sauermann P, Werner M, Schuessler B, Blick N, Muentener M, Strebel RT, Perucchini D, Scheiner D, Schaer G, John H, Reitz A, Hauri D, Schurch B. Experience with 100 cases treated with botulinum-A toxin injections in the detrusor muscle for idiopathic overactive bladder syndrome refractory to anticholinergics. *J Urol.* 2006 Jul;176(1):177-85.
[55] Brubaker L, Richter HE, Visco A, Mahajan S, Nygaard I, Braun TM, Barber MD, Menefee S, Schaffer J, Weber AM, Wei J; Pelvic Floor Disorders Network . Refractory idiopathic urge urinary incontinence and botulinum A injection. *J Urol.* 2008 Jul;180(1):217-22
[56] Flynn MK, Amundsen CL, Perevich M, Liu F, Webster GD. Outcome of a randomized, double-blind, placebo *J Urol.* 2009 Jun;181(6):2608-15
[57] Sahai A, Khan MS, Dasgupta P. Efficacy of botulinum toxin-A for treating idiopathic detrusor overactivity: results from asingle center, randomized, double-blind, placebo controlled trial. *J Urol.* 2007 Jun;177(6):2231-6.
[58] Rapp DE, Lucioni A, Katz EE, O'Connor RC, Gerber GS, Bales GT. Use of botulinum-A toxin for the treatment of refractory overactive bladder symptoms: An initial experience. *Urology* 2004;63:1071-5.
[59] Flynn MK, Webster GD, Amundsen CL. The effect of botulinum: A toxin on patients with severe urge urinary incontinence. *J Urol* 2004;172:2316-20.
[60] Kuo HC. Urodynamic evidence of effectiveness of botulinum A toxin injection in treatment of detrusor overactivity refractory to anticholinergic agents. *Urology* 2004;63:868-72.
[61] Kessler TM, Danuser H, Schumacher M, Studer UE, Burkhard FC. Botulinum A toxin injections into the detrusor: an effective treatment in idiopathic and neurogenic detrusor overactivity? *Neurourol Urodyn.* 2005;24(3):231-6.
[62] Werner M, Schmid DM, Schóssler B. Efficacy of botulinum-A toxin in the treatment of detrusor overactivity incontinence: A prospective nonrandomized study. *Am J Obstet Gynecol* 2005;192:1735-40.
[63] Schulte-Baukloh H, Weiss C, Stolze T, Herholz J, Stürzebecher B, Miller K, Knispel HH. Botulinum-A toxin detrusor and sphincter injection in treatment of overactive

bladder syndrome: objective outcome and patient satisfaction. *Eur Urol.* 2005 Dec;48(6):984-90

[64] Schulte-Baukloh H, Weiss C, Stolze T, Stürzebecher B, Knispel HH. Botulinum-A toxin for treatment of overactive bladder without detrusor overactivity: urodynamic outcome and patient satisfaction. *Urology.* 2005 Jul;66(1):82-7.

[65] Popat R, Apostolidis A, Kalsi V, Gonzales G, Fowler CJ, Dasgupta P. A comparison between the response of patients with idiopathic detrusor overactivity and neurogenic detrusor overactivity to the first intradetrusor injection of botulinum-A toxin. *J Urol.* 2005 Sep;174(3):984-9.

[66] Rajkumar GN, Small DR, Mustafa AW, Conn G. A prospective study to evaluate the safety, tolerability, efficacy and durability of response of intravesical injection of botulinum toxin type A into detrusor muscle in patients with refractory idiopathic detrusor overactivity. BJU Int 2005;96:848-52

[67] Khan S, Kessler TM, Apostolidis A, Kalsi V, Panicker J, Roosen A, Gonzales G, Haslam C, Elneil S, Fowler CJ, Dasgupta P. What a patient with refractory idiopathic *J Urol.* 2009 Apr;181(4):1773-8.

[68] Awad SA, Al-Zahrani HM, Gajewski JB, Bourque-Kehoe AA. Long-term results and complications of augmentation ileocystoplasty for idiopathic urge incontinence in women. *Br J Urol* 1998;81:569-73

[69] Venn SN, Mundy AR. Long-term results of augmentation cystoplasty *Eur Urol.* 1998;34 Suppl 1:40-2.

[70] Daher P, Zeidan S, Riachy E, Iskandarani F. Bladder augmentation and/or continent urinary diversion: 10-year experience. *Eur J Pediatr Surg.* 2007 Apr;17(2):119-23.

[71] Blaivas JG, Weiss JP, Desai P, Flisser AJ, Stember DS, Stahl PJ. Long-term followup of augmentation enterocystoplasty and continent diversion in patients with benign *J Urol.* 2005 May;173(5):1631-4.

[72] Reyblat P, Chan KG, Josephson DY, Stein JP, Freeman JA, Grossfeld GD, Esrig D, Ginsberg DA. Comparison of extraperitoneal and intraperitoneal augmentation enterocystoplasty for neurogenic bladder *World J Urol.* 2009 Feb;27(1):63-8.

[73] Gill IS, Rackley RR, Meraney AM, Marcello PW, Sung GT. Laparoscopic enterocystoplasty. *Urology.* 2000 Feb;55(2):178-81.

[74] Kang IS, Lee JW, Seo IY. Robot-assisted laparoscopic augmentation ileocystoplasty: a case report. *Int Neurourol J.* 2010 Apr;14(1):61-4.

[75] Yong SM, Dublin N, Pickard R, Cody DJ, Neal DE, N'Dow J. Urinary diversion and bladder reconstruction *Cochrane Database Syst Rev.* 2003;(1):CD003306. Review.

[76] Hamid R, Greenwell TJ, Nethercliffe JM, Freeman A, Venn SN, Woodhouse CR. Routine surveillance cystoscopy for patients with augmentation and substitution cystoplasty for benign urological conditions: is it necessary? *BJU Int.* 2009 Aug;104(3):392-5.

In: Urinary Incontinence
Editor: Eric Chung

ISBN: 978-1-62618-482-4

Chapter 10

Continence Appliances and Alternative Management Strategies

Karina So, Melissa O'Grady and Virginia Ip
Clinical Nurse Consultants, Sydney Local Health District, NSW, Australia

Abstract

The selection of appropriate continence appliances helps each patient achieve their goal of social continence optimising their health outcome. The aim is to support good clinical practice in the prevention and reduction of continence related problems including catheter-associated urinary tract infection (CA-UTI).

In this chapter we provide details, and the pros and cons of each of the eight categories of continence products identified by the International Continence Society Subcommittee (ICSS). This chapter will also detail some bladder training programs.

The eight categories are: absorbent pads, sheaths, body worn urinals, catheters, urine drainage equipment, mechanical devices, hand-held urinals and bed pads and commodes.

Bladder training programs can improve, or in some cases cure urinary incontinence. These programs are tailored to a patients' individual medical problems and more specifically their type of urinary incontinence. As such, it is imperative that bladder training programs be conducted under the supervision of a qualified health practitioner in order to maximise the therapeutic outcome for the patient. Other conservative strategies that we detail here include habit retraining, timed toileting and prompted voiding.

Good knowledge in product selection and other conservative strategies using the multi-disciplinary team approach is essential in the delivery of safe quality patient-centred continence care.

Continence Appliances

We know that when the elimination of urine is not under control it can cause psychological stress as well as complicate the management of the patients' illnesses. This could also have major economic consequences for patients and medical teams alike. Patients also often experience shame and embarrassment, this in turn can affect their self-esteem to such an extent that they begin to isolate themselves from society. Therefore it comes as no surprise that depression and anxiety are linked to incontinence as well as a reduced quality of life [1].

Incontinence is a known predictor of early admission to institutionalised care for the elderly because they or their families have difficulty coping with the incontinence at home.

Continence products can be used in a number of ways, firstly to improve a person's quality of life whilst they are awaiting another treatment for their incontinence; secondly while they are waiting for their other treatment to work; thirdly, when treatment has been unsuccessful or finally, when the patient declines other treatment options. They can also be used for children who are yet to gain continence or who will never achieve continence due to disability. The aim of these products is to keep people socially continent. Products can be unisex or gender specific.

As previously specified, the 8 categories according to ICSS are:-[2]:

1. Absorbent Products
2. Sheaths
3. Body worn urinals
4. Catheters
5. Urine drainage equipment
6. Mechanical devices
7. Hand-held urinals
8. Bed pads and Commodes

1. Absorbent Products

These are the most commonly used products to contain urinary incontinence. They are usually easy to manage independently for most people. The ICSS divides absorbent products into the sub-categories of disposable inserts, disposable pull-ups, disposable all-in-ones, disposable T-shaped pads and washable bodyworns [2].

Disposable Pads

Nowadays most disposable pads are composed of three layers. Closest to the wearer's skin is a water permeable top sheet, then an absorbent core made of wood pulp (Fluff pulp), super absorbent polymer (SAP) and thermoplastic fibres which are sometimes added to reduce breakdown of the core when wet. The outer coating consists of polypropylene (PP) and polyethylene (PE) and in some pads tapes, elastics and adhesives [3, 4]. SAP absorbs extremely large amounts of liquid relative to its own mass and maintains cohesion under pressure. This property of SAP allows the pads to be thin, but have a high absorbency [3, 4].

Sometimes the disposable products will have writing on the underside which dissolves when urine comes in contact with it, thus giving the user or their carer evidence of when the pad is reaching its containment threshold. Disposable products will often have elasticised hydrophobic cuffs in the groin area to direct leakage back into the pad away from the legs.

When the appropriate disposable pad is used, people with incontinence will be able to participate in everyday life to the extent of their capacity.

Disposable Inserts

Insert pads do not have a waterproof layer. In the past they have been rectangular in shape, but more often nowadays they are an hour glass to contour to the body more. The inserts can be used in conjunction with the bigger absorbent pads or briefs to increase the absorption capacity.

Disposable pads are held in place by the user's close fitting underpants or commercially available mesh pants. The smaller insert pads may have an adhesive strip on the underside which aids in securing the pad in place. Men with light urinary incontinence may select male disposable inserts which are similar to a pouch that encloses the penis and/or penis and scrotum.

Disposable Pull-ups

Pull-ups are an insert pad incorporated into a pair of disposable underwear. They are often used when children are being toilet trained. This type of product is becoming more popular among adults with incontinence and carer of people with dementia as they are accepted by this group as being like their normal underwear.

Disposable All-in-Ones

Disposable all-in-ones are commonly known as nappies or diapers. They have an elasticised waist and legs. The sides have self-adhesive or velcro tabs and incorporate the absorbent components of inserts.

Disposable T-Shaped Pads

These type of products are similar to all-in-ones, but rather than having tabs on the sides they have a velcro belt that is placed around the waist. The padding is brought up between the legs and secured in place on the belt.

Washable Bodyworns

Washable bodyworn pads come in all the above types and shapes, but can be washed and reused. They are bulkier than the disposable alternative as they don't incorporate the same technology in terms of water retention, but can be more economical both financially and environmentally.

However, they are only appropriate for people who are independent in doing their own laundry or who have a capable carer. The trend of people wanting more environmentally friendly products has seen more washable products on the market. Product development priorities need to include better washable pads for women [5].

2. Sheaths

Sheaths are fitted to the penis just like a condom except that the end of the sheath closest to the head of the penis is adapted so that a urine drainage bag can be fitted to collect urine. They are also known as condom urinals, uridomes or external male catheters [6]. There are two types of sheaths: one-piece where the adhesive is on the inside of the sheath and two - pieces where double-sided adhesive tape is positioned around the penis and then the sheath is rolled over the tape. Sheaths are made out of latex, non-latex or a silicone material.

Compared to pads they may be more readily accepted by men with moderate to severe incontinence or those who have mobility issues combined with frequency and urgency incontinence. They can also be used by men with overflow incontinence as they contain urine between intermittent catheterisations [2].

Sheaths may remain attached for nearly 24 hours only being removed when the user showers at which time a new sheath is applied. Some men, however, only use the sheaths at night or when going out. Sheaths, however, are not suitable in some instances, for example if the man has poor manual dexterity and is unable to fit the sheath (or their carer if they are fitting the sheath); if the man has a retracted or small penis; if they are confused, or have compromised penile skin or an allergy to any component of the sheath.

3. Body Worn Urinals

These products are rarely used but there are some companies who make these products for men with a retracted penis. They consist of a washable non-adhesive silicone or rubber sheath that is placed over the penis and firmly held in place against the pubis by a belt and straps. The sheath is then attached to a urine drainage bag. It needs to be expertly fitted to ensure comfort and prevent leakage. Another type of male body worn urinal is called a dribble pouch. They are similar to a colostomy bag and can be secured to the body with an adhesive flange (after shaving the skin) or with a belt. Problems with these types of devices are excoriation of the penile skin and leakage [2]. Use of a skin barrier product and conduct a thorough assessment to obtain the right sheath size could reduce potential problems.

4. Urinary Catheters

Urinary catheterisation should only be performed for the following reasons:

- To bypass obstruction and relieve retention.
- To determine residual urine volume.

- To manage vesico-rectal or vaginal fistula.
- To prevent urine coming into contact with wounds or pressure areas until they are healed.
- To drain the bladder for patients who are paralysed and / or sedated.
- To monitor haemodynamically unstable patients.
- To perform urodynamic studies.
- To irrigate the bladder.
- To instil medication

Long-term urinary catheterisation should be avoided whenever possible as the risk of catheter related complications is high and catheters are rarely unproblematic [7]. The frequency of catheter replacement can vary from 4 weeks to less than 3 months but this practice should be individualised according to the patients' needs and medical conditions. The interval between catheter replacement should not exceed the manufacturers' recommendations. Catheter related problems include urine leaks around the catheter, blockage, irritation and symptomatic infection.

Urine leakage around the catheter can occur due to blockage or bladder spasms. Frequent bladder spasm is uncomfortable and it may be triggered by urinary tract infection (UTI), blocked catheter or idiopathic detrusor overactivity. The first step here is to assess the need for the urinary catheter and remove when it is no longer required. Secondly, clinician can try to replace the current catheter with a smaller one and put less water in the catheter balloon. This works by decreasing the surface area of catheter in the bladder (as long as the catheter is not prone to blockage) and may even reduce bladder irritability.

Once a catheter sample of urine (CSU) has been collected from the new catheter and UTI has been excluded the patient may need a trial of anticholinergic medication if urethral leakage continues to cause distress [8].

Symptomatic UTIs can occur in up to 28% of catheterised patients [9]. When symptomatic UTI develops, the urinary catheter must be replaced before a specimen is taken from the new catheter and sensitivities determined before appropriate antibiotics are commenced [10]. All catheters will block if left in long enough, but blockages occur more frequently in some patients as they excrete more calcium, protein, and mucin in their urine which collects around the lumen of the catheter thereby obstructing the flow of urine from the catheter [11]. There are 3 types of catheterisation: - urethral, suprapubic and intermittent.

Urethral Catheterisation

Urethral catheters are usually inserted by a doctor or qualified nurse using aseptic technique. It should be used for short term bladder care only when the patient is not capable of or appropriate for intermittent catheterisation.

In some circumstances, it is used if the patient is not surgically fit to have suprapubic catheter insertion. Urethral catheters can be uncomfortable; they can affect a patient's body image and reduce the level of independence. For sexually active patients, it means that intercourse needs to be preceded by removing or adjusting their catheter [2]. Usually a nurse who is proficient in urethral catheterisation will perform the regular catheter replacement.

Suprapubic Catheterisation

Suprapubic catheterisation involves a catheter being inserted into the bladder via an incision in the lower abdominal wall by a urologist under a local or general anaesthetic in a hospital setting. It is the preferred method of long-term catheter care as it avoids the risk of urethral trauma or erosion. Other benefits include better access for catheter replacement in those with reduced mobility and reduced risk of UTIs related to faecal contamination and decreased risk of urethritis, epididymo-orchitis and prostatitis [12].

Intermittent Self Catheterisation (ISC)

Intermittent self catheterisation is a urethral catheterisation procedure performed by patient using a clean technique. This method is suitable for patient with a hypocontractile bladder and is the gold standard for long term bladder management. Several studies have shown patients who perform ISC have the lowest associated infection rate [13, 14] and can avoid the potential problems associated with urethral and suprapubic catheters. Intermittent self catheterisation is appropriate for motivated, dextrous, cognitively intact individuals. In some circumstances, patients may be agreeable to accept the assistance of a carer.

Selection of Indwelling Urethral Catheter (IUC)

When insertion of a two-way urethral catheter for short-term or long-term drainage is indicated, it is necessary to select the most appropriate catheter type, catheter size and catheter material to match the patients' medical or individual needs. Ideally, urethral catheter should be soft, smooth and small in size with integrated balloon to minimize the catheter related problems such as irritation, bladder spasm and ascending infection [15]. With advances in medical technology, there are a variety of urinary catheters to choose from. Catheter specifications include catheter material, catheter tip shape, length from the base of the balloon to the tip, balloon size, catheter size, catheter length and special properties. Decision on catheter selection should be dependent on individual patient circumstances so that the most appropriate catheter is used to optimize drainage from the urinary bladder and to minimize potential catheter related problems.

In 2010, The Infectious Diseases Society of America developed a set of guidelines in collaboration with a number of leading medical organisations in several major countries for the diagnosis, prevention, and management of persons with catheter-associated urinary tract infection (CA-UTI). Due to the frequent use of urinary catheter in hospitals and long-term care facilities, CA-UTI becomes the most common health care-associated infection worldwide [16]. The physical, psychological and social effects of CA-UTI to the catheterised patients are significant. One cannot underestimate the economic burden to the individual, the community and the government. In the last few years, some health care institutions have set up systems to prompt daily review on the need for IUC. Good clinical practice includes removal of urinary catheter as soon as clinically appropriate [16]. Use of IUC is the last alternative to be used only when the clinician has exhausted all other options. Conservative strategies to manage patient with voiding dysfunction or urinary incontinence are discussed in other parts of this chapter.

Catheter Specifications

Catheter size is colour coded and the colour indicator is located on the distal balloon channel. Same size urinary catheters do not have the same internal calibre or shape. Catheter intraluminal calibre is directly related to the rate of urine flow.

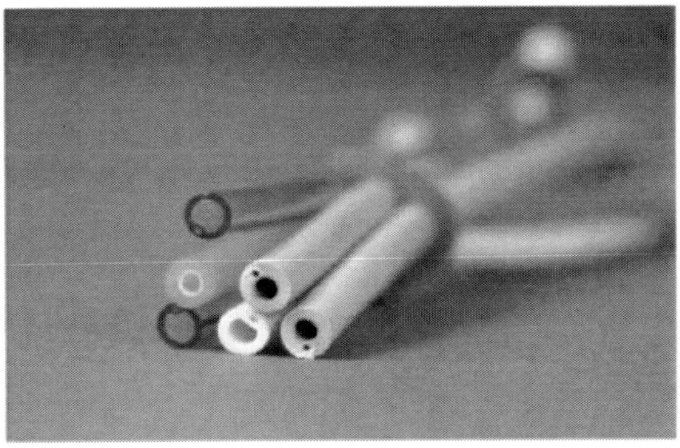

Picture 1.

Size (Fr)	12	14	16	18	20	22	24
Colour							

Different Catheter Tip and Various Lengths Measured From the Base of the Inflated Balloon

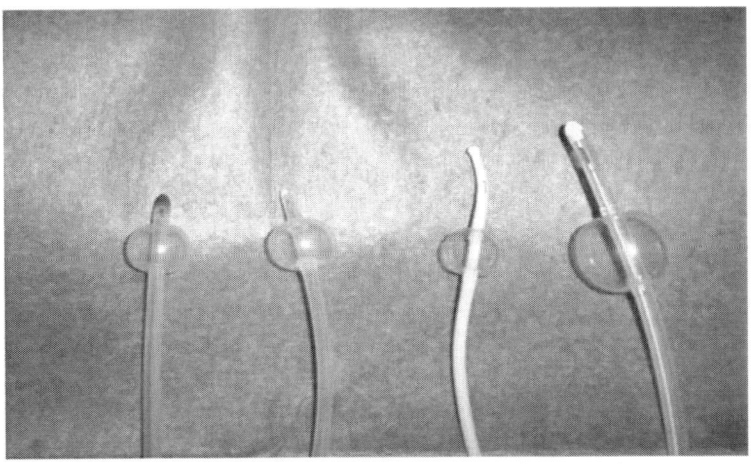

1 2 3 4

Picture 2.

Urinary Catheter examples:

1. Short tip catheter – two eyelets, 10 ml in balloon
2. Standard urinary catheter – two eyelets, 10 ml in balloon
3. Coude tip urinary catheter – single eyelet, 10 ml in balloon
4. 3-way urinary catheter – two eyelets, 30 ml in balloon

The Urinary Catheter Selection Guidelines Should Be Used as a General Guide for Adults Only

Whistle tip urinary catheter is usually inserted by urologist or urology registrar only. It is designed to drain blood clots due to severe haematuria.

Urinary Catheter Balloon Size

Paediatric catheter balloon size – 3ml, 5ml. Adult urinary catheter balloon size – 10ml, 20ml, 30ml and 60ml. Catheter with integrated balloon is a better design providing a uniform outer diameter reducing patient discomfort and irritation to the urethral epithelium on insertion and removal of the urinary catheter.

Urinary Catheter Length

Length range - 20 cm, 30 cm or 40cm.

When considering the length of urinary catheter, assessment of individual needs and physical characteristics should be conducted to identify the most appropriate catheter for the recommended drainage system. Female patients may prefer the shorter 20 cm urinary catheter.

Selection of Urinary Catheter for Patients with Special Clinical Conditions

The Australian Catheter Compass [19] is a useful tool developed recently to assist healthcare professionals selecting the appropriate urinary catheter for the patient. It offers guidance for medical practitioners or nurses in the clinical settings and facilitates discussion on the most appropriate catheter products available. Jahn et al. [20] conducted a systematic review on types of indwelling urinary catheters for long-term bladder drainage in adults. The group found that very few trials have compared types of urinary catheter for long-term catheter care and was unable to made practical conclusion.

Table 1.

Catheter size	Indication for use	Catheter type
12 – 14 Fr	clear urine, no mucus	2-way round tip catheter
16 Fr	clear urine, small thin mucus,	2-way round tip catheter
18 – 20 Fr	mild haematuria, small soft clots, some sediment, debris or thin mucus.	2- way round tip or open tip catheter
22 – 24 Fr	moderate haematuria, thin to small lumps of mucus, sediment and debris	3-way round tip catheter 2- way round tip or open tip catheter

Table 2. (Hooton et al. 2010)

Catheter variety	Clinical Indication
Soft curved Coude tip	Enlarged prostate.
Olive or Tieman tip	Enlarged prostate, short mild urethral stricture, bladder neck stricture
Open tip catheter	Chronic haematuria, excessive debris and sediment, vesico-rectal fistula.
Catheter with extra eyelet below the balloon	Vesical fistula. Regular urine bypassing urethral catheter.
Antimicrobial coated (Silver alloy or Nitrofurozone coated)	At risk of ascending urinary tract infection. May prevent bacteriuria in hospitalised patients with short-term catheterisation [17, 18]
Hydrophilic	No special medical indication

Selection of Urinary Catheter for Intermittent Self Catheterisation (ISC)

On selection of intermittent urinary catheter, health care practitioner needs to consider the physical, social, as well as the economic aspects of ISC care. Discussion on the pros and cons of ISC and the recommended catheter product should be appropriate to the patient specific activities of daily living. In reality, most patients who need to catheterise the bladder several times a day cannot afford to pay for disposable single-use intermittent urinary catheter unless the cost is covered by government scheme or private health insurance. Evidence has shown some support for use of multiple-use catheters by single patient using clean technique in outpatient and institutional settings. However, more studies are needed to find the best catheter sterilisation technique to reduce the risk of CA-UTI [16, 21-23].

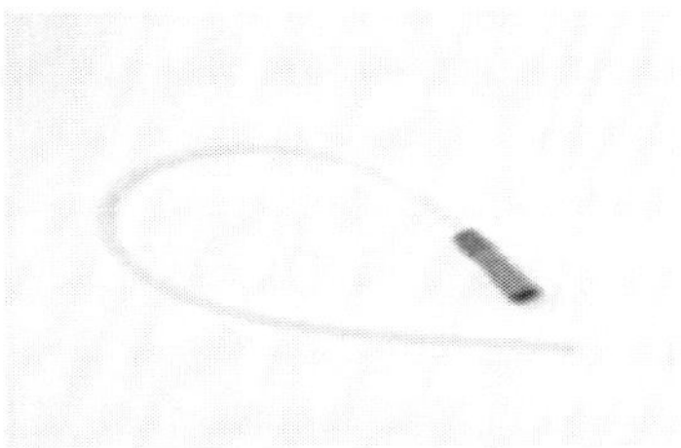

Picture 3.

Intermittent catheters use the same colour coding system to differentiate the sizes as the indwelling urinary catheters.

Nelaton Catheter Specifications

Nelaton catheter length: female catheter – 18 or 20cm, male catheter – 40cm

Nelaton Catheter Size and Material

Nelaton catheters come in a number of sizes ranging from 8 to 18 Fr. The degree of catheter stiffness is either soft or normal. It is made of medical grade thermo sensitive PVC material or silicone. Soft catheters may be selected by patients with good hand dexterity who have experienced discomfort on hard catheter insertion. In addition, the development of hydrophilic-coated catheters has offered more options for this group of patients. A recent Cochrane review [24] showed the group of patients performed ICS had a lower incidence of catheter associated bacteriuria when compared with the indwelling urethral catheterisation group. Motivated patients with proper assessment including catheter selection, education and discussion, training and support on ICS could be some of the key factors in achieving favourable bladder management outcome [16].

Nelaton Catheter Selection for Patients with Lower Urinary Tract Symptoms

Table 3.

Size	type and coating	Clinical indication
8	round tip	hypocontractile bladder
10, 12 and 14	round tip, Coude tip hydrophilic-coated	urinary retention, urethral stricture, bladder neck stricture. sensitive urethra
16, 18	round tip, Olive tip hydrophilic-coated Coude tip	urethral or bladder neck stricture

5. Urine Drainage Accessories

It is necessary for penile sheaths and urinary catheters to be attached to a collection device such as urine drainage bag or bottle. In addition, urinary catheters can be attached to a catheter valve. Urinary catheter should be attached to a sterile urine drainage bag to establish a closed system and only replaced when the catheter is changed [25]. Maintenance of a closed drainage system is universal practice [26] but the clinical protocol on the frequency of drainage bag replacement varies among institutions. A penile sheath is attached to a non-sterile leg bag or a bigger capacity bag, then removed and cleaned according to a care plan and the manufacturers' recommendations.

Catheter Drainage Systems

Catheter drainage system consists of either a continuous drainage or intermittent drainage. Continuous drainage of urine from the bladder requires the use of sterile bag which has different capacity, tubing length, shape, wear period, strap and outlet design. This system comes in 2 main types: leg bags and large capacity urine bags or bottles. Leg bags are appropriate for mobile patients as they only hold 350-1000mls and can be discreetly held in place with leg straps under clothes. They have a drainage port or tap to allow intermittent urine drainage into the toilet or a jug when the bag is nearly full. The patient needs to have manual dexterity to independently manage a leg bag. Non-ambulant patients should use the large capacity drainage bags. Ambulant patients with a leg bag overnight may attach a large capacity extension bag to establish a link system. In Australia, non-ambulant patients living at home with a urinary catheter may establish a closed system using a 4 litres bottle. The large capacity bags are suspended on a stand or hooked onto the bed and the bottles are self standing. Urine can be drained intermittently from the bladder using a catheter valve. Catheter valve is connected to the urinary catheter, IUC or SPC, and frequency of bladder emptying is control by the patient or care giver. Selection of appropriate drainage system is dependent on individual preference and professional advice based on clinical reason(s). The latest evidence continues to support the use of sterile urinary bag with urinary catheter and is endorsed by the experts [16, 26]. Comprehensive assessment prior to selection and product trial involves the physical, social, disease and financial aspects. The initial assessment and subsequent review assists the patient to find the most suitable product available.

Continuous Drainage System

Sterile bag products are recommended by the manufacturers to be replaced every 7 days. Some products are designed for longer wearing time.

Sterile drainage bag – Tubing length is either120 cm or 150cm.
Capacity range - 1500ml, 2000, 3000ml.
Shape – rectangle or pear
Outlet design - T-tap, lever tap, splash-proof switch.

Sterile leg bag - Tubing length – 5cm, 10cm, 25cm or 50cm
Capacity – 300cm, 500cm, 750cm, 800cm.
Outlet tap – T-tap, lever tap.

Intermittent Drainage System

This system allows the bladder to fill up with urine in the normal manner. Patients with normal bladder sensation and capacity are advised to drain urine when they experience an urge. In the absence of or reduced bladder sensation a patient should adhere to a strict timed regime to avoid bladder over distension.

Catheter Valves

A catheter valve is a small device that can be released intermittently to drain the bladder. A catheter valve has two common designs, flip-flow or lever tap with spring to allow automatic closure of the valve. They are particularly useful when attached to a suprapubic catheter (SPC) as the patient can try to pass urine and, if unsuccessful, the valve can then be released. At night the patient can attach the catheter valve to a urine drainage bag thus reducing the need to empty the bladder while asleep. A patient must fulfil the following criteria to be deemed suitable for intermittent drainage of urine using a catheter valve: -

1. good renal function
2. no ureteric reflux
3. a stable bladder
4. be cognitively intact
5. be motivated
6. has good manual dexterity
7. no vesical fistula
8. no haematuria [2].

6. Mechanical Devices – Women and Men

Women

There are two different types of mechanical devices available to reduce women's mild stress incontinence. These are intra-urethral devices and intra-vaginal devices. They may be useful for some women especially before contemplating surgery to address their stress incontinence or for those women who are not fit for surgery.

Intraurethral Devices

FemSoft is the only intra-urethral device currently available. It comprises of a cylinder made of a soft, compressible, mineral oil-filled silicone layer and an insertion probe. Prior to insertion the oil is in tip of the cylinder, but as the device is pushed into the urethra the fluid moves to the distal end allowing the device to pass through the urethra. Once in place the fluid flows back to the tip to hold the device in place at the bladder neck [2].

In the limited evaluation that intraurethral devices have had so far, although mild stress incontinence decreased a number of problems came to light, such as UTIs, haematuria, discomfort and migration into the bladder requiring cystoscopic removal [27].

Intra-Vaginal Devices

The purpose of using the intra-vaginal device is to support the bladder neck or the urethra in order to reduce stress incontinence. Studies have been done on 2 groups of intra-vaginal devices: tampons, pessaries and contraceptive diaphragms and devices exclusively designed to support the bladder neck.

The use of tampons, pessaries and contraceptive diaphragms are shown to be effective ways of reducing mild incontinence in some women when inserted prior to exercise. These devices exert mild pressure on the bladder neck to stop urine leakage [28]. However discomfort is one of the reasons that some women cannot tolerate using these devices. Further, intra-vaginal devices are not appropriate unless the user has good manual dexterity and accepts the idea of independently inserting a device into the vagina and is willing to remove or clean the device.

Intra-vaginal Devices Designed Specifically to Support the Bladder Neck

There are two categories of intra-vaginal devices to support the bladder neck: reusable and disposable.

Reusable Vaginal Devices

The Contiform intra-vaginal device is made of Santoprene, a non-allergic thermoplastic rubber shaped like a ring at the base with the back being higher than the front [29]. It is compressed and inserted into the vagina to the location behind the symphysis. The anterior part of the ring is situated underneath the urethra and the posterior part of the device resting behind the cervix. This device is not designed to reduce a prolapse [30]. It can be worn all day or simply during activities such as physical exercise, but it must be removed at night to be cleaned and before sexual intercourse. The device comes with a silicone ribbon to aid removal. It should be replaced every month or when it shows signs of deterioration (whichever comes first) [31].

In a study in which 37 women completed a trial of the Contiform, 54% was cured with the primary end point being < 2g urine leakage in 24hrs. Again, this device is not suitable for women with poor manual dexterity; a small vaginal introitus or a shortened or narrow vagina. Other contraindications for use include the device falling out when the woman coughs; or the user experiencing difficulty on device insertion or removal, and the woman being unprepared to insert a device into the vagina [30].

Mechanical Devices – Men

Mechanical devices for men compress the penis with a clamp or peri-penile strap aiming to occlude the urethra to prevent urinary leakage [2]. The penis is compressed ischemia and pain can occur especially when the device is used for prolonged periods. A trained health professional should fit and educate the user about the device.

Mechanical devices are suitable for men who have mild to moderate stress incontinence, mentally competent, and those who have good bladder and penile sensation, intact penile skin and good manual dexterity [32]. They are not a common continence device that men would select due to the pain experienced on fitting.

7. Hand-Held Urinals

Hand-held urinals can be used when users are not able to access a toilet due to reduced mobility, inflexibility, contractures or severe frequency and urgency. There are urinals that suit both men and women. Urinals are made of stainless steel, soft or hard plastic with different shape and capacity. Some soft ones are compactable, disposable and discreet. They can also be very useful for travel purposes. Most male urinals are made of hard plastic and have a spout into which the penis is placed. The urine then drains into a reservoir which is emptied as necessary. They can be used in many positions i.e. while in bed, in a wheelchair/chair or when standing. Some male urinals have a non-spill adaptor to reduce the risk of leakage during urination. Due to the anatomy of females, female urinals come in a variety of shapes and materials. Depending on the voiding position of patient, this product needs to be trialled to determine which shape prevents spillage and leakage [2].

8. Bed Pads and Commodes

If a person is not able to access a toilet due to mobility or safety issues, disability or medical condition, bed pans or commodes may offer a solution. A bed pan is a portable container for urine or faeces. It can be used on a bed, a chair or it is placed on a commode chair. A commode is a piece of equipment that look like a chair, and when the seat is lifted up there is a frame into which a bed pan can be placed. A mobile commode has wheels which can be placed over the toilet.

Behavioural Training Programs

Bladder Training / Retraining

The terms "Bladder Training" and "Bladder Retraining" are used interchangeably in literature reviews and involve the use of educational and behavioural interventions to re-establish urinary control in adults [33, 34]. For simplicity, we will use the term bladder training in our discussion. Bladder training was developed in the mid to late 1970s for people who were physically and cognitively able [34-36]. The intervention is effective in improving the quality of life of women with urge, stress or mixed incontinence [37]. Bladder training should be considered as the first-line treatment option for women with mild to moderate stress, urge or mixed urinary incontinence. This program is also suitable for men with similar urinary control problems. The aims of bladder training include:

- Increasing bladder capacity, therefore prolonging voiding intervals with reduced urinary frequency.
- Improving ability to control bladder urgency and reducing the incidence of urge incontinence.
- Building patient confidence to overcome long standing faulty habits .e.g. voiding "just in case".

A study by Franl et al. [38] showed that bladder training reduced the number of incontinent episodes by 57% for both urge and stress incontinence. In addition, the quantity of fluid loss was also reduced by 54%. Number of diurnal and nocturnal voluntary micturition was also reduced [33]. There are various bladder training programs which range from a strict toileting regime to a flexible toileting times.

Strict Toileting Regime

This method involves the establishment of strict voiding schedules starting from every hour during waking hours with restriction of voiding in between toileting times. Each week, the voiding interval is increased by 15 to 30 minutes per week depending on progress. For most patients, the desirable voiding interval is 3 to 4 hours and for most elderly patients, 2 to 3 hours are the optimal duration. When the optimal toileting regime has been established for individual patient, voiding is encouraged at scheduled times. Both patient and carers need to be diligent and apply self-control over bladder urgency.

Flexible Toileting Regime

In flexible toileting regime, the patient is advised to void when the sense of urge becomes intolerable. The training program incorporates the cognitive deferment technique. Here the patient is advised to defer the first urge of urination, starting with deferring for 5 to 10 minutes and gradually increasing this time to 30 minutes. Once the patient is able to defer 30 minutes or longer, he/she will be able to surpass the first urge and is allowed to void at the next urge. The flexible toileting regime is less stressful for the patient as they start from a more comfortable level. This regime is also more manageable especially for the older age group. Bladder training programs usually take 10-12 weeks to achieve therapeutic goal.

In order to maximum treatment outcome, the programs should be individualized, dependent on the patients' physical environment and personal capability. Patients who participate in bladder training programs require motivation and compliance in order to adhere to the program including the recording a bladder diary. The control of urge sensationcan be achieved by the following methods:

1. Relaxation: taking deep breathes, breathing slowly, and not rushing to the toilet.
2. Distraction: take the mind off about going to toilet by distracting. Consider doing an alternative task such phoning a friend, or counting backwards from 100.
3. Perineal pressure: Apply direct pressure on the perineum. Such as sitting on the arm of a chair or on a rolled up towel, or crossing the legs.
4. Pelvic floor muscle contraction is used to control the urge to urinate.

(Further reading: Pelvic Floor Muscle Training (PFMT) for management of urinary incontinence in women, Hay –Smith et. al in Abrams et al. (eds) 2008, p.1034-1055 and p.1079-1080. PFMT for management of urinary incontinence in men, same chapter p.1082 - 1087 and p.1094)

Bladder Diary

A Bladder Diary is similar to a fluid balance chart and is an invaluable diagnostic tool that also aids clinical assessment and outcome evaluation of patients with voiding dysfunction. Although it is called a 'Bladder Diary', the patient is required to record both fluid intake and urine output over a 24 hour period. Usually a 3-day Bladder Diary is needed for initial assessment and to monitor progress. The patient has to record the following information in the diary.

- Fluid intake – time of intake, type of fluid and amount
- Urine output – voiding time, amount, any leakage of urine
- Comment - urgency, urge incontinence, provoking factors such as leakage when bearing down

From the three days record, the clinician can confirm functional bladder capacity, frequency, voiding intervals, nocturia, and identify any trends and factors associated with incontinence. Periodic recording of 3- day Bladder Diary is also a useful tool in assessing progress. Table 4 is a diary of a 30 year old man undergoing bladder training because of urinary frequency and nocturia.

Table 4. A Bladder Diary

DATE	TIME	FLUID INTAKE	URINE OUTPUT	COMMENT
13/8/2010	1:30 am		200ml	
	5:00 am		200ml	
	8:50 am		250ml	Out of bed
	9:30 am	Coffee 50ml		
		Milkshake 400ml		
		Milk 100ml with cereal		
	10:00 am		75ml	
	10:30 to 11:30 am	Water 750ml		
	12 noon		375ml	Hold on x 30mins on train
	1:30pm	Coffee 250ml		
	2 to 3pm	Water 500ml		
	3:15pm		525ml	
	4:30pm	Coke 375ml		
	6:00pm	Coffee 250ml		
	6:15pm		550ml	
	7 to 8pm	Water 500ml		
	7:50pm		400ml	
	9:45pm		350ml	
	10:30pm		100ml	
Total		3,205 ml	3,025ml	

From this Bladder Diary, the clinician can identify the following concerns:

Fluid Intake

Total fluid intake is 3.2litre, with 29% being caffeine drink (Coffee and Coke = 925ml). The fluid intake is well over the recommended 1.5 to 2 litre limit per day.In this man, eExcessive fluid intake is likely the cause for urine frequency. Caffeine is a known stimulant responsible for 2% to 13% of lower urinary tract symptoms in younger men (20 to 49 years old) [39], and causes a significant increase in detrusor pressure during bladder filling phrase in women with detrusor instability [40].

Urine Output

Total urine output is just over 3 litres with minimal output at 75ml and maximal output at 550ml. Minimal voiding interval is 45 minutes and maximal voiding interval is 3 hours and 30 minutes. Urine frequency is 8 times during the day and 2 times at night.

Patient has a normal bladder capacity at 550mls. He was able to defer voiding for 30 minutes while he was travelling on the train.

From the information available in the Bladder Diary, the clinician can make the following recommendations to the patient:

- Reduce the fluid intake to 2 litres per day, space out through the day till 7pm.
- Reduce caffeine intake to 2 cups of coffee a day (no coffee at 6pm) initially, then stop having Coke at 4:30pm. The aim is to reduce the total caffeine intake.
- With a maximal bladder capacity of 550ml, patients should be encouraged to avoid going to the toilet at the first urge.
- He can also be encouraged to practice deferment technique which he is capable of.
- It is also advisable to continue to record urgency or urge incontinence in the Diary for review.

So we can see here how useful the 3-day Bladder Diary is in confirming initial findings and monitoring treatment progress. The Diary is an invaluable diagnostic, therapeutic and educational tool.

Additional voiding programs for the management of urinary incontinence in adults include habit retraining, timed voiding and prompted voiding.

Habit Retraining

This is one of the behavioural interventions to treat incontinence for people with cognitive and physical disabilities such as those residents in rehabilitation centre or long term institutional care. This two week training program requires motivated staff to check on the individual every hour for incontinence to identify individual's unique voiding pattern. Results are then used to design an individual toileting program that identifies the time when urinary incontinence may occur so that the resident can be prompted and toileted before the incontinence episodes. Burgio et al. [41] found that there was a mean increase in dryness from 30% of pants checks during baseline to 62% during the training phase. As the residents improved in their continence status, the staff can adjust the frequency of toileting appropriately.

Timed Voiding

Timed voiding is a toileting assistance program for the management of urinary incontinence for people with cognitive and physical disabilities. This is a common toileting program practised in residential care facilities. Staff attend a 'commode round' that is toileting at a fixed time interval, e.g. every 2 hours or soon after each meal. . This program is very rigid and may not meet individual needs.

A systematic review by Ostaszkiewicz et al. in 2004 [42] on timed voiding found a reduction in the number of incontinence episodes in two trials. However, fixed schedule of toileting was combined with other interventions in these trials and therefore the reviewers were not able to confirm the effects of timed voiding for the management of urinary incontinence.

Prompted Voiding

By using verbal prompts and positive reinforcement, this behavioural therapy aims to promote continence for people with or without dementia. Prompted voiding is commonly used in residential care settings. A review by Eustice et al. in 2000 [43] found there was a suggestive evidence of short-term benefit from prompted voiding. However, long-term benefit was not confirmed in the study.

Conclusion

To date there has been insufficient quality research conducted to measure the treatment effects of continence products and the treatment impacts on the psychological well-being of individuals. The care of patients with urinary incontinence often requires multidisciplinary and multi-faceted treatments. Comprehensive nursing assessment, individualized treatment programs and careful selection of the most appropriate continence products for each individual are essential aspects of good care.

Ongoing monitoring and evaluation of patients' health status is necessary to respond to their changing continence needs in order to optimise their quality of life and health outcomes.

References

[1] Miner, P.B., Economic and personal impact of fecal and urinary incontinence. *Gastroenterology*, 2004. 126(1): p. S8-S13.

[2] Cottenden, A., Bliss, D.; Buckley, B.; Fader, M.; Getliffe, K.; Paterson, J.; Pieters, R. and Wilde, M., Management with Incontinence Products. In: Abrams, P., Cardoszo, L.,

Khoury, S. and Wein, A. editors. "*Incontinence*" 4th eds., Plymouth, England: Health Publications Ltd. 2009. p.1519-1642.

[3] Fader, M.; Cottenden, A. and Getliffe, K. et al. Absorbent products for urinary/fecal incontinence: a comparative evaluation of key product designs. *Health Technol Assess.* 2008; 12(29): iii-iv, ix-185

[4] Horie, K.; Baron M.; Fox, R. B.; He, J.; Hess, M.; Kahovec, J.; Kitayama, T.; Kubisa, P.; Maréchal, E.; Mormann, M.; Stepto, R. F. T.;Tabak, D.; Vohlídal, J.; Wilks, E. S and Work, W. J., Definitions of terms relating to reactions of polymers and to functional polymeric materials (IUPAC Recommendations 2003). *Pure and Applied Chemistry*, 2004. 76(4): p. 889–906.

[5] Fader, M.; Bliss, D.; Cottenden, A.; Moore, K. and Norton C., Continence products: research priorities to improve the lives of people with urinary and/or fecal leakage. *Neurourology and Urodynamics*, 2010. 29(4): p. 640-644.

[6] Pomfret, I.J., Use of Continence Products. In: ed. C. Norton. *Nursing for Continence*, 2nd ed. Beaconsfield, UK. Beaconsfield Publishers Ltd. 1998.

[7] Maki, D.G.; Tambyah, P.A.; Engineering out the risk for infection with urinary catheters. *Emerging Infectious Diseases*, 2001. 7(2): p. 342-347.

[8] Landi, F.; Cesari, M.; Onder, G.; Zamboni, V.; Barillaro, C.; Lattanzio, F, et al., Indwelling urethral catheter and mortality in frail elderly women living in community. *Neurourology and Urodynamics*, 2004. 23(7): p. 697-701.

[9] Saint, S.; Veenstra, D.L.; Lipsky, B.A., The clinical and economic consequences of nosocomial central venous catheter related infection: are antimicrobial catheters useful? *Infection Control Hospital Epidemiology*, 2000. 21(6): p. 375-380.

[10] Cravens, D.D.; Zweig, S., Urinary catheter management. *American Family Physician*, 2000. 61: p. 369-376.

[11] Newman, S. and J. Lawler, Managing health care under New Public Management: A Sisyphean challenge for nursing. *Journal of Sociology*, 2009. 45(4): p. 419-432.

[12] Shekelle, P.G.; Morton, S.C.; Clark, K.A.; Pathak, M.; Vickrey, B.G., Systematic review of risk factors for urinary tract infection in adults with spinal cord dysfunction. *Journal of Spinal Cord Medicine*, 1999. 22(4): p. 258-272.

[13] Johansson, I.; Athlin, E.; Frykholm, L.; Bolinder, H. and Larsso, G., Intermittent versus indwelling catheters for older patients with hip fractures. *Journal of Clinical Nursing*, 2002. 11(5): p. 651-656.

[14] Saint, S.; Lipsky, B.A.; Preventing catheter-related bacteriuria: should we? Can we? How? *Archive of Internal Medicine*, 1999. 159(8): p. 800-808.

[15] Hart, S., Urinary catheterisation. *Nursing Standard*, 2008. 22: p. 44-48.

[16] Hooton, T.; Bradley, S.; Cardenas, D.; Colgan, R.; Geerlings, S.; Rice, J.; Saint, S.; Schaeffer, A.; Tambayh, P.; Tenke, P. and Nicolie, L., Diagnosis, Prevention, and Treatment of Catheter-Associated Urinary Tract Infection in Adults:2009 International Clinical Practice Guidelines from the Infectious Diseases Society of America. *Clinical Infectious Diseases*, 2010. 50(5): p. 625-663.

[17] Johnson, J. R.; Kuskowski, M.A. and Wilt, T.J., Systematic Review: Antimicrobial Urinary Catheters to Prevent Catheter-Associated Urinary Tract Infection in Hospitalized Patients. *Annals of Internal Medicine*, 2006. 144: p. 116-126.

[18] Schumm, K.L.; Lam, T.B., Types of urethral catheters for management of short-term voiding problems in hospitalized adults: a short version Cochrane review. *Neurourology Urodynamics*, 2008. 27(8): p. 738-746.

[19] Wicks, K., Catheter Compass, 2010. Available from Brightsky Australia.

[20] Jahn, P.; Preuss, M.; Kernig, A.; Seifert-Hühmer, A.; Langer, G., Types of indwelling urinary catheters for long-term bladder drainage in adults. *Cochrane Database Systematic Reviews*, 2007. (3).

[21] Kurtz M.J.; Van Zandt.K.; Burns J.L., Comparison study of home catheter cleaning methods. *Rehabilitation Nursing*, 1995. 20: p. 212-214, 217.

[22] Moore, K.N.; Burt, J.; Voaklander, D.C., Intermittent catheterisation in the rehabilitation setting: a comparison of clean and sterile technique. *Clinical Rehabilitation,* 2006. 20: p. 461-468.

[23] Moore, K.N.; Fader, M.; Getliffe, K., Long-term bladder management by intermittent catheterisation in adults and children. *Cochrane Database Systematic Review,* 2007.

[24] Niel-Weise B.S.; Van den Brorek, P.J., Urinary catheter policies for short-term bladder drainage in adults. *Cochrane Database Systematic Review*, 2005.

[25] Platt, R.; Polk, B.F.; Murdock, B.; Rosner, B., Reduction of mortality associated with nosocomial urinary tract infection. *Lancet*, 1983. 1(8330): p. 893-897.

[26] Gould, C., et al., Guideline for Prevention of Catheter-Associated Urinary Tract Infections 2009 •. *Infection Control and Hospital Epidemiology*, 2010. 31(4): p. 319-326.

[27] Brubaker, L., Harris,T.; Gleason D.; Newman, D. and North, B., The external urethral barrier for stress incontinence: a multicenter trial of safety and efficacy. Miniguard Investigators Group. *Obstetrics and Gynecology*, 1999. 93(6): p. 932-937.

[28] Nygaard, I., Prevention of exercise incontinence with mechanical devices. *Journal of Reproductive Medicine*, 1995. 40(2): p. 89-94.

[29] Morris, A.R.M.K.H., The Contiform incontinence device—efficacy and patient acceptability. *International Journal of Urogynaecology,* 2003. 14: p. 412-417.

[30] Allen, W.A.,; Leek, H.; Izurieta, A. and Moore, K.H., Update: the "Contiform" intravaginal device in four sizes for the treatment of stress incontinence *International Journal of Urogynaecology*, 2008. 19: p. 757-761.

[31] Contiform. Contiform Product information. Available from: http://www. contiform.com/whatBN.php.

[32] Moore, K.N., Schieman,S.; Ackerman, T.; Dzus, H.Y.; Metcalfe, J.B.; Voaklander, D.C., Assessing comfort, safety, and patient satisfaction with three commonly used penile compression devices. *Urology Journal*, 2004. 63(1): p. 150-154.

[33] Karon, S., a Team Approach to Bladder Retraining: A Pilot Study. *Urologic Nursing*, 2005. 25(4).

[34] Roe, B.; Ostaszkiewic, O.J.; Milne, J. and Wallace, S, Systematic reviews of bladder training and voiding programs in adults: a synopsis of findings from data analysis and outcomes using metastudy techniques. *Journal of Advance Nursing*, 2007. 57 (1): p. 15-31.

[35] Willington, F.L., Training and retraining for continence. *Nursing Times*, 1975. 71: p. 500 -503.

[36] Frewen, W.k., An objective assessment of unstable bladder of psychosomatic origin. *British Journal of Urology*, 1978. 50(4): p. 246-249.

[37] Wyman, J.F.; Fantl, J.A.; McClish, D.K.; Harkins, S.W.; Uebersax, J.S. and Ory, M.G., Quality of life following bladder training in older women with urinary incontinence. *International Urogynaecology Journal*, 1997. 8 (40): p. 223-229.

[38] Fantl, J.A.; Wyman, J.F.; McClish, D.K.; Harkins, S.W.; Elswick, R.K.; Taylor, J.R., et al., Efficacy of bladder training in older woman with urinary incontinence. *Journal of American Medical Association*, 1991(265): p. 609-613.

[39] Moon, T.D., Hagon, L.; Heisey, D.M., Urinary symptomatology in younger men. *Urology Journal*, 1997. 50 (5): p. 700-703.

[40] Creighton, S.M.; Stanton, l. Caffeine: Does it affect your Bladder? *British Journal of Urology,* 1990(66): p. 613-614.

[41] Burgio, L.; Engel, B.T.; McCormick, K.; Hawkins, A. and Scheve, Behavioural treatment for urinary incontinence in elderly inpatients: Initial attempts to modify prompting and toileting procedures. *Behavioural Therapy*, 1988. 19(3): p. 345- 357.

[42] Ostaszkiewicz, J.; Johnston, L.; Roe, B., Timed voiding for the management of urinary incontinence in adults. *Cochrane Database of Systematic Reviews*, 2004(1).

[43] Eustice S.; Roe, B. and Paterson. J., Prompted voiding for the management of urinary incontinence in adults. *Cochrane Database of Systematic Reviews,* 2000(2).

Special Section: Surgical Treatments for Female Urinary Incontinence

In: Urinary Incontinence
Editor: Eric Chung
ISBN: 978-1-62618-482-4

Chapter 11

Treatment of Overactive Bladder in Women

Joy A. Greer and Lily A. Arya
Hospital of the University of Pennsylvania, Division of Urogynecology, Department of OB-GYN, University of Pennsylvania, Philadelphia, PA, US

Abstract

Overactive bladder syndrome (OAB) affects more than 34 million people in the United States and increases with age and in symptom severity. The increasing costs of this disease both for the patient and society demand appropriate, effective therapy. Current therapeutic options for OAB include behavioral and physical therapy interventions, pharmacologic treatments, and nerve stimulation. Several new options for refractory OAB symptoms are showing initial promising results both in objective relief of symptoms and improved quality of life. Most studies investigating treatment options for OAB have evaluated short-term benefit only and have used variable outcome measures. Additional studies evaluating long-term effects, cost-effectiveness and comparative-effectiveness data on treatment options are needed to give clinicians and patients the best information possible.

Introduction

Overactive bladder (OAB) syndrome is defined as urinary urgency, usually accompanied by frequency and nocturia, with or without urgency urinary incontinence (UUI), in the absence of urinary tract infection or other obvious pathology [1]. In the United States, the prevalence of OAB is age-related, and more than 34 million people in the United States have OAB, on the basis of an estimated prevalence of 16.9% in adult women and 16% in adult men [2, 3]. Over time, OAB progresses to UUI with increasing severity of symptoms [4].

Appropriate treatment of OAB is necessary due to the increasing costs of the disease for the individual and society. The total estimated cost of OAB in the United States was $12.02

billion in 2000 [2], and women who have OAB, with or without urge incontinence, have significantly poorer scores on health-related quality of life, mental health, and quality of sleep when compared with age-matched controls after adjusting for other covariates, including comorbid illnesses [3].

Current therapeutic options for OAB range from behavioral and physical therapy interventions to pharmacologic treatments and nerve stimulation. The aim of this chapter is to discuss the existing and potential new therapy modalities for idiopathic OAB and UUI.

Pathophysiology

Urinary continence and micturition require an intact and functioning neuromuscular system. Central control of micturition resides in the pontine micturition center [5]. Peripheral control of micturition depends on combined action of several neurotransmitters regulating contraction of the smooth and striated muscles of the urinary bladder, urethra, and periurethral region [6]. Neurologically the urethral sphincter receives somatic innervation from the pudendal nerve, which arises from the anterior horn of the second through fourth sacral nerves. The urethra and the bladder receive innervation from the autonomic (sympathetic and parasympathetic) systems. The short preganglionic sympathetic fibers synapse in the sympathetic trunk and the long postganglionic fibers terminate in adrenergic receptors of the urethra and bladder neck. The sympathetic system stimulates beta receptors in the detrusor muscle of the bladder. The parasympathetic systems arise from the dorsolateral ganglion of the second through fourth sacral segments of the spinal cord and have long preganglionic fibers that synapse close to the bladder. These short postganglionic parasympathetic fibers end primarily on the muscarinic receptors of the detrusor muscle, urothelium, and suburothelium [7]. In the usual continent state, the bladder is functionally "turned off" and then "turned on" in appropriate circumstances, via positive feedback loops in the micturition reflex pathway, to eliminate urine [8]. When voiding occurs, bladder and perineal afferent activity is increased and stimulates efferent excitatory input to the bladder. This in turn stimulates the parasympathetic system and initiates a detrusor muscle contraction via muscarinic receptors, specifically M2 and M3. This positive feedback loop is mediated by supraspinal parasympathetic pathways through the pons and promotes efficient bladder emptying while minimizing residual urine in the bladder [5, 6, 9-11].

To maintain continence when voiding must be delayed, various visceral and somatic afferents and the recurrent inhibitory pathways inhibit the sacral preganglionic outflow to the bladder [5]. Afferent stimuli from pelvic organs such as the vagina, cervix and rectum can inhibit the sacral preganglionics to the bladder as well as increase urethral pressure through the visceral-visceral reflex otherwise called the guarding reflex [5]. Somatic afferents from the pudendal nerve assist with voiding inhibition and provide an important site that can be modulated by physiotherapy [12]. Contraction of the pelvic floor muscles can inhibit voiding by augmenting the guarding reflex through somatic efferents [5, 8].

OAB syndrome results from the inability of the bladder to store urine appropriately. The underlying mechanism is not well understood but is likely multi-factorial. Abnormalities in bladder receptors, peripheral and central innervation, myofascial components, and behavioral factors have all been implicated in the pathogenesis of OAB and UUI [6-9, 13-16]. Loss of central inhibitory controls of the positive feedback loop or sensitization of bladder afferent signaling leads to UUI [8, 17]. Recent studies show that afferent nerve sensitization and associated muscle dysfunction are fundamental elements of urgency-frequency syndrome and UUI [14, 18-21]. Experimental data from animals show that somatic afferent input to the spinal cord modulates the guarding and voiding reflexes that control continence and micturition [13]. Defects in other motor control factors have also been described in women with UUI. Women with SUI and UUI have been shown to have decreases in the maximal vaginal surface electromyography activity and vaginal pressure measurements [22]. Trigger points in the lower abdominal muscles have been implicated in increased urgency and frequency of micturition and may cause weakening or provocation of a partial contraction of the lower abdominal muscles [15]. In addition to postural and movement dysfunction, lower back pain, pelvic pain and breathing disorders have been strongly associated with urinary incontinence across age cohorts [16, 23, 24]. The contribution of musculoskeletal factors to the pathogenesis of UUI requires further investigation.

1. Behavioral Modification

First line treatment for OAB involves behavioral modification such as caffeine restriction, fluid manipulation if patients have excessive fluid intake, and bladder retraining through timed voiding [25]. For obese women, weight loss [26] is helpful in conjunction with exercise and behavioral modification to decrease OAB symptoms. Adding pelvic floor muscle exercises to behavioral therapy has resulted in significant decreases in urgency (52%), frequency (64%) and nocturia (32%) complaints [27] and improved overall treatment benefit [28]. Fantl et al. [29] also found that combinations of behavioral treatments were more effective than just one. Finally, a recent Cochrane Review [30] has also reported that OAB symptom improvement is greater when behavioral modification is combined with an antimuscarinic than either therapy alone [30].

2. Physiotherapy Treatment Options

2.1. Pelvic Floor Muscle Training

Pelvic floor muscle training (PMFT), commonly referred to as Kegel exercises, have been prescribed since 1948 [31] for the improvement of urinary incontinence symptoms. In brief, PMFT require tightening of the pelvic muscles and holding the contraction for a few seconds, followed by a rest period [32]. PMFT have been postulated to prevent urgency and UUI by inhibiting and aborting inappropriate detrusor contractions [33] as well as improving urge suppression by increasing pelvic floor muscle strength and endurance [34-36]. PMFT may also increase pudendal nerve activation, which in turn activates external urethral sphincter contraction to stimulate the guarding reflex [17, 34, 37-39]. (Figure 1).

Data from studies [27, 40] looking at PMFT for women with UUI suggest a benefit with decreased pad weights from urinary incontinence and decreased incontinent episodes per day. Significant decreases in urgency, frequency, nocturia, and leakage index urge score were also noted while these women were noted to have increased mean pelvic muscle strength following treatment.

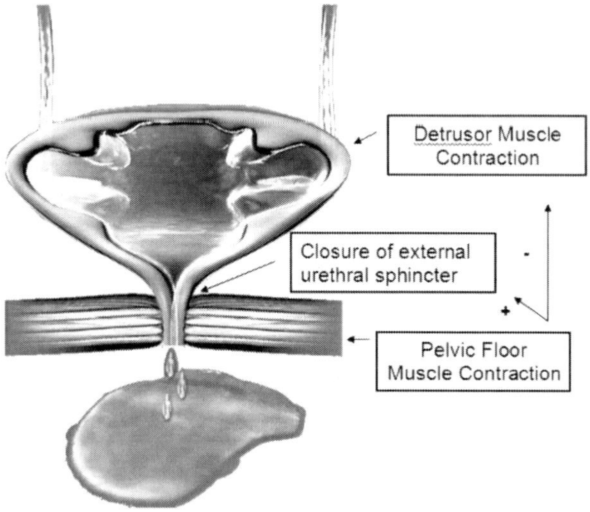

Figure 1. Pelvic Floor Muscle Training and Overactive Bladder.

Further scientific study of these techniques is certainly warranted because studies of PMFT in women with UUI are limited by a lack of placebo-controlled studies, small sample size, lack of adequate blinding and randomization, and the use of combined therapies. The advantages of PMFT are that these exercises are minimally invasive without side effects. Limitations include correct patient performance, compliance and long-term adherence.

2.2. Biofeedback

Pelvic floor biofeedback is a technique that uses surface perineal electrodes, vaginal cones, or rectal cones to monitor external urinary sphincter or levator ani muscle activity to augment PMFT. Biofeedback has been shown to be more effective than placebo or bladder training alone in reducing UUI [28, 32, 34]. Definitive data on the efficacy of biofeedback therapy alone for the treatment of UUI is lacking. Biofeedback in combination with behavioral training results in short-term improvement in OAB and UUI but the benefits are not maintained, possibly due to patient adherence or loss of gained pelvic floor muscle strength. Satisfaction with treatment for biofeedback combined with behavioral training is high even when objective measurements in reduction of UUI are comparable to control groups [35]. Limited evidence suggests that biofeedback may be helpful in specific groups of patients, such as women who have difficulty isolating and targeting appropriate muscle groups and who are visual rather than verbal learners. Biofeedback (as well as PMFT and behavioral changes) may be difficult in patients with cognitive impairment [34] and the technique requires patient motivation and long-term adherence to maintain efficacy [34].

2.3. Vaginal Electrical Stimulation

Vaginal electrical stimulation (VES) has been postulated to improve UUI by stimulating sympathetic input to the bladder, which in turn inhibits activation of the detrusor muscle by the parasympathetic nerves [5]. There is considerable variation in the devices, electrical parameters (10-20 Hz) and recommended frequency of treatment (twice weekly to twice daily) for VES [41, 42]. Relatively few studies have specifically examined the effectiveness of VES in a well-defined population of women with urge-predominant urinary incontinence, compared VES to placebo or other physiotherapy techniques, or used adequate sample size. Some studies have shown significant improvement in incontinence episodes and elimination of detrusor overactivity on urodynamic studies after VES [41-43], whereas other studies have not showed a significant difference between treatment and comparison arms [44, 45].

A significant placebo effect may exist in the use of VES in the treatment of OAB and UUI [41, 42]. Larger studies are required to determine the efficacy of VES, the optimal protocol for stimulation, and incremental benefit, if any, when VES is used in conjunction with PMFT or biofeedback.

2.4. Potential New Physiotherapy Techniques for UUI

A potential new modality for UUI is myofascial therapy. Myofascial therapy involves the treatment of trigger points and taut muscle bands and reeducation of the pelvic floor with stretching and strengthening exercises [14]. A trigger point has been described as a hyperirritable nodule located within a taut band of skeletal muscle, that when palpated, is tender and produces referred pain [46]. Myofascial physical therapy has been shown to modulate afferent nerve stimulation, reduce excitability and induce relaxation of the underlying muscles [47-51]. Myofascial physical therapy has been used successfully in women with urgency-frequency and bladder pain syndromes [14, 15, 52] with decreased urgency and frequency [14] suggesting that pelvic myofascial therapy may reduce UUI symptoms by reducing detrusor overactivity and inducing pelvic muscle relaxation. Given promising results of myofascial therapy in women with urgency-frequency syndrome, future studies investigating myofascial therapy in women with UUI may be beneficial.

3. Pharmacologic Therapies for OAB

3.1. Antimuscarinic

When behavioral measures and pelvic floor physical therapy are inadequate to control symptoms, pharmacologic treatment of OAB may be prescribed and its effects are well-established [30]. Medications focus on modulating detrusor muscle contractility through their effect on the nerve supply of the lower urinary tract [7]. Acetylcholine is the main neurotransmitter at the neuromuscular junction in the detrusor muscle, and it exerts its effect by stimulation of the muscarinic receptors [53].

The human body contains five subtypes of muscarinic receptors (M1-M5) which are found in many organs. Urinary smooth muscle and urothelium contain mainly M2 and M3 muscarinic receptors. While M3 receptors only account for approximately 20% of the receptors in the urinary tract, they are primarily responsible for bladder contraction [54]. Antimuscarinic receptors act during the filling-storage phase by inhibiting afferent input from the bladder and directly inhibiting smooth muscle contractility. Antimuscarinic medications are the most commonly used pharmacotherapy for OAB. Data from well designed randomized clinical trials on the efficacy of tricyclic antidepressants, α-adrenergic agonists, afferent nerve inhibitors, prostaglandin antagonists, β-adrenergic agonists, and calcium channel blockers for OAB as compared to antimuscarinics are lacking and these medications are not widely used [55].

Table 1. Dose, receptor selectivity, and adverse reactions * of antimuscarinic medications

Generic Name	Brand Name	Subtype of Muscarinic Blockage [61]	Dose	Adverse Reactions (>10%)
Darifenacin	Enablex	Relatively selective for M3	7.5-15 mg daily	Dry mouth (19% to 35%) Constipation (15% to 21%)
Fesoterodine	Toviaz	Similar block of M2 and M3	4-8 mg daily	Dry mouth (19% to 35%; dose related)
Oxybutinin IR	Ditropan *	Relatively selective for M3 and M1	5 mg two to four times daily	Dizziness (4% to 17%) Somnolence (2% to 14%) Dry mouth (29% to 71%; dose related) Constipation (7% to 15%) Nausea (2% to 12%) Impaired memory recall and immediate learning [92]
Oxybutinin ER	Ditropan XL †	Relatively selective for M3 and M1	5-30 mg daily	Dizziness (4% to 17%), somnolence (2% to 14%) Dry mouth (29% to 71%; dose related), constipation (7% to 15%) Nausea (2% to 12%) *Less than IR preparation*
Oxybutinin transdermal patch	Oxytrol	Relatively selective for M3 and M1	One patch every three to four days	Local skin irritation, pruritus (14%)
Oxybutynin transdermal gel	Gelnique	Relatively selective for M3 and M1	1g gel daily	None reported at rates > 10%
Solifenacin	Vesicare	Relatively selective for M3 and M1	5-10 mg daily	Dry mouth (11% to 28%; dose-related) Cconstipation (5% to 13%; dose-related)
Tolterodine IR	Detrol	Similar block of M3 and M2, relatively nonselective	1-2 mg twice daily	Dry mouth (35%)
Tolterodine ER	Detrol LA	Similar block of M3 and M2, relatively nonselective	2-4 mg daily	Dry mouth (23%)
Trospium IR	Sanctura	Similar block of M3 and M2, relatively nonselective	20 mg twice daily	Dry mouth (9% to 22%)
Trospium ER	Sanctura XR	Similar block of M3 and M2, relatively nonselective	60 mg daily	Dry mouth (9% to 22%)

* Adverse reaction data obtained from drug prescribing information unless otherwise noted. † Generic form also available.

In addition to being present in the urinary smooth muscle and urothelium, M2 and M3 receptors are also present in other tissues of the body (bowel, salivary glands, eye as well as cardiac smooth muscle). This has led to considerable difficulty in the development of purely uroselective drugs. Most of the widely used antimuscarinic medications used to treat OAB produce varying degrees of antimuscarinic side effects such as dry mouth, blurred vision, confusion, constipation [56] and rarely increased heart rate[7, 57] and can lead to discontinuation rates as high as 71% [58]. Six antimuscarinic medications to treat OAB and UUI are currently available in the United States and include oxybutynin [59-66], tolterodine [61, 63, 67], trospium [68-73], solifenacin [74-77], darifenacin [78-79], and festoterodine [80-86]. Table 1 summarizes each medication, dosage and adverse reaction profile (Table 1).

3.2. Antimuscarinics in the Elderly

While the prevalence of OAB increases with age, there are relatively little data on the central nervous system safety in the elderly due to a lack of reporting [87, 88] and the inadequacy of the prior clinical trials to appropriately screen for, measure, and document CNS symptoms [88]. Few trials have reported specifically on the efficacy of antimuscarinic medications in elderly populations, but older patients seem to have similar efficacy without an increase in serious adverse effects or side effect profiles were similar when compared with younger women [89-91]. While drug absorption is generally unchanging with age, drug distribution may change because of decreased muscle mass with decreased water content and renal impairment. Additionally, co-morbidities and other medications may make the blood-brain barrier more permeable in elderly patients increasing the rate of central nervous system side effects [87]. There is significant concern for cognitive side effects with oxybutinin [92] in the elderly; concerns also exist for the additive antimuscarinic effect of medications used to treat Parkinson's disease or dementia. Relatively few cognitive side effects have been reported in older women participating in clinical trials with the other antimuscarinics [87]: darfenicin, transdermal oxybutynin, tolterodine [92], trospium [90] and solifenacin [93]. Close monitoring is needed when prescribing these medications to older women.

3.3. β-3 Agonists

The β-3 agonists, mirabegron [94] and solabegron [95], potential new therapies for OAB, are currently in Phase II placebo-controlled trials. These drugs stimulate the β-3 androreceptors, the predominate receptors of the detrusor muscle [96, 97], to improve relaxation during the storage phase of micturition [97]. In animal models, the bladder capacity is increased without the negative side effect of decreasing detrusor muscle contraction with micturition [98, 99]. The results of these early trials show mirabegron to be more effective than placebo in treating OAB [100, 101]. Headache and gastrointestinal adverse events including dry mouth were reported less frequently for individuals receiving mirabegron than with tolterodine extended-release while dizziness and palpatations were slightly higher. Although small statistically significant changes in blood pressure and heart rate were noted, there was no increase in cardiovascular adverse events in the short-term studies completed thus far. Long-term safety data is needed [94]. Specific modulation of this site may be a target for overactive bladder therapy without the common side effects of antimuscarinic medications.

4. Botulinum-A Toxin

Injection of botulinum toxin into the detrusor muscle was first used for the treatment of neurogenic detrusor overactivity in 2000 [102]. Botulinum toxin A (Botox, Allergan) has recently been approved by the FDA for the treatment of neurogenic OAB. Botulinum toxin(BoNT/A) is a potent neurotoxic protein produced by the bacterium *Clostridium botulinum*. The toxin binds to the presynaptic terminals of motor neurons and impedes the fusion of synaptic vesicles with the neuronal membrane [103]. This interruption in the neuronal transmission of the efferent and afferent branches of the micturition reflex inhibits detrusor contractions by blocking the release of achetylcholine and other neurotransmitters. BoNT/A may also decrease sensory input to the bladder by down-regulating the neurotransmitter receptors of afferent neurons in the detrusor muscle [104]. BoNT/A not only has a direct effect on detrusor motor innervation but also modulates intrinsic bladder reflexes through a multimodal effect on sensory pathways. Such mechanisms may contribute to the efficiency of this treatment and partly explain how it affects abnormal detrusor contractions more markedly than voluntary bladder emptying [105]. In clinical practice, a single standardized technique for botulinum injection has not been developed. In a commonly used technique, the toxin is delivered via multiple injections into the detrusor muscle of the bladder under cystoscopic guidance using local anesthesia, with sparing of the trigone. Injections may need to be repeated in 3-12 months to maintain efficacy. Risks with the procedure include gross hematuria (6-10%) [106], urinary tract infection (7-22%) [106], pain, and increased post-void residual or urinary return requiring de novo intermittent self-catheterization to range from 5-21% in idiopathic OAB patients [107]. Neurologic side effects have also been reported and range up to 10% but are usually transient [108]. Systemic side effects such as diffuse muscle weakness have also been reported but are rare (1%) [109] and usually resolve within a few months.

Doses of 100 to 200 units of BoNT/A for refractory idiopathic OAB have been shown in placebo controlled trials to improve UUI episodes, maximum cystometrogram capacity, maximum detrusor pressure and quality of life [110, 111]. Brubaker et al. [110] reported significant improvement in symptoms were in 60% of women with sustained clinical effects for almost 1 year, but the trial was halted early due to unexpectedly high rates of urinary retention and urinary tract infections. More recently, BoNT/A injections have been showed to be more successful in patients with anticholinergic intolerability as compared to patients with poor medication efficacy (86% vs. 60%, P = 0.02) [112].

A Cochrane Review [113] evaluating BoNT/A for both neurogenic and idiopathic overactive bladder concluded that although the drug can improve symptoms of OAB, too little data exist on safety and efficacy compared with placebo and other treatments. Experts recommend use of the drug in treatment of refractory symptoms in neurogenic and idiopathic detrusor overactivity [114] but recommend caution because of the risk of voiding difficulty and duration of effect have not yet been accurately evaluated [115]. A clear consensus on the use of the drug in clinical practice including optimal dose, location and number and timing of initial and repeat injections has not yet emerged. The use of BoNT/A for idiopathic OAB is off-label and should be restricted to patients who have failed conservative therapies [116, 117].

5. Estrogen

The prevalence of OAB in postmenopausal women is high likely due to the effect of loss of estrogen on uogential tissue including thinning of mucosa, loss of sphincter muscle tone, and alteration of the urethrovesical angle [118]. Although oral estrogen use for the treatment of OAB has not been shown to be effective, several studies have found that vaginal estrogen improves symptoms of urgency and frequency in postmenopausal women [119-122].

In a randomized controlled trial [123] comparing 12 weeks of ultralow-dose estradiol-releasing vaginal ring (Estring; Pfizer, New York, NY) to oral oxybutynin chloride 5 mg twice daily for treatment of OAB symptoms in postmenopausal women, both treatments had significant decreases in number of voids and improved quality of life but these improvements were not statistically significant between groups. While discontinuation rates were the same, significantly more women in vaginal ring group desired to continue with the same therapy compared to women in the oxybutynin group. While results with vaginal estrogen are promising for some OAB symptoms, it has not yet been shown to decrease UUI episodes [120, 124].

6. Neuromodulation

A newer area of investigation for treatment of OAB symptoms involves neuromodulation of the nerves supplying the detrusor muscle and the pelvic floor muscles. These options are used when a patient has failed behavioral and at least one pharmacologic interventions to correct her OAB symptoms.

6.1. Peripheral Nerve Stimulation

Percutaneous tibial nerve stimulation (PTNS) delivers neuromodulation to the pelvic floor through the S2-S4 junction of the sacral nerve plexus via the less invasive route of the posterior tibial nerve. The tibial nerve is accessed via a fine needle electrode inserted slightly above the ankle. This anatomical area, long recognized as the bladder center, has projections to the sacral nerve plexus, creating a feedback loop that modulates bladder innervations [125, 126]. PTNS has been shown to be more effective than placebo with significantly decreased symptom severity score and increased health-related quality of life score [127, 128]. Significant decreases in daytime and nighttime voids, urinary urgency, UUI, along with increased mean voided volume were also seen [127]. PTNS has been more effective than drug therapy for OAB and UUI [125, 129]. Most trials [125, 127, 129] report the effects of 12 weekly 30-minute intervention sessions and may allow those patients with symptom improvement to continue treatment at individually based greater intervals for sustained relief of OAB symptoms [125]. Schreiner et al. [128] reported that according to the efficacy of the urge incontinence treatment, of every two patients treated, one is aided by electrical stimulation of the tibial nerve. MacDiarmid et al. [130] reported that the significant overactive bladder symptom improvement achieved with 12 weekly PTNS treatments was maintained through 12 months. In addition to the short term benefits, the durability of response demonstrates the effectiveness of PTNS as a viable, long-term therapy for overactive bladder.

6.2. Sacral Neuromodulation

Sacral neuromodulation (InterStim® – Medtronic, Minneapolis, MN, Figure 2) was approved the FDA for the treatment of urgency urinary incontinence in 1997 and received approval for urgency-frequency syndrome in 1999. Sacral neuromodulation (SNM) involves chronic stimulation of the S3 sacral nerve root to affect the reflexes between the bladder, urethral sphincter, and pelvic floor muscles [131]. Chronic therapy requires that an electrode is placed via the sacral foramen alongside a sacral nerve (usually S3). In a second procedure the electrode is connected by cables under the skin to an implanted programmable pulse generator that provides stimulation within set stimulation parameters. Implantation of the pulse generator is usually carried out only after a successful trial of either a percutaneous (skin surface) nerve evaluation (PNE) or Stage I procedure [132].

SNM is indicated for patients who have refractory UUI or urinary urgency-frequency syndrome and who do not have anticipated future needs for magnetic resonance imaging [131] and have responded with at least a 50% improvement in target symptoms for at least 3 days during the testing phase [133]. Eighty percent of patients who received SNM became dry or showed improvement in the main incontinence symptoms [134]. After 3 years of follow-up, Siegel et al. [133] reported that 59% of patients reported 50% or greater reduction in incontinence episodes per day and 46% of patients were completely dry.

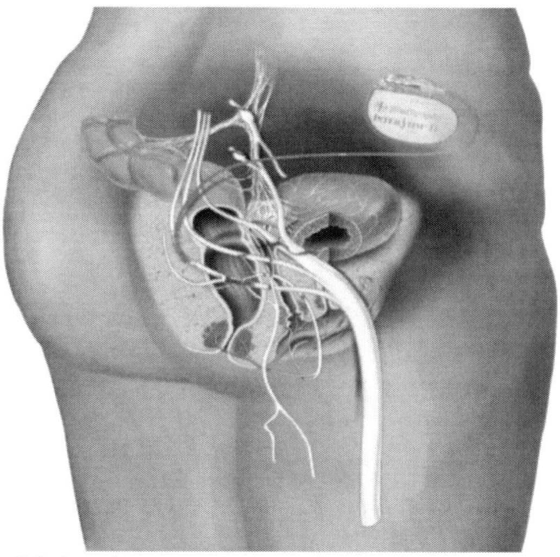

Used with permission from Medtronic.

Figure 2. Sacral Neuromodulation with InterStim®.

Heavy leaking episodes and the average number of pads replaced per day were also significantly decreased [133]. Similarly, a majority of patients with urgency-frequency also showed 50% or greater reduction in daily voids and improvement in the degree of urgency before voiding [133]. Amundsen et al. [135] assessed risk factors for SNM cure rates and reported that the cure rate inversely rated to age, having three or more chronic conditions and having a co-existent neurologic condition.

Common complications that have been reported with SNM include pain at the implant site (25%), lead migration (16%), wound problems (7%), adverse effect on bowel function (6%), infection (5%), and generator problems (5%). Overall, 33% of patients have required surgical revision of the SNM implant [134]. While significant success has been seen with SNM, many unanswered questions remain: the placement of the implant, unilateral versus bilateral leads, different methods of securing the leads, costs and benefits, and implant failure in some patients despite positive test phase results.

6.3. Magnetic Therapy

A more recent alternative to electrical stimulation of the pelvic floor muscles is extracoporeal magnetic innervation for the treatment of urinary incontinence [136]. Activation of sacral nerve roots by magnetic stimulation has been shown to acutely suppress uninhibited detrusor contractions [137-139]. Magnetic therapy is usually administered by either continuous or intermittent stimulation for 15 to 30 minutes in twice-weekly sessions for up to 8 weeks [137, 140, 141]. The stimulation can be administered either through an external magnet applied over the S3 sacral foramen or through a specialized chair using the Neocontrol system (Neotonus Inc., Marietta GA). Two randomized controlled trials [137, 141] including women with UUI and urge-predominant MUI compared magnetic stimulation to sham stimulation. Both these trials showed significant decreases in daily voids, mean leaks, and increased mean voided volume for the magnetic stimulation group without significant changes in the sham stimulation group.

7. Surgical Treatment

Surgical treatment for the management of OAB syndrome and UUI is very rare and is reserved for the most severe cases that have not responded to other more conservative options [30]. Beyond the PTNS, SNM and intravesical botulinum injections discussed above, other surgical options include augmentation cystoplasty, detrusor myectomy and urinary diversion [142]. Management of refractory OAB is very challenging and requires specialist expertise [142].

8. Cost-Effectiveness

Limited cost-effectiveness studies have been performed in the treatment of OAB and UUI with behavioral modifications or physiotherapy treatments [37, 143]. The costs of alleviating symptoms through PMFT or vaginal cone therapy were reported to be much higher compared with a simple nurse-led continence service [143].

Multiple investigators internationally have looked at the cost-effectiveness of various antimuscarinics in OAB treatment both in actual cost and quality-adjusted life years. Solifenacin has emerged as a more cost-effective therapy for OAB in the United States [144], Canada [145], the United Kingdom [146], Italy [147], and in four Nordic countries [148]. However, Arlandis-Guzman et al. [149] reported that in Spain, treatment with fesoterodine resulted in similar overall costs and greater quality-adjusted life year gain than treatment with either tolterodine or solifenacin. Finally, an older study [150] which did not include solifenacin, reported that in the UK, France and Austria, starting OAB treatment with oxybutynin controlled-release was a clinically more effective strategy and potentially the most cost-effective strategy when compared to immediate-release oxybutynin or tolterodine.

Padmanabhan et al. [151] compared the cost of BoNT/A to augmentation cystoplasty. BoNT/A was found to be cheaper over 5 years when the initial duration of benefit was greater than 5.1 months, and agumentation cystoplasty was cheaper when the cost of BoNT/A increased or the augmentation cystoplasty complication rate dropped below 14% [151]. One study [152] compared the cost-effectiveness of SNM to BoNT/A. SNM resulted in higher quality-adjusted life-year gain but at a higher cost than BoNT/A. SNM started to be cost-effective after 4 years and at 5 years was cost-effective compared to BoNT/A [152]. Arlandis et al. [153] also showed that in Spain, SNM was the more economical option at 10 years compared to BoNT/A and continued oral therapy.

Conclusion

While several non-pharmacologic and pharmacologic options for patients with OAB, most studies have evaluated short-term benefit only. Outcome measures have been highly variable across studies with relatively few studies including objective, subjective, and quality of life measures. The optimal placebo arm for non-pharmacologic trials has not been determined because blinding both the provider and the patient to treatment is difficult. Randomized controlled studies in which efficacy of different physiotherapy options are compared to each other as well as continuing long-term trials involving both behavioral modification and antimuscarinics are required to allow determination of optimal first line treatment methods for OAB and length of benefit after completing treatment course. Several new options for refractory OAB symptoms are showing initial promising results both in objective relief of symptoms and improved quality of life. Additionally, more cost-effectiveness and comparative-effectiveness data on these options are needed on non-pharmacologic OAB therapy to give clinicians and patients the best information possible.

References

[1] Haylen BT, de Ridder D, Freeman RM, Swift SE, Berghmans B, Lee J, et al. An International Urogynecological Association (IUGA)/ International Continence Society

(ICS) joint report on the terminology for female pelvic floor dysfunction. *Int. Urogynecol. J. Pelvic. Floor Dysfunct.* 2010 Jan; 21(1):5-26.

[2] Hu TW, Wagner TH, Bentkover JD, LeBlanc K, Piancentini A, Stewart WF, et al. Estimated economic costs of overactive bladder in the United States. *Urology* 2003 Jun; 61(6):1123-1128.

[3] Stewart WF, Van Rooyen JB, Cundiff GW, Abrams P, Herzog AR, Corey R, et al. Prevalence and burden of overactive bladder in the United States. *World J. Urol.* 2003 May; 20(6):327-336.

[4] Irwin DE, Milsom I, Chancellor MB, Kopp Z, Guan Z. Dynamic progression of overactive bladder and urinary incontinence symptoms: A systematic review. *Eur. Urol.* 2010 Jun 15.

[5] Chai TC, Steers WD. Neurophysiology of micturition and continence in women. *Int. Urogynecol. J. Pelvic Floor Dysfunct.* 1997; 8(2): 85-97.

[6] Andersson KE, Wein AJ. Pharmacology of the lower urinary tract: Basis for current and future treatments of urinary incontinence. *Pharmacol. Rev.* 2004 Dec; 56(4):581-631.

[7] Saks EK, Arya LA. Pharmacologic management of urinary incontinence, voiding dysfunction, and overactive bladder. *Obstet. Gynecol. Clin. North Am.* 2009 Sep; 36(3):493-507.

[8] Leng WW, Chancellor MB. How sacral nerve stimulation neuromodulation works. *Urol. Clin. North Am.* 2005 Feb; 32(1): 11-18.

[9] Andersson KE, Arner A. Urinary bladder contraction and relaxation: Physiology and pathophysiology. *Physiol. Rev.* 2004 Jul; 84(3): 935-986.

[10] Birder L, de Groat W, Mills I, Morrison J, Thor K, Drake M. Neural control of the lower urinary tract: Peripheral and spinal mechanisms. *Neurourol. Urodyn.* 2010; 29(1): 128-139.

[11] de Groat WC. Integrative control of the lower urinary tract: Preclinical perspective. *Br. J. Pharmacol.* 2006 Feb; 147 Suppl 2:S25-40.

[12] Junemann KP, Schmidt RA, Melchior H, Tanagho EA. Neuroanatomy and clinical significance of the external urethral sphincter. *Urol. Int.* 1987; 42(2):132-136.

[13] Fowler CJ, Griffiths D, de Groat WC. The neural control of micturition. *Nat. Rev. Neurosci.* 2008 Jun; 9(6):453-466.

[14] Weiss JM. Pelvic floor myofascial trigger points: Manual therapy for interstitial cystitis and the urgency-frequency syndrome. *J. Urol.* 2001 Dec; 166(6):2226-2231.

[15] Hains G, Hains F, Descarreaux M, Bussieres A. Urinary incontinence in women treated by ischemic compression over the bladder area: A pilot study. *J. Chiropr. Med.* 2007 Dec; 6(4):132-140.

[16] Eisenstein SM, Engelbrecht DJ, el Masry WS. Low back pain and urinary incontinence. A hypothetical relationship. *Spine* (Phila Pa 1976) 1994 May 15; 19(10):1148-1152.

[17] de Groat WC. A neurologic basis for the overactive bladder. *Urology* 1997 Dec; 50(6A Suppl):36-52; discussion 53-6.

[18] Schmidt RA, Jonas U, Oleson KA, Janknegt RA, Hassouna MM, Siegel SW, et al. Sacral nerve stimulation for treatment of refractory urinary urge incontinence. Sacral Nerve Stimulation Study Group. *J. Urol.* 1999 Aug; 162(2):352-357.

[19] Raz S, Smith RB. External sphincter spasticity syndrome in female patients. *J. Urol.* 1976 Apr; 115(4):443-446.

[20] Schmidt RA, Tanagho EA. Urethral syndrome or urinary tract infection? *Urology* 1981 Oct; 18(4):424-427.

[21] Kaplan WE, Firlit CF, Schoenberg HW. The female urethral syndrome: External sphincter spasm as etiology. *J. Urol.* 1980 Jul; 124(1):48-49.

[22] Gunnarsson M, Teleman P, Mattiasson A, Lidfeldt J, Nerbrand C, Samsioe G. Effects of pelvic floor exercises in middle aged women with a history of naive urinary incontinence: a population based study. *Eur. Urol.* 2002 May; 41(5):556-561.

[23] Finkelstein MM. Medical conditions, medications, and urinary incontinence. Analysis of a population-based survey. *Can. Fam. Physician* 2002 Jan; 48:96-101.

[24] Smith MD, Russell A, Hodges PW. Disorders of breathing and continence have a stronger association with back pain than obesity and physical activity. *Aust. J. Physiother.* 2006; 52(1):11-16.

[25] Wallace SA, Roe B, Williams K, Palmer M. Bladder training for urinary incontinence in adults. *Cochrane Database Syst. Rev.* 2004; (1)(1): CD001308.

[26] Subak LL, Whitcomb E, Shen H, Saxton J, Vittinghoff E, Brown JS. Weight loss: A novel and effective treatment for urinary incontinence. *J. Urol.*2005Jul; 174(1):190-195.

[27] Aslan E, Komurcu N, Beji NK, Yalcin O. Bladder training and Kegel exercises for women with urinary complaints living in a rest home. *Gerontology*2008;54(4):224-231.

[28] Wyman JF, Fantl JA, McClish DK, Bump RC. Comparative efficacy of behavioral interventions in the management of female urinary incontinence. Continence Program for Women Research Group. *Am. J. Obstet. Gynecol.* 1998 Oct; 179(4):999-1007.

[29] Fantl JA, Wyman JF, McClish DK, Harkins SW, Elswick RK, Taylor JR, et al. Efficacy of bladder training in older women with urinary incontinence. *JAMA* 1991 Feb 6; 265(5):609-613.

[30] Alhasso AA, McKinlay J, Patrick K, Stewart L. Anticholinergic drugs versus non-drug active therapies for overactive bladder syndrome in adults. *Cochrane Database Syst. Rev.* 2006 Oct 18; (4)(4):CD003193.

[31] Kegel AH. Progressive resistance exercise in the functional restoration of the perineal muscles. *Am. J. Obstet. Gynecol.* 1948 Aug; 56(2): 238-248.

[32] Vasconcelos M, Lima E, Caiafa L, Noronha A, Cangussu R, Gomes S, et al. Voiding dysfunction in children. Pelvic-floor exercises or biofeedback therapy: A randomized study. *Pediatr. Nephrol.* 2006 Dec; 21(12): 1858-1864.

[33] Godec C, Cass AS, Ayala GF. Bladder inhibition with functional electrical stimulation. *Urology* 1975 Dec; 6(6):663-666.

[34] Burgio KL, Locher JL, Goode PS, Hardin JM, McDowell BJ, Dombrowski M, et al. Behavioral vs drug treatment for urge urinary incontinence in older women: A randomized controlled trial. *JAMA* 1998 Dec 16; 280(23):1995-2000.

[35] Burgio KL, Goode PS, Locher JL, Umlauf MG, Roth DL, Richter HE, et al. Behavioral training with and without biofeedback in the treatment of urge incontinence in older women: A randomized controlled trial. *JAMA* 2002 Nov 13; 288(18):2293-2299.

[36] Borello-France D, Burgio KL, Goode PS, Markland AD, Kenton K, Balasubramanyam A, et al. Adherence to behavioral interventions for urge incontinence when combined with drug therapy: Adherence rates, barriers, and predictors. *Phys. Ther.* 2010 Jul 29.

[37] Dumoulin C, Hay-Smith J. Pelvic floor muscle training versus no treatment, or inactive control treatments, for urinary incontinence in women. *Cochrane Database Syst. Rev.* 2010 Jan 20; (1)(1):CD005654.

[38] Petros PE, Ulmsten UI. An integral theory of female urinary incontinence. Experimental and clinical considerations. *Acta Obstet. Gynecol. Scand. Suppl.* 1990; 153:7-31.

[39] de Groat WC, Fraser MO, Yoshiyama M, Smerin S, Tai C, Chancellor MB, et al. Neural control of the urethra. *Scand. J. Urol. Nephrol. Suppl.* 2001; (207)(207):35-43; discussion 106-25.

[40] Nygaard IE, Kreder KJ, Lepic MM, Fountain KA, Rhomberg AT. Efficacy of pelvic floor muscle exercises in women with stress, urge, and mixed urinary incontinence. *Am. J. Obstet. Gynecol.* 1996 Jan; 174(1 Pt 1): 120-125.

[41] Brubaker L, Benson JT, Bent A, Clark A, Shott S. Transvaginal electrical stimulation for female urinary incontinence. *Am. J. Obstet. Gynecol.* 1997 Sep; 177(3):536-540.

[42] Barroso JC, Ramos JG, Martins-Costa S, Sanches PR, Muller AF. Transvaginal electrical stimulation in the treatment of urinary incontinence. *BJU Int.* 2004 Feb; 93(3): 319-323.

[43] Siegel SW, Richardson DA, Miller KL, Karram MM, Blackwood NB, Sand PK, et al. Pelvic floor electrical stimulation for the treatment of urge and mixed urinary incontinence in women. *Urology* 1997 Dec; 50(6): 934-940.

[44] Amaro JL, Gameiro MO, Kawano PR, Padovani CR. Intravaginal electrical stimulation: A randomized, double-blind study on the treatment of mixed urinary incontinence. *Acta Obstet. Gynecol. Scand.* 2006; 85(5): 619-622.

[45] Wang AC, Wang YY, Chen MC. Single-blind, randomized trial of pelvic floor muscle training, biofeedback-assisted pelvic floor muscle training, and electrical stimulation in the management of overactive bladder. *Urology* 2004 Jan; 63(1):61-66.

[46] Lucas N, Macaskill P, Irwig L, Moran R, Bogduk N. Reliability of physical examination for diagnosis of myofascial trigger points: A systematic review of the literature. *Clin. J. Pain* 2009 Jan; 25(1):80-89.

[47] Arroyo-Morales M, Olea N, Martinez MM, Hidalgo-Lozano A, Ruiz-Rodriguez C, Diaz-Rodriguez L. Psychophysiological effects of massage-myofascial release after exercise: a randomized sham-control study. *J. Altern. Complement. Med.* 2008 Dec; 14(10): 1223-1229.

[48] Hadlock T, Lindsay R, Edwards C, Smitson C, Weinberg J, Knox C, et al. The effect of electrical and mechanical stimulation on the regenerating rodent facial nerve. *Laryngoscope* 2010 Jun; 120(6): 1094-1102.

[49] Manni L, Albanesi M, Guaragna M, Barbaro Paparo S, Aloe L. Neurotrophins and acupuncture. *Auton. Neurosci.* 2010 May 7.

[50] Weerapong P, Hume PA, Kolt GS. The mechanisms of massage and effects on performance, muscle recovery and injury prevention. *Sports Med.* 2005; 35(3): 235-256.

[51] Moyer CA, Rounds J, Hannum JW. A meta-analysis of massage therapy research. *Psychol. Bull.* 2004 Jan; 130(1):3-18.

[52] FitzGerald MP, Anderson RU, Potts J, Payne CK, Peters KM, Clemens JQ, et al. Randomized multicenter feasibility trial of myofascial physical therapy for the

treatment of urological chronic pelvic pain syndromes. *J. Urol.* 2009 Aug; 182(2): 570-580.

[53] Wein AJ. Diagnosis and treatment of the overactive bladder. *Urology* 2003 Nov; 62(5 Suppl 2):20-27.

[54] Abrams P, Andersson KE, Buccafusco JJ, Chapple C, de Groat WC, Fryer AD, et al. Muscarinic receptors: their distribution and function in body systems, and the implications for treating overactive bladder. *Br. J. Pharmacol.* 2006Jul; 148(5):565-578.

[55] Roxburgh C, Cook J, Dublin N. Anticholinergic drugs versus other medications for overactive bladder syndrome in adults. *Cochrane Database Syst. Rev.* 2007 Oct 17;(4)(4):CD003190.

[56] Meek PD, Evang SD, Tadrous M, Roux-Lirange D, Triller DM, Gumustop B. Overactive bladder drugs and constipation: a meta-analysis of randomized, placebo-controlled trials. *Dig. Dis. Sci.* 2011 Jan; 56(1): 7-18.

[57] Schiffers M, Sauermann P, Schurch B, Mehnert U. The effect of tolterodine 4 and 8 mg on the heart rate variability in healthy subjects. *World J. Urol.* 2010 Oct; 28(5):651-656.

[58] Gopal M, Haynes K, Bellamy SL, Arya LA. Discontinuation rates of anticholinergic medications used for the treatment of lower urinary tract symptoms. *Obstet. Gynecol.* 2008 Dec; 112(6):1311-1318.

[59] Anderson RU, Mobley D, Blank B, Saltzstein D, Susset J, Brown JS. Once daily controlled versus immediate release oxybutynin chloride for urge urinary incontinence. OROS Oxybutynin Study Group. *J. Urol.* 1999 Jun; 161(6):1809-1812.

[60] Andersson KE, Chapple CR. Oxybutynin and the overactive bladder. *World J. Urol.* 2001 Nov; 19(5):319-323.

[61] Hegde SS. Muscarinic receptors in the bladder: From basic research to therapeutics. *Br. J. Pharmacol.* 2006 Feb; 147 Suppl 2:S80-7.

[62] Zobrist RH, Quan D, Thomas HM, Stanworth S, Sanders SW. Pharmacokinetics and metabolism of transdermal oxybutynin: In vitro and in vivo performance of a novel delivery system. *Pharm. Res.* 2003 Jan; 20(1):103-109.

[63] Diokno AC, Appell RA, Sand PK, Dmochowski RR, Gburek BM, Klimberg IW, et al. Prospective, randomized, double-blind study of the efficacy and tolerability of the extended-release formulations of oxybutynin and tolterodine for overactive bladder: Results of the OPERA trial. *Mayo. Clin. Proc.* 2003 Jun;78(6):687-695.

[64] Dmochowski RR, Sand PK, Zinner NR, Gittelman MC, Davila GW, Sanders SW, et al. Comparative efficacy and safety of transdermal oxybutynin and oral tolterodine versus placebo in previously treated patients with urge and mixed urinary incontinence. *Urology* 2003 Aug; 62(2):237-242.

[65] Staskin DR, Dmochowski RR, Sand PK, Macdiarmid SA, Caramelli KE, Thomas H, et al. Efficacy and safety of oxybutynin chloride topical gel for overactive bladder: a randomized, double-blind, placebo controlled, multicenter study. *J. Urol.* 2009 Apr; 181(4):1764-1772.

[66] Diokno A, Ingber M. Oxybutynin in detrusor overactivity. *Urol. Clin. North Am.* 2006 Nov; 33(4):439-45, vii.

[67] van Kerrebroeck PE, van Voskuilen AC, Heesakkers JP, Lycklama a Nijholt AA, Siegel S, Jonas U, et al. Results of sacral neuromodulation therapy for urinary voiding

dysfunction: Outcomes of a prospective, worldwide clinical study. *J. Urol.* 2007 Nov;178(5):2029-2034.

[68] Cardozo L, Chapple CR, Toozs-Hobson P, Grosse-Freese M, Bulitta M, Lehmacher W, et al. Efficacy of trospium chloride in patients with detrusor instability: A placebo-controlled, randomized, double-blind, multicentre clinical trial. *BJU Int.* 2000 Apr; 85(6):659-664.

[69] Staskin DR, Rosenberg MT, Sand PK, Zinner NR, Dmochowski RR. Trospium chloride once-daily extended release is effective and well tolerated for the treatment of overactive bladder syndrome: An integrated analysis of two randomised, phase III trials. *Int. J. Clin. Pract.* 2009 Dec; 63(12): 1715-1723.

[70] Sand PK, Dmochowski RR, Zinner NR, Staskin DR, Appell RA. Trospium chloride extended release is effective and well tolerated in women with overactive bladder syndrome. *Int. Urogynecol. J. Pelvic. Floor Dysfunct.* 2009 Dec; 20(12):1431-1438.

[71] Dmochowski RR, Rosenberg MT, Zinner NR, Staskin DR, Sand PK. Extended-release trospium chloride improves quality of life in overactive bladder. *Value Health* 2010 Mar-Apr; 13(2):251-257.

[72] Staskin D, Kay G, Tannenbaum C, Goldman HB, Bhashi K, Ling J, et al. Trospium chloride has no effect on memory testing and is assay undetectable in the central nervous system of older patients with overactive bladder. *Int. J. Clin. Pract.* 2010 Aug; 64(9): 1294-1300.

[73] Staskin DR. Trospium chloride: distinct among other anticholinergic agents available for the treatment of overactive bladder. *Urol. Clin. North Am.* 2006 Nov; 33(4):465-73, viii.

[74] Cardozo L, Lisec M, Millard R, van Vierssen Trip O, Kuzmin I, Drogendijk TE, et al. Randomized, double-blind placebo controlled trial of the once daily antimuscarinic agent solifenacin succinate in patients with overactive bladder. *J. Urol.* 2004 Nov; 172 (5 Pt 1):1919-1924.

[75] Simpson D, Wagstaff AJ. Solifenacin in overactive bladder syndrome. *Drugs Aging* 2005;22(12):1061-1069.

[76] Ho CH, Chang TC, Lin HH, Liu SP, Huang KH, Yu HJ. Solifenacin and tolterodine are equally effective in the treatment of overactive bladder symptoms. *J. Formos. Med. Assoc.* 2010 Oct; 109(10):702-708.

[77] Chapple CR, Martinez-Garcia R, Selvaggi L, Toozs-Hobson P, Warnack W, Drogendijk T, et al. A comparison of the efficacy and tolerability of solifenacin succinate and extended release tolterodine at treating overactive bladder syndrome: Results of the STAR trial. *Eur. Urol.* 2005 Sep; 48(3):464-470.

[78] Haab F, Stewart L, Dwyer P. Darifenacin, an M3 selective receptor antagonist, is an effective and well-tolerated once-daily treatment for overactive bladder. *Eur. Urol.* 2004 Apr; 45(4):420-9; discussion 429.

[79] Zinner N. Darifenacin: a muscarinic M3-selective receptor antagonist for the treatment of overactive bladder. *Expert. Opin. Pharmacother.* 2007 Mar; 8(4):511-523.

[80] Chapple C, Van Kerrebroeck P, Tubaro A, Haag-Molkenteller C, Forst HT, Massow U, et al. Clinical efficacy, safety, and tolerability of once-daily fesoterodine in subjects with overactive bladder. *Eur. Urol.* 2007 Oct; 52(4):1204-1212.

[81] Nitti VW, Dmochowski R, Sand PK, Forst HT, Haag-Molkenteller C, Massow U, et al. Efficacy, safety and tolerability of fesoterodine for overactive bladder syndrome. *J. Urol.* 2007 Dec; 178(6):2488-2494.

[82] Goldman HB, Morrow JD, Gong J, Tseng LJ, Schneider T. Early onset of fesoterodine efficacy in subjects with overactive bladder. *BJU Int.* 2011 Feb; 107(4):598-602.

[83] Corcos J, Angulo JC, Garely AD, Carlsson M, Gong J, Guan Z, et al. Effect of fesoterodine 4 mg on bladder diary and patient-reported outcomes during the first week of treatment in subjects with overactive bladder. *Curr. Med. Res. Opin.* 2011 May; 27(5): 1059-1065.

[84] Kaplan SA, Schneider T, Foote JE, Guan Z, Carlsson M, Gong J. Superior efficacy of fesoterodine over tolterodine extended release with rapid onset: A prospective, head-to-head, placebo-controlled trial. *BJU Int.* 2011 May; 107(9):1432-1440.

[85] Herschorn S, Swift S, Guan Z, Carlsson M, Morrow JD, Brodsky M, et al. Comparison of fesoterodine and tolterodine extended release for the treatment of overactive bladder: A head-to-head placebo-controlled trial. *BJU Int.* 2010 Jan; 105(1):58-66.

[86] Scarpero H, Sand PK, Kelleher CJ, Berriman S, Bavendam T, Carlsson M. Long-term safety, tolerability, and efficacy of fesoterodine treatment in men and women with overactive bladder symptoms. *Curr. Med. Res. Opin.* 2011 May; 27(5):921-930.

[87] Pagoria D, O'Connor RC, Guralnick ML. Antimuscarinic drugs: review of the cognitive impact when used to treat overactive bladder in elderly patients. *Curr. Urol. Rep.* 2011 May 24.

[88] Paquette A, Gou P, Tannenbaum C. Systematic review and meta-analysis: do clinical trials testing antimuscarinic agents for overactive bladder adequately measure central nervous system adverse events? *J. Am. Geriatr. Soc.* 2011 Jul; 59(7):1332-1339.

[89] Zinner N, Noe L, Rasouliyan L, Marshall T, Runken MC, Seifeldin R. Impact of solifenacin on quality of life, medical care use, work productivity, and health utility in the elderly: an exploratory subgroup analysis. *Am. J. Geriatr. Pharmacother.* 2009 Dec; 7(6): 373-382.

[90] Sand PK, Johnson Ii TM, Rovner ES, Ellsworth PI, Oefelein MG, Staskin DR. Trospium chloride once-daily extended release is efficacious and tolerated in elderly subjects (aged >/= 75 years) with overactive bladder syndrome. *BJU Int.* 2011 Feb; 107(4): 612-620.

[91] Sand P, Zinner N, Newman D, Lucente V, Dmochowski R, Kelleher C, et al. Oxybutynin transdermal system improves the quality of life in adults with overactive bladder: a multicentre, community-based, randomized study. *BJU Int.* 2007 Apr; 99(4): 836-844.

[92] Kay G, Crook T, Rekeda L, Lima R, Ebinger U, Arguinzoniz M, et al. Differential effects of the antimuscarinic agents darifenacin and oxybutynin ER on memory in older subjects. *Eur. Urol.* 2006 Aug; 50(2): 317-326.

[93] Wagg A, Wyndaele JJ, Sieber P. Efficacy and tolerability of solifenacin in elderly subjects with overactive bladder syndrome: A pooled analysis. *Am. J. Geriatr. Pharmacother.* 2006 Mar; 4(1):14-24.

[94] Tyagi P, Tyagi V, Chancellor M. Mirabegron: a safety review. *Expert. Opin. Drug Saf.* 2011 Mar; 10(2):287-294.

[95] Hicks A, McCafferty GP, Riedel E, Aiyar N, Pullen M, Evans C, et al. GW427353 (solabegron), a novel, selective beta3-adrenergic receptor agonist, evokes bladder

relaxation and increases micturition reflex threshold in the dog. *J. Pharmacol. Exp. Ther.* 2007Oct; 323(1): 202-209.

[96] Drake MJ. Emerging drugs for treatment of overactive bladder and detrusor overactivity. *Expert. Opin. Emerg. Drugs* 2008 Sep; 13(3): 431-446.

[97] Tyagi P, Thomas CA, Yoshimura N, Chancellor MB. Investigations into the presence of functional Beta1, Beta2 and Beta3-adrenoceptors in urothelium and detrusor of human bladder. *Int. Braz. J. Urol.* 2009 Jan-Feb; 35(1):76-83.

[98] Takasu T, Ukai M, Sato S, Matsui T, Nagase I, Maruyama T, et al. Effect of (R)-2-(2-aminothiazol-4-yl)-4'-{2-[(2-hydroxy-2-phenylethyl) amino]ethyl} acetanilide (YM178), a novel selective beta3-adrenoceptor agonist, on bladder function. *J. Pharmacol. Exp. Ther.* 2007 May; 321(2): 642-647.

[99] Vij M, Robinson D, Cardozo L. Emerging drugs for treatment of urinary incontinence. *Expert. Opin. Emerg. Drugs* 2010 Jun; 15(2):299-308.

[100] Dose-ranging study of once-daily mirabegron (Ym178), A novel selective beta3-adrenoreceptor agonist, in patients with overactive bladder (OAB). European Urology Association *Annual Conference;* April 2010; Elsevier BV; 2010.

[101] Clinical proof of concept study(blossom) shows novel beta 3 adrenoceptor agonist YM178 is effective and well tolerated in the treatment of symptoms of overactive bladder (Abs 674). *European Urology Association Annual Conference*; 12 March 2008; Elservier BV; 2008.

[102] Schurch B, Stohrer M, Kramer G, Schmid DM, Gaul G, Hauri D. Botulinum-A toxin for treating detrusor hyperreflexia in spinal cord injured patients: A new alternative to anticholinergic drugs? Preliminary results. *J. Urol.* 2000 Sep; 164(3 Pt 1):692-697.

[103] Cruz F, Dinis P. Resiniferatoxin and botulinum toxin type A for treatment of lower urinary tract symptoms. *Neurourol. Urodyn.* 2007 Oct; 26(6 Suppl): 920-927.

[104] Karsenty G, Denys P, Amarenco G, De Seze M, Game X, Haab F, et al. Botulinum toxin A (Botox) intradetrusor injections in adults with neurogenic detrusor overactivity/neurogenic overactive bladder: A systematic literature review. *Eur. Urol.* 2008 Feb; 53(2):275-287.

[105] Vianello A, Proietti S, Giannantoni A. Effect of botulinum neurotoxin on the urinary bladder: novel insights on mechanism of action. *Minerva Urol. Nefrol.* 2010 Sep; 62(3):259-271.

[106] Kuo HC, Liao CH, Chung SD. Adverse events of intravesical botulinum toxin a injections for idiopathic detrusor overactivity: risk factors and influence on treatment outcome. *Eur. Urol.* 2010 Dec;58(6):919-926.

[107] Dmochowski R, Chapple C, Nitti VW, Chancellor M, Everaert K, Thompson C, et al. Efficacy and safety of botulinum toxin A for idiopathic overactive bladder: A double-blind, placebo controlled, randomized, dose ranging trial. *J. Urol.* 2010 Dec; 184(6): 2416-2422.

[108] Bauer RM, Gratzke C, Roosen A, Hocaoglu Y, Mayer ME, Buchner A, et al. Patient-reported side effects of intradetrusor botulinum toxin type A for idiopathic overactive bladder syndrome. *Urol. Int.* 2011 Feb; 86(1): 68-72.

[109] Dowson C, Khan MS, Dasgupta P, Sahai A. Repeat botulinum toxin-A injections for treatment of adult detrusor overactivity. *Nat. Rev. Urol.* 2010 Dec; 7(12):661-667.

[110] Brubaker L, Richter HE, Visco A, Mahajan S, Nygaard I, Braun TM, et al. Refractory idiopathic urge urinary incontinence and botulinum A injection. *J. Urol.* 2008 Jul; 180(1): 217-222.

[111] Sahai A, Khan MS, Dasgupta P. Efficacy of botulinum toxin-A for treating idiopathic detrusor overactivity: results from a single center, randomized, double-blind, placebo controlled trial. *J. Urol.* 2007 Jun; 177(6): 2231-2236.

[112] Makovey I, Davis T, Guralnick ML, O'Connor RC. Botulinum toxin outcomes for idiopathic overactive bladder stratified by indication: Lack of anticholinergic efficacy versus intolerability. *Neurourol. Urodyn.* 2011 Aug 8.

[113] Duthie J, Wilson DI, Herbison GP, Wilson D. Botulinum toxin injections for adults with overactive bladder syndrome. *Cochrane Database Syst. Rev.* 2007 Jul 18;(3)(3): CD005493.

[114] Apostolidis A, Dasgupta P, Denys P, Elneil S, Fowler CJ, Giannantoni A, et al. Recommendations on the use of botulinum toxin in the treatment of lower urinary tract disorders and pelvic floor dysfunctions: A European consensus report. *Eur. Urol.* 2009 Jan; 55(1):100-119.

[115] Giannantoni A, Mearini E, Del Zingaro M, Porena M. Six-year follow-up of botulinum toxin A intradetrusorial injections in patients with refractory neurogenic detrusor overactivity: clinical and urodynamic results. *Eur. Urol.* 2009 Mar;55(3):705-711.

[116] Carr LK. Botulinum toxin A should not be first-line therapy for overactive bladder. *Can. Urol. Assoc. J.* 2011 Jun; 5(3):204-205.

[117] Saks EK, Arya LA. Pharmacologic managment of overactive bladder. *The Female Patient* 2010 November 2010; 35(11):24-29.

[118] Schaffer J, Fantl JA. Urogenital effects of the menopause. *Baillieres Clin. Obstet. Gynaecol.* 1996 Sep;10(3):401-417.

[119] Lose G, Englev E. Oestradiol-releasing vaginal ring versus oestriol vaginal pessaries in the treatment of bothersome lower urinary tract symptoms. *BJOG* 2000 Aug; 107(8): 1029-1034.

[120] Cardozo LD, Wise BG, Benness CJ. Vaginal oestradiol for the treatment of lower urinary tract symptoms in postmenopausal women--a double-blind placebo-controlled study. *J. Obstet. Gynaecol.* 2001 Jul; 21(4): 383-385.

[121] Zullo MA, Plotti F, Calcagno M, Palaia I, Muzii L, Manci N, et al. Vaginal estrogen therapy and overactive bladder symptoms in postmenopausal patients after a tension-free vaginal tape procedure: a randomized clinical trial. *Menopause* 2005 Jul-Aug; 12(4): 421-427.

[122] Long CY, Liu CM, Hsu SC, Chen YH, Wu CH, Tsai EM. A randomized comparative study of the effects of oral and topical estrogen therapy on the lower urinary tract of hysterectomized postmenopausal women. *Fertil. Steril.* 2006 Jan; 85(1):155-160.

[123] Nelken RS, Ozel BZ, Leegant AR, Felix JC, Mishell DR,Jr. Randomized trial of estradiol vaginal ring versus oral oxybutynin for the treatment of overactive bladder. *Menopause* 2011 Sep; 18(9):962-966.

[124] Cardozo L, Lose G, McClish D, Versi E. A systematic review of the effects of estrogens for symptoms suggestive of overactive bladder. Acta *Obstet. Gynecol. Scand.* 2004 Oct; 83(10):892-897.

[125] Peters KM, Macdiarmid SA, Wooldridge LS, Leong FC, Shobeiri SA, Rovner ES, et al. Randomized trial of percutaneous tibial nerve stimulation versus extended-release

tolterodine: results from the overactive bladder innovative therapy trial. *J. Urol.* 2009 Sep; 182(3): 1055-1061.

[126] Kohli N, Rosenblatt PL. Neuromodulation techniques for the treatment of the overactive bladder. *Clin. Obstet. Gynecol.* 2002 Mar; 45(1): 218-232.

[127] Peters KM, Carrico DJ, Perez-Marrero RA, Khan AU, Wooldridge LS, Davis GL, et al. Randomized trial of percutaneous tibial nerve stimulation versus sham efficacy in the treatment of overactive bladder syndrome: results from the SUmiT trial. *J. Urol.* 2010 Apr; 183(4): 1438-1443.

[128] Schreiner L, dos Santos TG, Knorst MR, da Silva Filho IG. Randomized trial of transcutaneous tibial nerve stimulation to treat urge urinary incontinence in older women. *Int. Urogynecol. J. Pelvic Floor Dysfunct.* 2010 Sep; 21(9):1065-1070.

[129] Fall M, Lindstrom S. Transcutaneous electrical nerve stimulation in classic and nonulcer interstitial cystitis. *Urol. Clin. North Am.* 1994 Feb; 21(1):131-139.

[130] MacDiarmid SA, Peters KM, Shobeiri SA, Wooldridge LS, Rovner ES, Leong FC, et al. Long-term durability of percutaneous tibial nerve stimulation for the treatment of overactive bladder. *J. Urol.* 2010 Jan; 183(1): 234-240.

[131] Occhino JA, Siegel SW. Sacral nerve modulation in overactive bladder. *Curr. Urol. Rep.* 2010 Sep;11(5):348-352.

[132] Herbison GP, Arnold EP. Sacral neuromodulation with implanted devices for urinary storage and voiding dysfunction in adults. *Cochrane Database Syst. Rev.* 2009 Apr 15; (2)(2): CD004202.

[133] Siegel SW, Catanzaro F, Dijkema HE, Elhilali MM, Fowler CJ, Gajewski JB, et al. Long-term results of a multicenter study on sacral nerve stimulation for treatment of urinary urge incontinence, urgency-frequency, and retention. *Urology* 2000 Dec 4; 56(6 Suppl 1):87-91.

[134] Brazzelli M, Murray A, Fraser C. Efficacy and safety of sacral nerve stimulation for urinary urge incontinence: A systematic review. *J. Urol.* 2006 Mar; 175(3 Pt 1):835-841.

[135] Amundsen CL, Romero AA, Jamison MG, Webster GD. Sacral neuromodulation for intractable urge incontinence: are there factors associated with cure? *Urology* 2005 Oct; 66(4): 746-750.

[136] Yokoyama T, Fujita O, Nishiguchi J, Nozaki K, Nose H, Inoue M, et al. Extracorporeal magnetic innervation treatment for urinary incontinence. *Int. J. Urol.* 2004 Aug; 11(8): 602-606.

[137] Fujishiro T, Takahashi S, Enomoto H, Ugawa Y, Ueno S, Kitamura T. Magnetic stimulation of the sacral roots for the treatment of urinary frequency and urge incontinence: an investigational study and placebo controlled trial. *J. Urol.* 2002 Sep; 168(3): 1036-1039.

[138] Sheriff MK, Shah PJ, Fowler C, Mundy AR, Craggs MD. Neuromodulation of detrusor hyper-reflexia by functional magnetic stimulation of the sacral roots. *Br. J. Urol.* 1996 Jul; 78(1): 39-46.

[139] McFarlane JP, Foley SJ, de Winter P, Shah PJ, Craggs MD. Acute suppression of idiopathic detrusor instability with magnetic stimulation of the sacral nerve roots. *Br. J. Urol.* 1997 Nov; 80(5):734-741.

[140] Yamanishi T, Yasuda K, Suda S, Ishikawa N, Sakakibara R, Hattori T. Effect of functional continuous magnetic stimulation for urinary incontinence. *J. Urol.* 2000 Feb; 163(2): 456-459.

[141] But I, Faganelj M, Sostaric A. Functional magnetic stimulation for mixed urinary incontinence. *J. Urol.* 2005 May; 173(5):1644-1646.

[142] Wein A editor. Campbell-Walsh Urology, 10th. ed. Philadelphia, PA: Elsevier Saunders; 2011.

[143] Williams KS, Assassa RP, Gillies CL, Abrams KR, Turner DA, Shaw C, et al. A randomized controlled trial of the effectiveness of pelvic floor therapies for urodynamic stress and mixed incontinence. *BJU Int.* 2006 Nov;98(5):1043-1050.

[144] Ko Y, Malone DC, Armstrong EP. Pharmacoeconomic evaluation of antimuscarinic agents for the treatment of overactive bladder. *Pharmacotherapy* 2006 Dec; 26(12): 1694-1702.

[145] Herschorn S, Vicente C, Piwko C. Canadian cost-effectiveness analysis of solifenacin compared to oxybutynin immediate-release in patients with overactive bladder. *J. Med. Econ.* 2010; 13(3):508-515.

[146] Cardozo L, Thorpe A, Warner J, Sidhu M. The cost-effectiveness of solifenacin vs fesoterodine, oxybutynin immediate-release, propiverine, tolterodine extended-release and tolterodine immediate-release in the treatment of patients with overactive bladder in the UK National Health Service. *BJU Int.* 2010 Aug; 106(4):506-514.

[147] Pradelli L, Iannazzo S. Solifenacin in the treatment of overactive bladder syndrome in Italian patients: pharmacoeconomic evaluation. *J. Med. Econ.* 2009 Mar; 12(1):25-35.

[148] Milsom I, Axelsen S, Kulseng-Hansen S, Mattiasson A, Nilsson CG, Wickstrom J. Cost-effectiveness analysis of solifenacin flexible dosing in patients with overactive bladder symptoms in four Nordic countries. *Acta Obstet. Gynecol. Scand.* 2009; 88(6):693-699.

[149] Arlandis-Guzman S, Errando-Smet C, Trocio J, Arumi D, Rejas J. Cost-effectiveness analysis of antimuscarinics in the treatment of patients with overactive bladder in Spain: A decision-tree model. *BMC Urol.* 2011 May 20; 11:9.

[150] Guest JF, Abegunde D, Ruiz FJ. Cost Effectiveness of controlled-release oxybutynin compared with immediate-release oxybutynin and tolterodine in the treatment of overactive bladder in the UK, France and Austria. *Clin. Drug Investig* 2004; 24(6): 305-321.

[151] Padmanabhan P, Scarpero HM, Milam DF, Dmochowski RR, Penson DF. Five-year cost analysis of intra-detrusor injection of botulinum toxin type A and augmentation cystoplasty for refractory neurogenic detrusor overactivity. *World J. Urol.* 2011 Feb; 29(1): 51-57.

[152] Leong RK, de Wachter SG, Joore MA, van Kerrebroeck PE. Cost-effectiveness analysis of sacral neuromodulation and botulinum toxin A treatment for patients with idiopathic overactive bladder. *BJU Int.* 2011 Aug; 108(4):558-564.

[153] Arlandis S, Castro D, Errando C, Fernandez E, Jimenez M, Gonzalez P, et al. Cost-effectiveness of sacral neuromodulation compared to botulinum neurotoxin A or continued medical management in refractory overactive bladder. *Value Health* 2011 Mar-Apr; 14(2):219-228.

Conflict-of-Interest: None

Disclosures: None

Disclaimers: Joy A. Greer, MD, LCDR, MC, USN - LCDR Greer is a military service member. This work was prepared as part of her official duties. Title 17, USC, ¶105 provides that 'Copyright protection under this title is not available for any work of the United States Government.' Title 17, USC, ¶ 101 defines a U.S. Government work as a work prepared by a military service member or employee of the U.S. Government as part of that person's official duties. The views expressed in this article are those of the authors and do not necessarily reflect the official policy or position of the Department of the Navy, Department of Defense, nor the U.S. Government.

In: Urinary Incontinence
Editor: Eric Chung

ISBN: 978-1-62618-482-4

Chapter 12

Suburethral Sling Surgery for Management of Female Stress Urinary Incontinence

Cristina Jácome, Daniela Oliveira and Alda Marques
School of Health Sciences, University of Aveiro (ESSUA), Aveiro, Portugal

Abstract

Urinary incontinence (UI), defined as an involuntary loss of urine, can be divided into three types: stress, urge and mixed UI. Stress UI (SUI) is the most prevalent, affecting one third of adult women worldwide. Conservative therapies are the first option to manage SUI, however, when these techniques are ineffective, surgery is indicated. Several surgical procedures have been reported in the literature to treat SUI, however the suburethral slings have been recently described. Suburethral slings for female SUI can be classified according to the materials used, i.e., as biological, where autologous fascial sling is included, or synthetic, where retropubic, transobturator and mini-slings are commonly used. This book chapter aims to describe these suburethral sling procedures and review the literature about its efficacy and safety in the management of female SUI.

1. Introduction

Urinary incontinence is defined as an involuntary loss of urine [1]. This condition affects a significant number of women across different age groups and its prevalence varies between 25%-45% in young and adult women [2, 3] and 75% in elderly women [4]. Urinary incontinence (UI) may be further defined according to the patient's symptoms in stress, urge and mixed UI [1]. Stress UI (SUI), which is the most common type, is the complaint of involuntary loss of urine when intra-abdominal pressure is raised (e.g., sport activities, coughing or sneezing) [5]. It occurs at least weekly in one third of adult women worldwide

[6] and its prevalence is likely to increase due to the continuing rise of risk factors associated to it, such as age or obesity [7].

According to the international recommendations, SUI can be treated with conservative methods, such as lifestyle interventions and physical, behavioral and pharmacological therapies, or with surgical techniques [8, 9]. Surgical management aims to restore the woman's lower urinary tract function as closely as possible to normal [10]. In some cases this technique is more likely to treat SUI than conservative methods [6, 11]. The conservative methods are recommended as a first-line management for SUI however, when these interventions fail, surgical techniques, which have shown to be effective in the treatment of this condition, should be considered [10, 11].

There are two main groups of surgical techniques for SUI: the urethral/bladder neck-stabilizing procedures and the urethral sphincter augmentation [12]. The first group includes vaginal wall suspension, needle and suprapubic procedures, laparoscopic, suburethral retropubic space slings and suburethral obturator foramen procedures; the second group includes intramural urethral injectables, bulking agents, extra-urethral retropubic and circumferential variable resistance devices [12].

In the past, surgical procedures for SUI management, have been used to support and/or compress the bladder neck and return it to a more 'anatomical position' (e.g., needle procedures and laparoscopic), thus preventing motion and providing a 'backboard' for pressure transmission and compression [13]. However, a greater understanding of the pathogenesis of SUI through the integral theory led to a turnover on surgical procedures [14]. This theory suggests that continence depends on urethral closure related to an interplay of the pubourethral ligaments, a suburethral vaginal hammock and the pubococcygeus muscles [14]. Thus, integral theory was the basis for the introduction of suburethral sling techniques in the surgery management, which main aim is to give additional support at the mid-urethra, restoring continence [15, 16].

In the last decade, different types of suburethral slings were developed and are generally classified as biological or synthetic, based on the material used [17]. Mainly due to the progress of these sling procedures and the improvement of the surgical techniques, suburethral slings are currently considered the first surgical approach for SUI management [10]. Given its importance, suburethral slings will therefore be discussed in detail in this chapter.

2. Suburethral Sling Surgery for SUI

Since the beginning of the 20th century, suburethral sling procedures have been developed for the treatment of female SUI [18]. The first description of this surgical technique, using graccilis muscle around the urethra, was in 1907 by Von Giordano, however it only gained increased clinical use in 1978 with McGuire and Lytton [19]. In sling surgery, strips of material surrounding the urethra and connecting to the rectus muscle or to the ileopectineal ligaments are applied, resulting in a tightening of the sling and increasing the bladder support [17].

The materials that have been used for encircle the urethra can be either biological or synthetic [17]. Biological suburethral slings may be prepared from patient's fascial tissue, human donor tissue or animal tissue [20]. Autologous fascial sling is the most common and established biological sling option for SUI [20]. Synthetic suburethral sling include materials such as Teflon, Mersilene tape, lyodura, polytetrafluoroethylene, Marlex mesh and silastic [17]. In the literature, there are several types of synthetic slings, however the tension-free vaginal tape (TVT) and transobturator vaginal tape result in more effective outcomes [7]. More recently, mini-slings procedures, an innovated sling surgery option to treat SUI, have been developed [21].

2.1. Autologous Fascial Sling

According to the European Association of Urology (2010), autologous fascial sling is recommended as an effective long-lasting treatment for SUI (grade of recommendation A for surgical treatment [8]), contributing to high cure rates of this type of UI [22].

Autologous slings have been developed from human tissue, specifically from abdominal rectus or tensor fascia lata, contributing for a significantly decreased risk of rejection when compared to synthetic slings [23]. A harvested strip of this material is placed transvaginally at the proximal urethra level and then is secured superiorly to the abdominal rectus muscle with permanent sutures [22].

A research study (2006) comparing short-term results of pubovaginal autologous sling and transobturator sling in 20 women average age 52.5±11.8 years old, concluded that transobturator technique was less effective for treating female SUI than autologous pubovaginal sling [24]. Another study (2005), aiming to compared TVT with an autologous rectus fascial sling, verified that 12 months after surgery the cure rate of the autologous sling procedure was significantly higher than the TVT (92.8% versus 87.0%, respectively) [25]. Therefore, autologous sling procedures have been reported to be effective in the literature. Furthermore this procedure is not associated with significant morbidity (including low risk of erosion and infection), the long-term complication rate is low and it is related with high patient satisfaction [26]. However, a recent research study (2011) aiming to evaluate the efficacy of the autologous fascia rectus sling in treating female SUI, verified that 29.2% of women experienced complications related with this surgery such as postoperative urgency [19]. Other side effects associated with autologous sling have been described in the literature, such as permanent urinary retention, urinary tract infections and voiding dysfunctions [22, 27]. Hence, to overcome these complications, a less invasive technique with synthetic material has been developed. However, more evidence is needed to compare the effectiveness of these two types of slings [17].

2.2. Synthetic Suburethral Slings

A number of advantages are documented in using synthetic sling materials. Firstly, the use of synthetic slings minimize the morbidity and the time-consuming associated with autologous slings [28]. Synthetic materials maintain their strength over time, are durable and readily available in any required size [18, 28]. Another relevant characteristic is that synthetic materials are associated with minimal risk of causing a body inflammatory response and erosion [18, 28].

Synthetic materials can be classified into four types: i) macroporous, monofilament, with pore size greater than 75 μm; ii) microporous with pore size less than 10 μm; iii) macroporous, with multifilamentous or microporous components and iv) submicron pore size [10]. The macroporous monofilament is relatively resistant to infection and inflammation and therefore, is currently used in SUI standard care [29].

In the mid-1990s, Ulmsten and Petros developed the first polypropylene mid-urethra tension-free sling, the TVT [30]. There are currently three main types of synthetic sling procedures, including the retropubic synthetic sling, the transobturator synthetic sling and the single-incision synthetic sling.

2.2.1. Retropubic Synthetic Sling

Retropubic approach involves the insertion of two needles blindly through the retropubic space from the vagina to the abdomen (bottom-to-top route) [30] or from the abdomen to the vagina (top-to-bottom route) [31]. Nevertheless, most data regarding the retropubic approach relate to a bottom-up approach, namely, the TVT. In this procedure, the sling is placed at the level of the mid-urethra to reinforce the pubourethral ligaments and allows fixation of the urethra to the pubic bone (Figure 4).

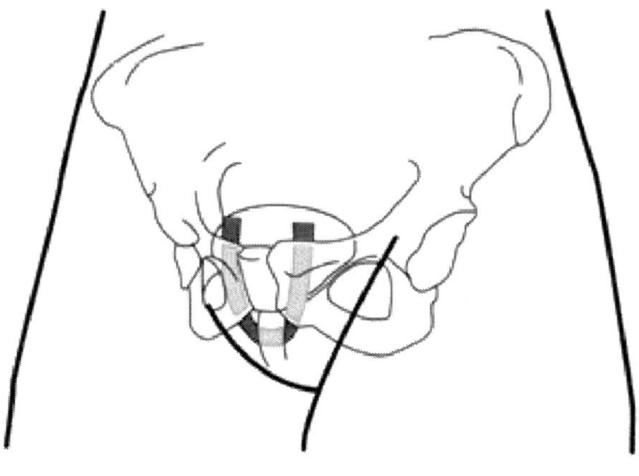

Figure 4. The tension-free vaginal tape (TVT) surgery.

Most studies have shown that the TVT procedure is effective, presenting cure rates between 81% and 93% at up to 5 years of follow-up [32-34]. In a three-center prospective observational cohort study, Nilsson et al. (2008), evaluated the long term effectiveness and safety of the TVT. After a follow-up of 11 years, they reported 90% objective cure rate and 77% subjective cure rate [35], verifying that TVT maintain its efficacy over time.

Tension-free vaginal tape has been compared with others surgical methods and no significant differences have been found. Tension-free vaginal tape was compared with autologous rectus fascia sling and demonstrated similar outcomes and complication rates. However, as autologous fascial sling is a more complex surgery, resulted in a longer operative time and longer hospital stay [32, 36]. A prospective randomized trial (2008) aiming to compare the long-term efficacy of laparoscopic Burch colposuspension with TVT for the treatment of SUI, found after a follow-up of 4–8 years, success rates of 43% and 52%, respectively [37]. Furthermore, in a study by Bai et al. (2005), after a follow-up of 12 months, the TVT had similar efficacy to laparoscopic Burch (87.4% vs. 87%) [25].

Due to the long-term high cure rate and simplicity, TVT is recommended as a treatment option for SUI if conservative management has failed (grade of recommendation A) [8, 10]. Tension-free vaginal tape is one of the most common surgical treatment for SUI and it is estimated that more than 1 million cases have been performed worldwide [38]. Although cure rates are excellent with the TVT, complications associated with the blind passage of needles through the retropubic space have been reported. The most common complications documented were bladder perforation, pelvic haematoma and storage lower urinary tract symptoms [15, 39]. To overcome some of these complications, transobturator approach has been developed.

2.2.2. Transobturator Synthetic Sling

Transobturator synthetic sling preserves the same principles of mid-urethral, tension-free placement of a synthetic sling material, maintaining the mid-urethral support. Transobturator approach involves trocar passage between the vaginal incision, through the obturator membrane and obturator internus muscle to a groin incision below the adductor muscle insertion (Figure 5). It can be applied using two techniques, outside-in and inside-out [40, 41].

The outside-in technique was developed by Delorme et al. (2003) to avoid the blind passage of trocars through the retropubic space and therefore, minimize complications seen with earlier retropubic procedures for SUI [40]. In this surgical procedure, the sling passes beneath the urethra and out through the obturator foramen (an oval opening in the pelvis surrounded by the bodies and rami of the pubis and ischium) to the skin surface [40]. Despite the outside-in being a safe technique, some adverse events were identified, namely urethra and bladder injuries [42, 43]. Therefore, de-Leval (2003) described the inside-out technique, where the needle is passed in a reverse route, i.e., is inserted from the vaginal incision and goes out through the obturator foramen [41]. Lee et al. (2008), in a prospective study, compared the efficacy and safety of inside–out and outside–in transobturator procedures. After a minimum follow-up of 12 months, similar cure rates (86% vs. 92%, respectively) were found [44]. A systematic review confirmed these data and showed that inside–out transobturator procedures was related to less complications, such as bladder injuries and voiding difficulties [45]. Both transobturator sling techniques have been shown to be effective procedures for SUI, with cure rates between 85% and 92% [44, 46-49].

The theory behind the introduction of transobturator route was related to being a safer procedure than TVT, with less risk of complications. According to a meta-analysis published in 2008, transobturator approach compared to retropubic, is associated with fewer bladder perforations, pelvic haematoma and storage lower urinary tract symptoms [39]. Two recent meta-analyses showed that retropubic technique has higher objective cure rates than transobturator [13, 50]. Despite transobturator approach being associated with less voiding dysfunction, blood loss and bladder perforation than TVT (0.3% versus 5.5%, RR 0.14, 95% CI 0.07 to 0.26), groin pain was significantly higher in the transobturator approach [13, 50].

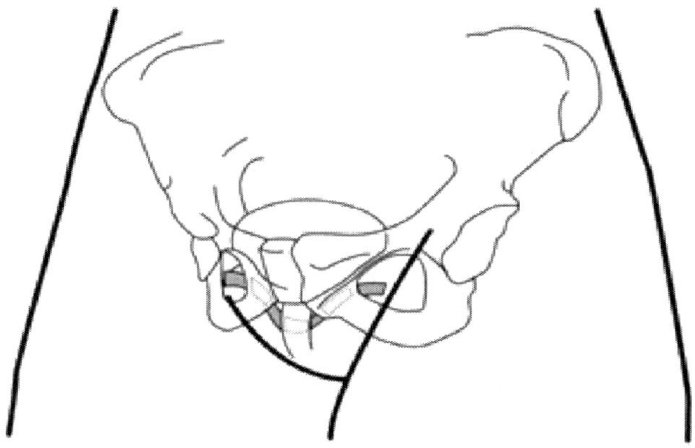

Figure 5. Transobturator synthetic sling surgery.

2.2.3. Single-Incision Mini-Slings

In 2006, single-incision mini-slings were introduced for the treatment of female SUI, with the concept of using a small piece of polypropylene mesh that could be introduced via a single vaginal incision [51]. The main aim of this less invasive technique was to offer similar efficacy as mid-urethral slings with reduced morbidity [51]. Since these surgical procedures do not have any exit incisions and avoid both blind retropubic and groin muscle trajectories, the risk of vascular or visceral injury is minimized [52-54]. These slings have the potential to be used in a true outpatient setting (using local anesthetic without sedation) [51]. A number of single-incision mini-slings are currently used in clinical practice, being the TVT-Secur (Ethicon, Edinburgh, UK) [55] and the MiniArc (American Medical Systems, Minnetonka, MN, USA) [56], the most widely used.

2.2.3.1. TVT-Secur

The TVT-Secur device consists of a polypropylene tape (the same as used with TVT and transobturator) of 8 cm long and 1 cm wide, coated at both ends with an absorbable fleece material composed of Vicryl, Polyglactin 910, and Poly-p-dioxanon to provide fixation [57]. The TVT-Secur is placed via one single incision at the level of the anterior vaginal wall and no needles are required to pass through the abdomen or groin [51, 57]. However, there is a metal blade/trocar attached to the ends of the mesh to pass it into either the obturator fascia and muscle or the retropubic space [51]. This device can potentially be implanted under local anesthesia as it is a less-invasive technique, using minimal vaginal dissection as well as avoidance of retropubic space and obturator foramen [58]. There have been several studies using the TVT-Secur sling, reporting objective cure rates of 87.5%, 88.6% and 89.5% at 6, 12, and 24 months follow-up respectively [53]; of 81% with a mean follow-up of 15±3 months [59] and of 76% at 24 months follow-up [60]. In a prospective study, Cornu and Haab (2011) have also showed a cure rate of 93.5% at short-term evaluation and of 40% at the last follow-up (30.2±9.8 months) [60].

The TVT-Secur sling can either be fixed in a U-shaped position into the connective tissue of the urogenital diaphragm or in a hammock position into the obturator internus muscle [16, 53, 61]. Nevertheless, recent evidence suggests that U-shaped position appears to be safer and more effective than the hammock position in the treatment of SUI [58, 61, 62].

A number of randomized control trials have been published comparing the efficacy of TVT-Secur with mid-urethral slings in the treatment of SUI. Andrada Hamer et al. (2011), in a prospective randomized multicenter study, found that subjective cure rate was significantly lower in a group of patients treated with TVT-Secur (72%) than a group of patients treated with TVT (92%) [63]. Tommaselli et al. (2010), compared the transobturator sling with the TVT-Secur and no differences in terms of cure rate at 12 months follow-up were found (81.6% vs. 83.8%, respectively) [64]. In another randomized control study with a larger sample (2011), the objective cure rate of the TVT-Secur was significantly lower (83.6%) than the transobturator sling (97.6%) [65]. Wang et al. (2011), aimed to compare efficacy of TVT, transobturator sling and TVT-Secur and observed that cure rates were similar between the TVT (93.8%) and the transobturator sling (91.7%) groups, but were significantly lower in the TVT-Secur (67.6%) [66]. Regarding safety of the TVT-Secur, none of these described randomized control trials showed a decreased in adverse events with the TVT-Secur, as it could be expected from this less invasive technique. Therefore, the lower success rates of TVT-Secur when compared with mid-urethral slings may be due to a potential long learning curve effect, i.e., improvement in surgical outcomes with increasing surgeon experience, reported in a number of studies [21, 58, 60, 61, 65].

2.2.3.2. MiniArc

The MiniArc involves a minimally invasive procedure similar to the TVT-Secur. The MiniArc sling kit comprises a 8.5 cm monofilament macroporous polypropylene mesh with small, integrated polypropylene self-fixating tips, a curved needle that fits into the self-fixating tip for placement of the sling [56]. The surgical procedure with MiniArc uses a single-incision approach and self-fixating anchoring tips in the obturator internus muscle and membrane [67]. The polypropylene mesh tape is placed in a similar position to the transobturator sling (hammock position) without the passage of needles through the groin, obturator space or medial adductor muscles [54, 56]. The procedure can be completed under local, monitored anesthesia or general anesthesia [56].

Observational studies about MiniArc in the treatment of SUI have shown cure rates between 77.8 and 91.4% at 12 months [54, 56, 68]. In a prospective observational study, Pickens et al. (2011) reported 12-months outcomes for 120 women who had undergone surgical intervention with the MiniArc [69]. In this study, 113 patients (94%) were "cured" at 1 month after surgery and 101 (93.5%) one year after. The adverse events included bladder perforations in 3 patients and postoperative urinary retention in 2 patients [69]. Ridder et al. (2010), in a retrospective cohort study, aiming to compare MiniArc sling with the transobturator sling, found that 91% of the patients had a negative cough test 6 weeks after surgery with both procedures [67]. At 1 year follow-up, 89% of the patients treated with transobturator sling and 85% treated with MiniArc maintained a negative cough test, which suggest that MiniArc sling and the transobturator sling were equally effective in the treatment of SUI. MiniArc procedure is rarely associated with intraoperative complications, nevertheless, vaginal wall perforation, bleeding and bladder perforation have been reported [54, 67, 68]. Postoperative adverse events included urinary retention, de novo urge, groin pain, urinary tract infection, constipation, vaginal infection and dyspareunia [54, 67, 68].

Initial Level 1 evidence for MiniArc comes from the Basu and Duckett trial (2010), which have conducted a prospective randomized control trial comparing MiniArc with TVT in the treatment of SUI [70]. The results from this trial showed that MiniArc was associated with a significantly higher failure rate compared with TVT at 6 weeks and 6 months. The complication rate was low and similar in the two procedures. Oliveira et al., (2011) in a study with 90 patients treated randomly with transobturator sling, TVT-Secur or Mini-Arc, found a cure rate of 83% after transobturator sling, 67% after TVT-Secur and 87% after Mini-Arc [71]. In this study, the pain score was lower after Mini-Arc and more complications occurred after the transobturator sling. The evidence about the use of MiniArc showed that this single-incision sling is safe and short-term effective to treat female SUI.

Although single-incision mini-slings may offer success rates for SUI associated with low morbidity, more studies are needed to show that these procedures are equivalent to conventional suburethral sling procedures [16, 51].

Conclusion

Stress UI is a condition experienced by a significant number of women at all ages that can be managed through surgical procedures. Suburethral sling surgery is currently the first option for UI surgery mainly because is associated with low patient morbidity, provides durable cure and it is easy to perform [10, 11].

During the past decade, suburethral sling surgery has had a significant evolution in terms of the technique of sling placement and also in the materials used. The materials used can be biological or synthetic. The most common type of biological sling is the autologous that may be made from the patient's own fascial tissue, namely abdominal rectus or tensor fascia lata [20]. Several studies reported that autologous sling is an effective and safe surgery with improved rates of continence in short and long-term [24-26]. However, recently it was found that postoperative complications, namely urgency, may be associated with this type of sling [19, 22, 27]. To minimize the complications associated with biological suburethral slings, synthetic materials emerged [18, 28]. There are several types of synthetic slings, however the most common are the retropubic synthetic sling, the obturator synthetic sling and the single-incision synthetic sling. Retropubic synthetic sling, namely TVT, is associated with high cure rates of SUI over time [32-35], nevertheless obturator synthetic sling was related to less side effects [45]. Single-incision mini-slings are a less invasive procedure, theoretically with fewer complications than retropubic and transobturator slings, however, studies about these type of procedures are still scarce.

The current evidence suggests that suburethral sling procedures are effective and safe, nevertheless, prospective randomized comparative studies of the various types of slings with standard techniques and with long-term follow-ups are needed to draw definite recommendations about its use in the management of female SUI.

Acknowledgments

The authors would like to acknowledge Lígia Pinto for the illustrations that accompanied this chapter.

References

[1] Abrams P, Andersson KE, Birder L, Brubaker L, Cardozo L, Chapple C, et al. Fourth international consultation on incontinence recommendations of the international scientific committee: Evaluation and treatment of urinary incontinence, pelvic organ prolapse, and fecal incontinence. *Neurourology and Urodynamics.* 2010;29(1):213-40.

[2] Carls C. The prevalence of stress urinary incontinence in high school and college-age female athletes in the midwest: implications for education and prevention. *Urologic Nursing.* 2007; 27(1):21-4,39.

[3] Buckley BS, Lapitan MCM. Prevalence of Urinary Incontinence in Men, Women, and Children-Current Evidence: Findings of the Fourth International Consultation on Incontinence. *Urology.* 2010;76(2):265-70.

[4] Boyington JEA, Howard DL, Carter-Edwards L, Gooden KM, Erdem N, Jallah Y, et al. Differences in Resident Characteristics and Prevalence of Urinary Incontinence in Nursing Homes in the Southeastern United States. *Nursing Research.* 2007;56(2):97-107.

[5] Haylen B, de Ridder D, Freeman R, Swift S, Berghmans B, Lee J, et al. An International Urogynecological Association (IUGA)/International Continence Society (ICS) joint report on the terminology for female pelvic floor dysfunction. *International Urogynecology Journal.* 2010;21(1):5-26.

[6] Nygaard IE, Heit M. Stress Urinary Incontinence. *The American College of Obstetricians and Gynecologists.* 2004;104(3):607-20.

[7] Firouz D. Surgical Treatment of Female Stress Urinary Incontinence, Decades Learned Lessons. *European Urology.* 2010;58(2):239-41.

[8] Schröder A, Abrams P, Andersson K-E, Artibani W, Chapple CR, Drake MJ, et al. *Guidelines on Urinary Incontinence;* 2010.

[9] Scottish Intercollegiate Guidelines Network. Management of urinary incontinence in primary care - *A national clinical guideline;* 2004. Available from: http://www.sign.ac.uk/guidelines/fulltext/79/index.html.

[10] National Collaborating Centre for Women's and Children's Health. Urinary incontinence: the management of urinary incontinence in women. London: *Royal College of Obstetricians and Gynaecologists Press;* 2006. Available from: http://www.nice.org.uk/nicemedia/live /10996/30281/30281.pdf.

[11] Holroyd-Leduc JM, Straus SE. Management of Urinary Incontinence in Women. *JAMA: The Journal of the American Medical Association.* 2004;291(8):986-95.

[12] Abrams P, Hilton P, Lucas M, Smith T. A proposal for a new classification for operative procedures for stress urinary incontinence. *BJU International.* 2005;96(3):232-3.

[13] Ogah J, Cody J, Rogerson L. Minimally invasive synthetic suburethral sling operations for stress urinary incontinence in women. *Cochrane Database of Systematic Reviews.* 2009;7(4).

[14] Petros P, Ulmsten U. An integral theory of female urinary incontinence. Experimental and clinical considerations. *Acta Obstetricia Et Gynecologica Scandinavica Supplement.* 1990;153:7-31.

[15] Bullock TL, Ghoniem G, Klutke CG, Staskin DR. Advances in female stress urinary incontinence: mid-urethral slings. *BJU International.* 2006;98:32-40.

[16] Fong EDM, Nitti VW. Review article: Mid-urethral synthetic slings for female stress urinary incontinence. *BJU International.* 2010;106(5):596-608.

[17] Bezerra C, Bruschini H, Cody J. Traditional suburethral sling operations for urinary incontinence in women. *Cochrane Database of Systematic Reviews.* 2005(3).

[18] Bukkapatnam R, Rodríguez LV. Synthetic Sling Options for Stress Urinary Incontinence. *Current Urology Reports.* 2004;5(5):374-80.

[19] Athanasopoulos A, Gyftopoulos K, McGuire EJ. Efficacy and Preoperative Prognostic Factors of Autologous Fascia Rectus Sling for Treatment of Female Stress Urinary Incontinence. *Urology.* 2011;78(5):1034-8.

[20] National Institute for Health and Clinical Excellence. Insertion of biological slings for stress urinary incontinence in women. London: National Institute for Health and Clinical Excellence; 2006. Available from: www.nice.org.uk/IPG154distributionlist.

[21] Cornu J-N, Haab F. Mini-slings for Female Stress Urinary Incontinence: Not Yet at the Age of Reason. *European Urology.* 2011;60(3):481-2.

[22] Albo ME, Richter HE, Brubaker L, Norton P, Kraus SR, Zimmern PE, et al. Burch Colposuspension versus Fascial Sling to Reduce Urinary Stress Incontinence. *New England Journal of Medicine.* 2007;356(21):2143-55.

[23] McBride AW, Ellerkmann RM, Bent AE, Melick CF. Comparison of long-term outcomes of autologous fascia lata slings with Suspend Tutoplast fascia lata allograft slings for stress incontinence. American *Journal of Obstetrics and Gynecology.* 2005;192(5):1677-81.

[24] Silva-Filho A, Cândido E, Noronha A, Triginelli S. Comparative study of autologous pubovaginal sling and synthetic transobturator (TOT) SAFYRE sling in the treatment of stress urinary incontinence. *Archives of Gynecology and Obstetrics.* 2006;273(5):288-92.

[25] Bai SW, Sohn WH, Chung DJ, Park JH, Kim SK. Comparison of the efficacy of Burch colposuspension, pubovaginal sling, and tension-free vaginal tape for stress urinary incontinence. *International journal of gynaecology and obstetrics: the official organ of the International Federation of Gynaecology and Obstetrics.* 2005;91(3):246-51.

[26] Latini JM, Lux MM, Kreder KJ. Efficacy and Morbidity of Autologous Fascia Lata Sling Cystourethropexy. *The Journal of urology.* 2004;171(3):1180-4.

[27] Chaikin DC, Rosenthal J, Blaivas JG. Pubovaginal fascial sling for all types of stress urinary incontinence: long-term analysis. *The Journal of urology.* 1998;160(4):1312-6.

[28] Serels S. Thoughts on midurethral synthetic slings. *Current Urology Reports.* 2007;8(5):359-63.

[29] Boublil V, Ciofu C, Traxer O, Sebe P, Haab F. Complications of urethral sling procedures. *Current Opinion in Obstetrics & Gynecology.* 2002;14(5):515-20.

[30] Ulmsten U, Petros P. Intravaginal Slingplasty (IVS): An Ambulatory Surgical Procedure for Treatment of Female Urinary Incontinence. *Scandinavian Journal of Urology and Nephrology.* 1995;29(1):75-82.

[31] Deval B, Levardon M, Samain E, Rafii A, Cortesse A, Amarenco G, et al. A French Multicenter Clinical Trial of SPARC for Stress Urinary Incontinence. *European Urology.* 2003;44(2):254-9.

[32] Guerrero KL, Emery SJ, Wareham K, Ismail S, Watkins A, Lucas MG. A randomised controlled trial comparing TVTTM, PelvicolTM and autologous fascial slings for the treatment of stress urinary incontinence in women. *BJOG: An International Journal of Obstetrics & Gynaecology.* 2010;117(12):1493-503.

[33] Tseng L-H, Wang AC, Lin Y-H, Li S-J, Ko Y-J. Randomized comparison of the suprapubic arc sling procedure vs tension-free vaginal taping for stress incontinent women. *International Urogynecology Journal.* 2005;16(3):230-5.

[34] Ward K, Hilton P. Tension-free vaginal tape versus colposuspension for primary urodynamic stress incontinence: 5-year follow up. *BJOG An International Journal of Obstetrics and Gynaecology.* 2008;115(2):226-33.

[35] Nilsson CG, Palva K, Rezapour M, Falconer C. Eleven years prospective follow-up of the tension-free vaginal tape procedure for treatment of stress urinary incontinence. *International Urogynecology Journal and Pelvic Floor Dysfunction.* 2008;19(8):1043-7.

[36] Sharifiaghdas F, Mortazavi N. Tension-free vaginal tape and autologous rectus fascia pubovaginal sling for the treatment of urinary stress incontinence: a medium-term follow-up. *Medical Principles and Practice.* 2008;17(3):209-14.

[37] Jelovsek JE, Barber MD, Karram MM, Walters MD, Paraiso MFR. Randomised trial of laparoscopic Burch colposuspension versus tension-free vaginal tape: long-term follow up. *BJOG: An International Journal of Obstetrics & Gynaecology.* 2008;115(2):219-25.

[38] Deng DY, Rutman M, Raz S, Rodriguez L. Presentation and Management of Major Complications of Midurethral Slings: Are Complications Under-reported? *Neurourology and Urodynamics.* 2007;26(1):46-52.

[39] Novara G, Galfano A, Boscolo-Berto R, Secco S, Cavalleri S, Ficarra V, et al. Complication Rates of Tension-Free Midurethral Slings in the Treatment of Female Stress Urinary Incontinence: A Systematic Review and Meta-Analysis of Randomized Controlled Trials Comparing Tension-Free Midurethral Tapes to Other Surgical Procedures and Different Devices. *European Urology.* 2008;53(2):288-309.

[40] Delorme E, Droupy Sp, Tayrac Rd, Delmas V. [Transobturator tape (Uratape). A new minimally invasive method in the treatment of urinary incontinence in women.]. *Progrès en urologie : journal de l'Association française d'urologie et de la Société française d'urologie.* 2003;13(4):656-9.

[41] Leval Jd. Novel Surgical Technique for the Treatment of Female Stress Urinary Incontinence: Transobturator Vaginal Tape Inside-Out. *European Urology. 2003*;44(6):724-30.

[42] Sung VW, Schleinitz MD, Rardin CR, Ward RM, Myers DL. Comparison of retropubic vs transobturator approach to midurethral slings: a systematic review and meta-analysis. *American Journal of Obstetrics and Gynecology.* 2007;197(1):3-11.

[43] Barry C, Lim Y, Muller R, Hitchins S, Corstiaans A, Foote A, et al. A multi-centre, randomised clinical control trial comparing the retropubic (RP) approach versus the transobturator approach (TO) for tension-free, suburethral sling treatment of urodynamic stress incontinence: the TORP study. *International Urogynecology Journal and Pelvic Floor Dysfunction.* 2008;19(2):171-8.

[44] Lee K-S, Choo M-S, Lee Y, Han J-Y, Kim J-Y, Jung B, et al. Prospective comparison of the 'inside–out' and 'outside–in' transobturator-tape procedures for the treatment of

female stress urinary incontinence. *International Urogynecology Journal.* 2008;19(4):577-82.

[45] Latthe PM, Singh P, Foon R, Toozs-Hobson P. Two routes of transobturator tape procedures in stress urinary incontinence: a meta-analysis with direct and indirect comparison of randomized trials. *BJU International.* 2010;106(1):68-76.

[46] Abdel-fattah M, Ramsay I, Pringle S, Hardwick C, Ali H. Evaluation of transobturator tapes (E-TOT) study: randomised prospective single-blinded study comparing inside-out vs. outside-in transobturator tapes in management of urodynamic stress incontinence: Short term outcomes. *European Journal of Obstetrics & Gynecology and Reproductive Biology.* 2010;149(1):106-11.

[47] Zullo MA, Plotti F, Calcagno M, Marullo E, Palaia I, Bellati F, et al. One-Year Follow-up of Tension-free Vaginal Tape (TVT) and Trans-obturator Suburethral Tape from Inside to Outside (TVT-O) for Surgical Treatment of Female Stress Urinary Incontinence: A Prospective Randomised Trial. *European Urology.* 2007;51(5): 1376-84.

[48] Liapis A, Bakas P, Creatsas G. Monarc vs TVT-O for the treatment of primary stress incontinence: a randomized study. *International Urogynecology Journal.* 2008;19(2):185-90.

[49] Lee K-S, Han DH, Choi YS, Yum SH, Song SH, Doo CK, et al. A Prospective Trial Comparing Tension-Free Vaginal Tape and Transobturator Vaginal Tape Inside-Out for the Surgical Treatment of Female Stress Urinary Incontinence: 1-Year Follow-up. *The Journal of urology.* 2007;177(1):214-8.

[50] Novara G, Artibani W, Barber MD, Chapple CR, Costantini E, Ficarra V, et al. Updated Systematic Review and Meta-Analysis of the Comparative Data on Colposuspensions, Pubovaginal Slings, and Midurethral Tapes in the Surgical Treatment of Female Stress Urinary Incontinence. *European Urology.* 2010;58(2):218-38.

[51] Moore R, Serels S, Davila G, Settle P. Minimally Invasive Treatment for Female Stress Urinary Incontinence (SUI): A Review Including TVT, TOT, and Mini-Sling. *Surgical Technology International.* 2009;18:157-73.

[52] Meschia M, Barbacini P, Baccichet R, Buonaguidi A, Maffiolini M, Ricci L, et al. Short-term outcomes with the Ajust™ system: a new single incision sling for the treatment of stress urinary incontinence. *International Urogynecology Journal.* 2011;22(2):177-82.

[53] Bernasconi F, Napolitano V, Natale F, Leone V, Lijoi D, Cervigni M. TVT SECUR™ System: Final results of a prospective, observational, multicentric study. *International Urogynecology Journal.* 2012:23(1):93-8.

[54] Kennelly MJ, Moore R, Nguyen JN, Lukban JC, Siegel S. Prospective Evaluation of a Single Incision Sling for Stress Urinary Incontinence. *The Journal of urology.* 2010;184(2):604-9.

[55] Molden S, Lucente V. New minimally invasive slings: TVT Secur. *Current Urology Reports.* 2008;9(5):358-61.

[56] Moore R, Mitchell G, Miklos J. Single center. Retrospective study of the technique, safety, and 12-month efficacy of the MiniArcTM single-incision sling: a new minimally invasive procedure for treatment of female SUI. *Surgical Technology International.* 2009;18:175-81.

[57] Gorlero F, Lijoi D, Glorio M, Mistrangelo E, Nicoletti A, Ferrero S, et al. A new technique for surgical treatment of stress urinary incontinence: the TVT-secur. *Minerva Ginecologica.* 2008;60(6):459-68.

[58] Gagnon L-O, Tu LM. Better Short-term Outcomes With the U-Method Compared With the Hammock Technique for the Implantation of the TVT-SECUR Under Local Anesthesia. *Urology.* 2010;75(5):1060-4.

[59] Martan A, Svabík K, Masata J, Koleska T, El-Haddad R, Pavlikova M. Correlation between changes in ultrasound measurements and clinical curative effect of tension-free vaginal tape-SECUR* procedure. *International Urogynecology Journal.* 2009;20(5):533-9.

[60] Shin YS, Cha JS, Cheon MW, Kim YG, Kim MK. Efficacy and Safety of the TVT-SECUR® and Impact on Quality of Life in Women with Stress Urinary Incontinence: A 2-Year Follow-Up. *Korean Journal of Urology.* 2011;52(5):335-9.

[61] Lee K-S, Lee Y-S, Seo JT, Na YG, Choo M-S, Kim JC, et al. A Prospective Multicenter Randomized Comparative Study Between the U- and H-type Methods of the TVT SECUR Procedure for the Treatment of Female Stress Urinary Incontinence: 1-Year Follow-Up. *European Urology.* 2010;57(6):973-9.

[62] Liapis A, Bakas P, Creatsas G. Comparison of the TVT SECUR System "hammock" and "U" tape positions for management of stress urinary incontinence. *International Journal of Gynecology & Obstetrics.* 2010;111(3):233-6.

[63] Andrada Hamer M, Larsson P-G, Teleman P, Etén-Bergqvist C, Persson J. Short-term results of a prospective randomized evaluator blinded multicenter study comparing TVT and TVT-Secur. *International Urogynecology Journal.* 2011;22(7):781-7.

[64] Tommaselli G, Di Carlo C, Gargano V, Formisano C, Scala M, Nappi C. Efficacy and safety of TVT-O and TVT-Secur in the treatment of female stress urinary incontinence: 1-year follow-up. *International Urogynecology Journal.* 2010;21(10):1211-7.

[65] Hinoul P, Vervest HAM, den Boon J, Venema PL, Lakeman MM, Milani AL, et al. A Randomized, Controlled Trial Comparing an Innovative Single Incision Sling With an Established Transobturator Sling to Treat Female Stress Urinary Incontinence. *The Journal of urology.* 2011;185(4):1356-62.

[66] Wang Y-j, Li F-p, Wang Q, Yang S, Cai X-g, Chen Y-h. Comparison of three mid-urethral tension-free tapes (TVT, TVT-O, and TVT-Secur) in the treatment of female stress urinary incontinence: 1-year follow-up. *International Urogynecology Journal.* 2011;22(11):1369-74.

[67] De Ridder D, Berkers J, Deprest J, Verguts J, Ost D, Hamid D, et al. Single incision mini-sling versus a transobutaror sling: a comparative study on MiniArc™ and Monarc™ slings. *International Urogynecology Journal.* 2010;21(7):773-8.

[68] Gauruder-Burmester A, Popken G. The MiniArc® Sling System in the Treatment of Female Stress Urinary Incontinence. *International Brazilian Journal of Urology.* 2009;35(3):334-43.

[69] Pickens RB, Klein FA, Mobley Iii JD, White WM. Single Incision Mid-urethral Sling for Treatment of Female Stress Urinary Incontinence. *Urology.* 2011;77(2):321-4.

[70] Basu M, Duckett J. A randomised trial of a retropubic tension-free vaginal tape versus a mini-sling for stress incontinence. BJOG: An *International Journal of Obstetrics & Gynaecology.* 2010;117(6):730-5.

[71] Oliveira R, Botelho F, Silva P, Resende A, Silva C, Dinis P, et al. Exploratory Study Assessing Efficacy and Complications of TVT-O, TVT-Secur, and Mini-Arc: Results at 12-Month Follow-Up. *European Urology*. 2011;59(6):940-4.

In: Urinary Incontinence
Editor: Eric Chung
ISBN: 978-1-62618-482-4

Chapter 13

Concomitant Pelvic Organ Prolapse and Stress Urinary Incontinence: Concepts and Management Strategies

Rachel Esler[1] and Vincent Tse[2]
[1]Department of Urology, Concord Repatriation General Hospital, University of Sydney, Australia
[2]Clinical Senior Lecturer, University of Sydney, Australia

Introduction

Both pelvic organ prolapse (POP) and stress urinary incontinence (SUI) are common conditions affecting females, with the incidence of both increasing with age. POP and SUI can present in isolation or concomitantly, with a wide variation of clinical manifestations. It is well recognized that SUI can be functionally masked by POP, resulting in incontinence in women following POP surgery. To deal with this issue many have advocated the use of prophylactic incontinence procedures in women undergoing POP repair. Similarly, 40-60% of women presenting with SUI will require a concurrent procedure for POP at the time of incontinence surgery [1]. In both scenarios there is a risk of over-treatment and the associated complications. There are a number of controversial issues in this area, relating both to the practice of prophylactic SUI surgery in the treatment of primary POP as well as the prophylactic treatment of POP in patients presenting with primary SUI. Evidence for the use of prophylactic procedures in both instances remains limited, however we will discuss the issues with the available evidence.

Epidemiology and Risk Factors for SUI and POP

In the aging female, POP and SUI are both common. Currently in the United States, 11% of women will undergo surgery for POP or SUI before the age of 80 years [2]. It is likely that the absolute number of women with POP and SUI is much greater, with the majority not treated surgically. It is estimated that up to 50% of parous women have some degree of POP, although many are asymptomatic. [3] As the population ages and more women remain active into their seventh and eighth decades, the demand for interventions, both operative and non-operative, is likely to increase.

The structure and function of the pelvic floor is inherently linked to the development of both SUI and POP. Any condition that leads to pelvic floor dysfunction leads to an increased risk of both conditions. Age, hereditary, chronic cough, multiparity, vaginal and traumatic deliveries, history of hysterectomy and connective tissue disorders have all been implicated in the pathogenesis of pelvic floor dysfunction. Obesity is the primary modifiable risk factor. The Women's Health Initiative identified that a BMI of greater than 30kg/m2 conferred a 40-75% increased risk of prolapse [4]. It is also noted that although parity is a risk factor, nulliparity does not provide absolute protection. POP and associated loss of pelvic organ support can lead to incontinence and voiding dysfunction. Commonly SUI is noted in the context of early (grade 1-2) prolapse, with progression to bladder outlet obstruction, overactive bladder or latent SUI in more severe disease (grade 3-4 prolapse). It has been shown that 4% of women with grade 1-2 POP have urethral obstruction, compared to 58% with grade 3-4 POP [5].

Clinical Presentation

Presentation with POP and SUI covers a spectrum of complaints. The three main presentations are 1) Concurrent POP + SUI, 2) Symptomatic POP without urinary symptoms (including those with latent or occult SUI), and 3) Symptomatic SUI with no or asymptomatic POP. The initial assessment of patients presenting with these complaints is vital, as the correct diagnosis and identification of the presence of concomitant disease can alter the surgical approach and hence outcomes markedly.

The presentation of POP is variable, which is not surprising given the spectrum of disease. It may be symptomatic or asymptomatic, with a range of symptoms and degree of bother that varies between individuals. The correlation between severity of POP and degree of bother is poor. Presenting complaints may include bulge, pelvic pressure, bladder complaints including incontinence and retention, bowel complaints including constipation, straining or faecal incontinence, vaginal mucosal erosions at the most dependent point of the prolapse due to constant contact with undergarments, or sexual dysfunction. Thorough clinical history including the presence of risk factors as listed above is imperative. A history of SUI that has resolved with progression of POP should raise suspicion for occult SUI. Meticulous physical examination is required to correctly evaluate the location and extent of prolapse to ensure the correct mode of repair is utilized. The POP-Q measurement system allows for uniformity in assessment and nomenclature. Similarly the identification of associated voiding dysfunction will potentially alter the surgical approach. Urodynamic assessment is essential to identify SUI, bladder stability, bladder outlet obstruction and with the careful reduction of advanced prolapse, the presence of occult SUI. There is no universally accepted technique for reducing POP for urodynamic assessment, with speculums, pessaries, tampons and vaginal packs all successfully used to reduce the prolapse. Care should be taken to ensure that the urethra is not obstructed by any of these techniques, resulting in a false negative result. It is also important to identify any complications from POP, specifically mucosal ulceration, infections, incomplete bladder emptying resulting in OAB, infections or upper tract deterioration, or most severely and very rarely, evisceration.

Management

The approach to managing such patients involves a therapeutic ladder based on the severity of symptoms, degree of bother, and the patient's general health, wishes and expectations. Options include observation, pelvic floor muscle exercises, pessary use and surgical intervention. [6]

Conservative Management

Non-operative interventions aim to minimize the severity of symptoms and bother experienced by the patient, and to defer or avoid surgical intervention where possible. This is appropriate in women with mild symptoms, who decline or are unfit for surgery, or as an adjunct to surgical repair. Non-operative interventions should also be considered as a first line treatment in patients who have symptoms that are inconsistent with their physical findings (ie. severe symptoms with mild prolapse) or atypical presentations (ie. back pain that may or may not be caused by POP). Conservative treatment should also aim to identify and treat coinciding conditions and factors that exacerbate POP and SUI. Patients should be encouraged to lose weight, exercise regularly and cease smoking. Chronic cough and other conditions creating an elevated intra-abdominal pressure should be optimally treated. Constipation should be thoroughly assessed and treated and consideration should be made for referral for colorectal cancer screening if necessary. In patients with a history of straining it is prudent to identify pelvic floor dysfunction and inappropriate straining with referral for independent assessment as required.

Pelvic floor muscle training (PFMT) aims to improve the support of the pelvic floor by increasing the strength and endurance of the pelvic floor musculature. There is evidence for the use in urinary and faecal incontinence, although there is no direct evidence for its use in POP. [7] Naturally, any likely benefit will depend on the severity of symptoms and extent of anatomical distortion, with little likelihood of benefit in advanced prolapse. It may however still provide some symptomatic improvement. For optimal utilization of PFME the intervention of a dedicated pelvic floor physiotherapist is recommended, both to teach the technique and to provide adequate follow-up to the patients. Pessaries have proven useful in women with POP who are not fit for definitive management or who wish to avoid surgery. [8] They are not appropriate in women with significant vaginal mucosal ulceration or in women who develop erosions during pessary use. They are generally well tolerated, but do require a degree of dexterity to insert and remove, or alternatively regular medical follow-up for insertion and removal to avoid complications. Pessary use can be associated with the development of new urinary symptoms, including SUI (with the unmasking of occult SUI) or

OAB secondary to bladder neck compression. The simultaneous use of a topical oestrogen preparation should also be considered depending on the degree of vaginal mucosal atrophy.

It should be noted, however, that there is no randomized evidence for the use of conservative therapy in the treatment of POP. [3]

Surgical Management

The aims of operative interventions for SUI and POP are to restore normal anatomy and function, and to achieve durable relief of symptoms. There are a wide range of approaches and interventions used for POP repair including vaginal, abdominal, laparoscopic and, rarely, trans-anal approaches. Repairs can utilize native tissue or synthetic meshes in a vast variety of forms. The type and approach of repair will depend of a number of factors, including the primary presenting symptom (SUI and/or POP), degree and anatomical site of POP, the presence of SUI or occult SUI, patient age, general health and level of activity, and surgeon experience and preference. [9] Whilst a detailed review of surgical techniques is beyond the scope of this chapter, the following points should be noted. Abdominal sacrocolpopexy was associated with a lower recurrence rate and less dyspareunia than a vaginal approach, although abdominal approach was associated with a longer operating time, longer recovery and higher cost than vaginal approach. [10] As such an abdominal approach is a reasonable option in a patient who is young, fit and sexually active, whereas a vaginal approach may be the less morbid option in a more elderly, less active woman. The use of synthetic mesh in transvaginal repairs remains topical, especially given the recent Food and Drug Administration (FDA) warning issued in July 2011. Current Cochrane data concluded that the use of transvaginal mesh has not been shown to improve functional outcomes, but may result in superior anatomical outcome and reduced recurrence rate in the anterior vaginal compartment. The FDA warns that transvaginal mesh repairs may expose the patient to a greater risk of mesh erosion, need for mesh excision and pain. The current recommendation is to carefully consider the use of mesh in individual patients.

Approaches to Address Concomitant SUI and POP

The International Continence Society Research Society (ICS-RS) recently discuss the issue of SUI surgery at the time of POP repair. It was noted that multiple approaches are being employed by pelvic floor reconstructive surgeons with literature supporting each of these approaches. Some perform a SUI operation in all patients undergoing POP repair, many are selective and do it only in patients with symptoms or signs of SUI (including occult SUI), and some would stage the two procedures and elect to perform POP repair only and see if they require SUI surgery afterwards. [10] The literature is also scarce on the issue of addressing asymptomatic POP at time of SUI surgery.

"To Sling or Not to Sling: That Is the Question" at Time of Prolapse Surgery

There have been many trials, with a myriad of study designs and methodology, undertaken recently to address this question. 10-15% of continent patients undergoing POP repair will develop bothersome SUI post-operatively. [11] If a prophylactic SUI procedure is undertaken 10% (8-16%) will develop new voiding symptoms such as urgency, urge incontinence or urinary retention. [12] Although on meta-analysis of the Cochrane data it was noted that new symptoms of overactive bladder and voiding dysfunction were noted in 12% of patients undergoing POP repair alone and that there was no clear increase in these symptoms in women undergoing concurrent SUI procedures. The method of reducing prolapse to look for occult stress incontinence had also not been standardized, furthering complicating interpretations of studies involving occult incontinence. [13]

From a clinical practice point of view, the dilemma of whether to perform a concomitant anti-incontinence procedure at time of POP repair is inherent in the lack of high-level current clinical data, and thus generates three different approaches stated above. There are pros and cons with each approach and the ICS-RS did not reach a concensus on which is the most correct. Indeed it is possible that given the same stage POP and severity of concomitant SUI in two different patients, the approach taken may be different. This may be due to other factors such as patient age, other urodynamic parameters such as detrusor contractility and peak flow rates, or patient preference of one approach over another, based on her understanding of the nature, risks and benefits of each option. These parameters are often overlooked in the recent large trials which mainly focus on randomization of various patient groupings to whether to have a concomitant sling or not. In any case, to assist the clinician to make a better informed decision on which of the 3 approaches to take for any individual patient, it would be prudent to be aware of some of the more current literature on this topic and recognize which approach each study supports with an understanding of the strengths and weaknesses in each.

There is limited evidence to support the concurrent repair of SUI and POP. Borstad et al. [14] randomized patients with symptomatic SUI and POP to POP repair with concurrent TVT, versus POP repair alone followed 3 months later by a TVT if indicated. 41/94 (44%) of the subjects did not require a TVT as they were either cured of their SUI (29%) or they have non-bothersome SUI after their POP had been repaired (15%). This paper may support the staged approach as a significant proportion of patient did not end up needing the sling, because either the POP repair had addressed the SUI, or the residual SUI post-POP repair did not bother the patient who initially most likely complained of POP symptoms more than the SUI symptoms. The disadvantages of the staged approach is that the patient may need to return to hospital a second time for the anti-incontinence procedure, with its associated psycho-socio-ecomonical impact.

The CARE study, which randomized abdominal sacrocolpopexy (ASC) to either be performed with or without Burch culposuspension in patients without significant SUI, showed that concomitant surgery is superior than ASC alone, with 24.5% of the ASC-alone group developing bothersome SUI, versus 6.1% in the concomitant repair group. [15] This study may support the 'sling-them-all' approach but when delving into the details of the study, there are weaknesses: (1) even though it is well-conducted, one cannot be sure whether these results can be extrapolated to transvaginal prolapse repairs which are done much more commonly in clinical practice than ASC in most centres, and (2) whether the results of this study can apply to sling procedures in addition to Burch culposuspension.

In contrast to the CARE study, Constantini et al. published a similar study recently showing that a concomitant Burch procedure at time of ASC for grade 3 or 4 prolapse may not necessarily be beneficial. In their study, more strict criteria were placed than the CARE trial: they only included women with a negative stress test before and after prolapse reduction, no preoperative history of incontinence symptoms, a negative symptoms questionnaire, and no leakage during urodynamics tests were considered eligible for the study; whereas the CARE included patients who reported either absent or rare SUI on the MESA questionnaire. The Constantini study showed that prophylactic Burch suspension during ASC for high-grade POP as prophylaxis for postoperative incontinence seems to emerge as overtreatment, as incontinence developed de novo in 35% of continent patients treated with colposuspension combined with sacropexy, at a mean follow-up of 39.5 months. [16] They explained that a difference in surgical technique, study design and patient inclusion and exclusion criteria, as well as a variation in follow-up intervals, between the CARE trial and their own, may have led to the very different results. This very fact illustrates that it can be difficult to organize 'the perfect trial' to address this issue of concomitant SUI surgery with POP repair due to the myriad of variables involved. Hence, based on these two trials, using a 'sling-them-all' approach at time of ASC may represent over-treatment and may not necessary eliminate urinary incontinence on longer-term follow-up.

At the International Continence Society Annual Meeting in August 2011, the OPUS trial was reported by Wei. It attempted to replicate the concept of the CARE study, but to focus on the utility of a retropubic mid-urethral synthetic sling (TVT) at time of transvaginal POP surgery in patients without symptoms of SUI. [17] 337 patients with a mean age of 63 years were randomized with 96% of them completing 12 month follow-up. The prophylactic TVT resulted in superior continence rates at 3 and 12 months. This benefit is balanced by the number needed to treat to prevent an additional case of symptomatic incontinence being 6.3 at 12 months, as well as an increased risk of bladder perforation and bleeding complications in the TVT group. Serious adverse events did not differ.

Using a urodynamic approach, two centres published on management of the urethra at time of prolapse repair. Ballert et al. compared the risk of concomitant sling surgery in patients with symptomatic or urodynamically proven SUI (including occult SUI) and the risk of requiring a sling later in those who have no evidence of any SUI either clinically or on urodynamics. They found that the risk of intervention for sling obstruction in the concomitant group was 8.5% and that of requiring a sling in those without symptomatic or urodynamic SUI, was similar at 8.3%. [18] Based on this similar risk, they recommend concomitant sling in those with clinical or urodynamic SUI only, advocating that this approach also eliminate the need for a second hospital admission later for sling surgery. One needs to bear in mind that there are variations across the world as far as socioeconomic costs are concerned, and that in some countries, there may be minimal or no direct financial cost to the patient while the cost may be very high in another country. [3] So it seems unreasonable to assume that a second hospital visit for delayed sling procedure is always inappropriate.

The second study using a urodynamic approach comes from Schierlitz et al. focused on the issue of occult stress incontinence and whether a mid-urethral sling (TVT) should be performed at time of POP repair for high-stage urogenital prolapse. [19] Eighty women were randomized to 43 no sling and 37 with concomitant sling, with median follow-up at 31 months. Four of 43 (9.3%) patients requested a TVT in the non-TVT group, 17 of 43 (39.5%) with USI remained asymptomatic and 12/43 (27.9%) women with occult USI in the no TVT group had no USI on repeat urodynamic testing following vaginal repair of the prolapse. These results showed that in occult SI and POP a clinician would need to insert 12 TVT slings to prevent one case needing a sling post-POP surgery. Furthermore 39/43 women in the non TVT group, who were asymptomatic, did not require any further surgical intervention in the longer term. They concluded that routine use of a mid-urethral sling at time of POP repair for occult incontinence is not desirable. Although this study did not look at results and complications stratified by age, it would be interesting to see if the more elderly group are more susceptible to obstructive complications. This trial supports the staged approach in concomitant occult SUI with POP, which is different to the recommendation from Ballert et al.

It is the authors' view that the potential harm and adverse outcomes in treating all women prophylactically outweighs the potential benefit to a smaller percentage of patients who will develop de novo SUI. If patients are adequately warned about this possibility pre-operatively this is rarely a problem. This is particularly applicable to the elderly whose presenting symptoms don't often correlate with urodynamic findings [20]; and more importantly, they are often more susceptible to, and have lower levels of reserve in coping with, sling complications, such as obstruction or de novo overactive bladder symptoms which may require further surgery, and drugs with anticholinergics side-effects, respectively.

SUI as Predominant Presenting Symptom with Concomitant POP

There is paucity of data to guide in the management of women who present with SUI and are found to have a degree of asymptomatic POP. There are reports to demonstrate that procedures done for urodynamic stress incontinence may, by altering vaginal axis and pelvic anatomy, increases the likelihood of subsequent pelvic organ prolapse. [21] For example, it is well-established that colposuspension may predispose to posterior compartment prolapse and upper anterior vaginal prolapse (high cystocele). [22] With respect to the mid-urethral sling, there is no published data as yet that it predisposes to prolapse. [23] As there is lack of data to address this scenario, management will be guided by the degree and site of prolapse and the bothersomeness and reduction in quality of life that the patient perceives. Although there are no published studies, it is intuitive that if there is clinical suspicion of a prolapse causing obstruction (eg. a large asymptomatic cystocele), it may be prudent to perform urodynamic assessment to exclude outlet obstruction, and carry out a concomitant prolapse repair at the time of sling surgery to reduce the risk of further obstruction at the vesicourethral angle. As data is lacking, the clinician must balance the potential morbidity of treatment with the intended clinical outcome, and in particular the informed consent should include a discussion on the nature, benefits and risks of native tissue or mesh use if a POP repair is performed concomitantly. [1]

Conclusion

As data continue to emerge with respect to concomitant use of SUI surgery in POP repair, it is important to note that there is a trend away from SUI surgery in all POP repairs, but rather focusing on a selective or staged approach, with the latter particularly relevant to occult incontinence. In regards to concomitant POP repair at time of SUI surgery where the latter is the leading symptom, there is still not enough high level data to develop a clinical algorithm. In general, whichever approach one takes in whichever scenario, it will be vital to spend time in counseling the patient with the pros and cons of each option as every individual has a different set of pathophysiological, social and economic circumstances in which she presents to the clinician. Only by taking this careful, well-informed and all-round approach would the patient appreciate the clinician's role in her management and benefit maximally from the treatment option that she eventually chooses.

References

[1] Latini J, Kreder K. Associated pelvic organ prolapse in women with stress urinary incontinence: when to operate? *Curr. Opin. Urol.* 2005; 15:380-385.

[2] Olsen AL, Smith VJ, Bergstrom JO, et al. Epidemiology of surgically managed pelvic organ prolapse and urinary incontinence. *Obstet. Gynecol.* 1997; 89:501-506.

[3] Adams E, Thompson A, Maher C, Hagen S. Mechanical devices for pelvic organ prolapse in women. *Cochrane Database Syst. Rev.* 2004; 2:CD004010.

[4] Hendrix SL, Clark A, Nygaard I et al. Pelvic Organ Prolapse in the Women's Health Initiative: gravity and gravidy. *Am. J. Obstet. Gynecol.* 2002; 186:1160-6.

[5] Romanzi LJ, Chaikin DC, Blaivas JG. The effect of genital prolapse on voiding. *J. Urol.* 199; 161:581-586.

[6] Weber A, Richter H. Pelvic Organ Prolapse. *Am. J. Obstet. Gynecol.* 2005; 106: 615-634.

[7] Maher C, Feiner B, Baessler K, et al. Surgical management of pelvic organ prolapse in women (review). *Cochrane Database Syst. Rev.* 2010; 4:CD004014.

[8] Adams E, Thompson A, Maher C, Hagen S. Mechanical devices for pelvic organ prolapse in women. *Cochrane Database Syst. Rev.* 2004; 2:CD004010.

[9] Meschia M, Pifarotti P, Spennacchio M et al. A randomized comparison of tension-free vaignal tape and endopelvic fascia plication in women with genital prolapse and occult stress urinary incontinence. *Am. J. Obstet. Gynecol.* 2004; 190:609-13.

[10] Goldman H. SUI Surgery at the Time of Vaginal POP Repair : Is a Surgical Algorithm Possible or Desirable? *Neurourol. Urodyn.*,2011,30 : 758-761.

[11] Maher C, Feiner B, Baessler K, et al. Surgical management of pelvic organ prolapse in women (review). *Cochrane Database Syst. Rev.* 2010; 4:CD004014.

[12] Groutz A, Gold R, Pauzner D et al. Tension-free Vaginal Tape (TVT) for the treatment of occult stress urinary incontinence in women undergoing prolapse repair: A prospective study of 100 consecutive cases. *Neurourol. Urodyn.* 2004; 23:632-5.

[13] Liang CC, Chang YL, Chang SD et al. Pessary test to predict postoperative urinary incontinence in women undergoing hysterectomy for prolapse. *Obstet. Gynecol.* 2004; 104:795-800.

[14] Borstad E, Abdelnoor M, Staff AC, Kulseng-Hanssen S. Pelvic organ prolapse and stress urinary incontinence in women: Combined surgical treatment. *Int. Urogyn. J. Pelvic. Floor Dysfunct.* 2010; 21(2): 179.

[15] Brubaker L, Nygaard I, Richter HE et al. Two-year Outcomes Following Sacrocolpopexy With and Without Burch to Prevent Stress Urinary Incontinence. *Obstetrics and Gynecology*, 2008; 112:49-55.

[16] Costantini E, Zucchi A, Giannantoni A et al. Must Colposuspension be Associated with Sacropexy to Prevent Postoperative Urinary Incontinence? *European Urology* 51 (3) : 788-794.

[17] Wei J. A Mid Urethral Sling Prevents Incontinence Among Women Undergoing Vaginal Prolapse Repair – the OPUS Trial. *Neurourol. Urodyn.* 30 (6) : 809-10.

[18] Ballert KN, Biggs GY, Isenalume A et al. Managing the Urethra at Transvaginal Pelvic Organ prolapse repair : A urodynamic approach. *J. Urol.* 181: 679-84.

[19] Schierlitz L, Dwyer P, Rosamilia A, et al. A prospective randomised controlled trial comparing vaginal prolapse repair with and without tension free vaginal tape (TVT) in women with severe genital prolapse and occult stress incontinence: long term follow up. Abstract 2, International Continence Society Annual Meeting 2010, *Neurourol. Urodyn.* vol. 29.

[20] Bromage SJ, Dorkin TJ, Chan L, Tse V. Urodynamics in the octogenarian female: is it worthwhile? *Int. Urogynecol. J.* 2010 Sep; 21(9): 1117-21.

[21] Robinson D, Cardozo L. The Effect of Continence Surgery on Urogenital Prolapse. *BJU International* 93 : 25-30.

[22] Kiiholma P, Makinen J, Chancellor MB, et al. Modified Burch colposuspension for stress urinary incontinence in females. *Surg. Gynaecol. Obstet.* 1993; 176:111-5.

[23] Kuuva N, Nilsson CG. A Nationwide Analysis of Complications Associated with the Tension Free Vaginal Tape (TVT) Procedure. *Acta Obstet. Gynaecol. Scand.* 2002; 81:72-7.

Special Section: Male Urinary Incontinence

In: Urinary Incontinence
Editor: Eric Chung ISBN: 978-1-62618-482-4

Chapter 14

Post-Prostatectomy Stress Urinary Incontinence: Pathophysiology and Diagnosis

Eric Chung*
Department of Urology, Princess Alexandra Hospital, risbane QLD, Australia

Abstract

Post prostatectomy urinary incontinence (PPI) is not uncommon despite the advances in surgical techniques and technologies. While in the past, the damage and subsequent atrophy of the external urethral sphincter was thought to be the primary cause, recent understandings of the pathophysiological changes that occurred with radical prostatectomy have highlighted other aetiological factors and mechanisms leading to the development of PPI. Amongst the possible causative factors are dysfunction of the bladder neck, shortened urethral length and changes in the urethral axis as well as intra-operative damage to both nerve and pelvic floor musculature. Recent studies have also demonstrated that both sphincteric urethral prolapse and urethral hyper-mobility also contribute to PPI. Furthermore underlying detrusor changes following radical prostatectomy would account for the development of urge and urge incontinence in these men. This chapter reviews the mechanisms and diagnosis of PPI.

Introduction

Despite significant advances in surgical techniques and technologies, stress urinary incontinence post radical prostatectomy (RP) remains a common complication. Post prostatectomy incontinence (PPI) can occur in upwards of 60% of men in the initial months post RP [1]. While most of the PPI resolve in the subsequent months following conservative

* Corresponding author: Dr Eric Chung - Department of Urology, Princess Alexandra Hospital, Ipswich Rd, Brisbane, QLD 4103, Australia. (T): +617-33242468. (F):+617-33242546. ericchg@hotmail.com.

measures such as pelvic floor physiotherapy, 5-10% of men continue to experience PPI 12 months post RP [2]. The presence of PPI markedly impairs the quality of life of these men and is associated with significant social and economic burden [3]. In fact, most men consider the need to wear incontinence pads a greater problem to them than post RP erectile dysfunction [4].

Presently there is no existing consensus on the exact mechanisms underlying PPI and whether any preoperative risk factors play a significant part [5]. The key mechanism of urinary incontinence and predicting factors of recovery of continence may differ in elapsed time post RP, even with standardization of surgical approach and technique. Given that various factors on urinary incontinence post RP is dependent upon the time course, the postoperative outcomes may be different, according to when PPI was evaluated. This makes the clarification of the mechanism of incontinence post RP difficult.

The most common cause of PPI in men is iatrogenic injury to the external urethral sphincter (EUS) resulting in intrinsic sphincter deficiency (ISD) [6]. The term ISD does not address and fully reflect the complex pathophysiology of PPI [7]. Urinary continence is depended upon a stable detrusor; healthy urothelium and urethral wall, functional smooth and striated muscles of the sphincter components; intact neurovascular supply; and robust pelvic floor musculature and supporting fascias. Therefore any damage to these structures result in PPI. The following chapter reviews the mechanisms and diagnosis of post-prostatectomy urinary incontinence.

Mechanisms of PPI

1. Pre-Operative Factors

The incidence of stress urinary incontinence in men is far less common than in women. This is partly attributable to the several anatomical differences. The prostatic tissue provides an anatomical obstruction to the lower urinary tract in men and also indirectly contributes to part of the prostate-membranous urethral sphincter. The prostate itself functions to maintain the shape of the bladder neck and allows the preprostatic sphincter to assume its role in maintaining continence.

Furthermore the male urethra is longer and therefore increases the resistance to urinary flow. Nonetheless several preoperative factors have been shown to play a significant part in the development of PPI.

First, age is an important predisposing factor in the development and progression of voiding dysfunction. Aging is associated with reduced elasticity of the muscle of bladder and pelvic floor and many studies have showed that aging males have limited ability for nerve recruitment leading to higher rates of PPI [8]. Furthermore, the incidence of detrusor overactivity is more common in the older men, who are more likely to have prostate cancer diagnosis and undergo RP.

Previous transurethral resection or irradiation of the prostate can also inadvertently damage the EUS and/or pelvic supporting structures leading to higher risk of voiding dysfunction. Another study showed that obesity is associated with higher rate of PPI due to the downward pressure of their intra-abdominal viscera on vesicourethral anastomosis following RP [9].

2. Intra-Operative Factors

2.1. Damage to Urethral Sphincter Complex: Striated and Smooth Muscle Components

The male urinary sphincter complex consists of both internal and external sphincters. The proper function of the urethral sphincter requires the combined efforts of an intact and functional urothelium, urethral wall, smooth and striated muscle components, and the correct positioning and appropriate mobility of the urethra [10]. The internal sphincter is composed of the bladder neck and prostate, with the vesical or bladder neck sphincteric system in continuity with the preprostatic sphincter, a relationship that plays an important role in maintaining continence mechanism at the level of bladder neck. The preprostatic sphincter is in continuity with the middle circular layer of the bladder and consists of circularly oriented fibers that lie beneath prostatomembranous urethra [11]. At the junction of the inferior bladder and proximal urethra, the urothelium becomes a key component of the internal sphincter. Under normal conditions, the elastic properties of the proximal urethral walls produce coaptation of the urothelium and this provides the primary resistance to the flow of urine out of the bladder to maintain urinary continence [12].

There is a controversy in the literature regarding the course and structure of the external urethral sphincter (EUS) complex. Nevertheless, there is a general agreement that the urethral sphincter is a distinct muscular structure and is not part of the pelvic floor musculature [13, 14]. The external urethral complex is composed of three distinct muscle layers and two distinct muscle types. The outer, horseshoe (or omega) shaped striated muscle is often referred to as the rhabdosphincter [15]. The rhabdosphincter inserts on the apex and the anterior surface of the prostate [16] and does not converge dorsally. The thickness of the muscle is greater at the ventral and ventrolateral aspect and becomes thinner at the posterolateral aspect of the sphincter.

The fibers of the rhabdosphincter arch across the front and pass around the urethra, uniting with the muscle of that opposite side behind the urethra via the tendinous median raphe and the caudal part of the sphincter is continuous with the central perineal tendon and the cephalad part of the posterior prostatic fascia [17]. Dorsally connective tissue and elastic fibers can also be found. The orientation of the muscle fibers is unclear and might be horizontal or vertical [18, 19]. This discrepancy may have to do with the variable axis of the urethral lumen with respect to the vertical axis of the human body and how histological sections are taken. The longitudinal oriented puboprostatic muscle, an extramural muscle from the levator system, lies on either side of the rhabdosphincter and provides reinforcement to the activity of the sphincter complex.

In contrast, the inner layer of the external urethral complex consists of smooth muscle fibers and is commonly referred to as the *musculus sphincter urethrae glaber* [20]. The posterior aspect of this smooth muscle urethral sphincter and the prostate apex is close to the anterior surface of the rectum. The inner muscle layer of this smooth muscle sphincter surrounds the urethra completely and consists of smooth muscle fibers and elastic tissue [17]. The smooth muscle layer can be subdivided into an inner, longitudinal-oriented layer and an outer, more circumferential-oriented layer. Although the superficial smooth muscle layer completely encircles the urethra, the deeper longitudinal layer is only found at the ventral and posterior aspect of the urethra [11]. Nonetheless these smooth muscle layers are intermingling, which suggests that sphincteric activity is a result of combined activity of all layers.

Excessive excision, traction, and thermal injury to the urethral sphincter during apical dissection, as well as tension on the constructed vesicourethral anastomosis from stump recession, urinoma, or clot formation, are all potential contributory factors to EUS dysfunction and PPI. The causes of intrinsic sphincter deficiency could be direct injury to the smooth or striated muscles lining the sphincteric segment of the urethra or damage to the nerve innervating these sphincteric muscles. The EUS complex is innervated by the autonomic branches of the pelvic plexus, which run with the neurovascular bundle (NVB) and partly derived from branches of the pudendal nerve [21, 22]. Another potential problem that can be encountered intra-operatively is the difficulty in identifying the tissue plane between EUS and prostatic tissue as almost a third of the prostate tissue overlaps onto the EUS. Furthermore the disruption and loss of the posterior insertion of the rhabdosphincter during RP could result in pelvic descent of the sphincteric complex. Rocco [23] underlined the role of the posterior restoration of the rhabdosphincter fibers (to create its original length) to improved urinary continence after RP.

Some authors consider the posterior tendinous insertion of the median dorsal raphe and the adjacent tissue as a fulcrum for the contraction of the sphincter complex, which allows movement of the urethra in the dorsal and caudal. This contraction combined with the contraction of the puboperinealis muscle results in a double-sling mechanism for closure of the urethra [24]. While the reconstruction of this posterior fulcrum during RP could theoretically hasten the recovery of urinary continence [25], no definite evidence has been conclusively shown [26, 27].

Caudal misalignment of the sphincter complex as a result of injury or increased laxity of the surrounding support structures can also affect the sphincteric mechanism and thus continence. Misalignment of the urethra post RP may reduce the effectiveness of coaptation of the urethra wall, even when the tone of the encasing muscle fibers is properly maintained [12].

2.2. Dissection of Pubo-Prostatic Ligament and Pubo-Perinealis Muscle

Puboprostatic ligaments are paired fibrous bands originating from visceral endopelvic fascia and ventral aspect of the prostate base, and insert on to the distal third of the posterior surface of pubic bone adjacent and anterior to the urethral sphincter [28]. In contrast, Santorini described the extension of the detrusor fibers beyond the bladder neck in males and that the outer straight fibers on the anterior wall of the bladder spread around the prostate and are clustered again in the pubis [29], hence the term puboprostatic ligaments are interchangeable with pubovesical ligaments. While this histological findings are obvious in newborn infant, it becomes less distinct in adult male and remains unknown if the so-called puboprostatic ligaments are part of muscle or not, connecting the base of the bladder to pubis or the prostate to the symphysis. Nonetheless the puboprostatic ligaments together with the tendinous arch of the pelvic fascia form the anterior urethral support mechanism [30] and stabilize the bladder neck, help secure the membranous urethra to the pubic bone and play a critical role in maintaining continence as well as initiating micturition [31, 32]. However the preservation of puboprostatic ligaments is often difficult to achieve in open RP [33].

2.3. Alteration of Urethral Length, Axis and Location

One of the common sequela of RP that may affect urinary sphincter activity is the reduction in the membranous urethra length resulting from its excision at the level of the prostate. The shape of the apical prostate varies substantially and directly influences the length of urethra from the apex of prostate [34]. Many studies have described a decrease in functional urethra length following RP and that a longer functional urethra was documented among continent patients compared to the incontinent patients. Paparel [35] reported that a longer preoperative or postoperative membranous urethral length was associated with superior continence ($p<0.01$) and that membranous urethral length loss ratio was significantly associated with postoperative continence ($p=0.02$). Lee [34] showed that there was a greater risk of significant shortening of the urethra and therefore potentially greater risk of urinary incontinence when the prostatic parenchyma covered the membranous urethra on the anterior and/or posterior side. Schlomm [36] reported a significantly higher continence rates at 50.1% (vs. 30.9%) 1 week after catheter removal ($p<0.01$) following preservation of full functional urethra length with strict apical dissection and anatomic restoration of the Mueller's ligaments. It appeared that the combination of a full functional urethra length preparation and improved preservation of the anatomic fixation of the urethral sphincter complex resulted in significantly higher early urinary continence outcomes. However the study is limited by the nonrandomized nature and the asymmetric number of patients in the study groups. Similarly, Nguyen [37] found that men in the longer urethral sphincter group (more than 14 mm) and those with total reconstruction of the continence mechanism were associated with earlier return of urinary continence compared to the group with shorter sphincter (less than 14 mm) and anterior reconstruction only.

Another important component of the sphincteric muscular complex is the vertically or longitudinal oriented muscle component of the urethral musculature. This inner muscular layer is close to the urethral lumen and many surgeons performing RP would retract the prostate during apical dissection to gain maximum urethral length. However it remains uncertain whether preservation of a long inner smooth muscular urethral component has any effect on postoperative urinary incontinence. Significant overlap makes the preservation of both long and short urethral sphincters difficult and should be considered during apical dissection and transection of the urethra at the apex.

The variability in postoperative measurements is likely related to the differences in anatomic landmarks. It appeared that the recovery of urinary continence was faster in patients in whom a urethral stump was preserved by intra-prostatic dissection during RP [38]. Hakimi [39] showed that longer stretched (distance from the perineal membrane to the prostate apex on stretch) and cut (urethral stump length) urethral lengths appeared to correlate with earlier return of urinary continence. The membranous urethral length on endo-rectal coil MRI correlates strongly with International Consultation on Incontinence Questionnaire (ICIQ) score ($p=0.07$).

The extent of damage to urethral support structures, such as the levator ani muscle can lead to urethral hypermobility and prevent the urethral support structures to be pulled forward and upward to stop urine flow. Urethral movement is a normal anatomical function in men during voiding and is different to the urethral hypermobility responsible for female incontinence. Urethral mobility which can be evaluated using voiding cystourethrography could prove to be a good predictor early urinary continence. The anatomical location and fiber characteristics of the levator ani muscle suggest that these fibers actively assist in urethral closure, particularly during events that cause increase in intra-abdominal pressure [40]. Myers [41] suggested that levator ani have important roles in maintaining urinary continence in male patients and indicated that the puboperineales, which form the anteromedial part of the levator ani, are positioned where they can pull the urethra forward and upward to stop the urinary stream quickly. Therefore it is likely that greater urethral movement signaled lesser preservation of nerve function and greater injury to the levator ani muscle during the operation. Jeong [42] found that younger patients with higher vesico-urethral anastomosis and a greater percentage of nerve sparing have a shorter time to continence. Vesico-urethral anastomosis location above the upper margin of the symphysis pubis represents an independent predictor of recovery of urinary continence and the higher the vesico-urethral anastomosis in the pelvic cavity, the earlier the recovery of urinary continence.

The role of postoperative urethral and periurethral fibrosis in patients post RP has been of recent interest. Tuygun [43] classified fibrosis as either involving the urethra and/or extending concentrically into periurethral tissue. Unfortunately the fibrotic process is not always circumferential and high-grade fibrosis in periurethral tissue may spare the urethra. Paparel [35] reported that patients with a high grade postoperative periurethral fibrosis have worse postoperative continence rate (HR 0.64, $p=0.16$). It is postulated that periurethral fibrosis impedes the recovery of continence mechanism after RP by altering the elasticity of the external sphincter. Nishida [44] found an inverse correlation between the length of urethral movement and urinary incontinence volume rate on day 7 after catheter removal. A statistically significant difference was observed in men with greater than 2mm of length of urethral movement compared to men with shorter urethral length (<2mm) on voiding cystourethrography with regard to early continence rate. At present there is no standardized definition or classification of postoperative urethral fibrosis. Furthermore, postoperative urethral fibrosis measured by endo-rectal coil MRI cannot be considered as a standard diagnostic modality and the statistically correlation between high grade of postoperative periurethral fibrosis and worse postoperative continence was not been conclusively demonstrated.

2.4. Neurovascular Compromise

The urethral sphincter is innervated by autonomic branches of the inferior hypogastric plexus, which partly runs with the NVB and partly derives from the branches of the pudendal nerve [21, 22].

The pelvic plexus contains the sympathetic fibers from T11-L2 ganglia (responsible for ejaculation), parasympathetic fibers from pelvic and splanchnic nerves and ventral rami of S2-4 (responsible for erection and bladder control). The pelvic plexus lies within a fibro-fatty, rectangular and sagitally oriented plate between the bladder and rectum. The anterior part of the pelvic plexus innervates the bladder, prostate, seminal vesicles, and vasa deferentia, and the most inferior part of this plexus becomes the cavernous nerves [45]. Nerve fibers surround predominantly the lateral aspect the bladder neck, proximal prostate, and the seminal vesicles in a cage-like fashion [45].

These nerves are located posterolateral to the seminal vesicles and travelled very close to the tip of seminal vesicle [46]. Therefore meticulous and careful surgical dissection around the seminal vesicles and/or seminal vesicle-sparing RP could improve the postoperative urinary continence and potency rates [47]. There is very minimal distance separating the nerves from pelvic structures and it has been reported that these nerve fibers are in direct contact (0mm) to the seminal vesicles and the prostate base, a distance of 4mm to the bladder neck, and 2 mm to the levator ani musculature [48, 49].

The branches designated as cavernous nerves destined for the urinary sphincters are mainly located posteriorly in the pelvic plexus [48]. Furthermore, the cavernous nerves and the pelvic plexus were found to be only 0-7mm lateral to the prostate pedicles [49]. The neural anatomy may vary substantially lateral to the prostate. These nerve fibers enter the urethral sphincter posterolaterally from both sides, mainly at the 5 and 7 o'clock position and the 3 and 9 o'clock positions [45]. The distance from the prostatic apex to the point, where the nearest pudendal neural branch enters the sphincter was measured to be 3-13 mm [50].

Since the NVB is found lateral to the urethra at the 2 and 10 o'clock position, dissection of the lateral parts of the DVC might be harmful to the CN, the autonomic innervation of the urethral sphincter [51]. Recent studies confirmed that NVB is not a distinct structure and consists of multiples finely dispersed nerve fibers lateral to the prostate gland [52]. It appears that the NVB develops during the embryonic phase of gestation as a distinct structure and later becomes dispersed over the lateral surface of the prostate during its development [46]. In addition, the development of benign prostatic hyperplasia may add substantially to the dispersion and distribution of the nerves over the lateral surface of the prostate. Nonetheless, approximately two thirds of these nerves are located on the posterolateral aspect and the remaining third lie on the anterolateral surface of the prostate [46, 48]. It is believed that the nerves fibers running anteriorly in the NVB mainly innervate the levator ani and the prostate while the more posteromedially located nerve fibers mainly innervate the corpora cavernosa [48]. Neurovascular bundle sparing was reported to result in an improved continence rate [53] and its relationship to intraurethral pressure has been previously demonstrated [50].

By preserving the pelvic plexus and branches providing autonomic and/or motor innervations to the rhabdosphincter during nerve sparing RP, earlier recovery of sphincteric function can be anticipated following functional recovery of these nerves [54]. Considering the recovery of erectile function after nerve sparing RP, the postulated time required for functional recovery from neuropraxic injury, along with anatomical integrity, the return of neural control of the urethra sphincter may required time too. Moreover the meticulous care in surgical technique of sparing the NVB may help decrease iatrogenic mechanical injury to the rhabdosphincter.

2.5. Pelvic Floor Musculature

The innermost muscle of the anterior pelvis is the levator ani complex. The levator ani muscle consists of two-strap liked muscles that originate from the pubis, flank the prostatourethral junction on each side, and attach to the perineal body dorsal to the urethra, and anterior to the anorectal junction [40]. The anterior part of the levator ani complex is the puboperinealis and puborectalis muscles [55]. Voluntary contraction of the puboperinealis and puborectalis muscles pulls the urethra forward and upward, resulting in a closure of the urethra and termination of urinary stream.

On the other hand, the rectourethralis muscle is a Y-shaped muscular structure that is dorsal to the membranous urethra, surrounded by both sides of the levator ani and located distal (>1cm) to the urethral sphincter complex [56, 57]. However several studies have demonstrated that there is no contact of this muscle with the urethra itself, suggesting that the term rectourethralis is perhaps a misnomer [58]. Nonetheless, the rectourethralis muscles, together with puboperinealis, puborectalis and levator ani fascia (LAF), distal portion of Denonvilliers fascia (DF) as well as the tendinous median raphe from the rhabdosphincter form a complex posterior attachment and support for the membranous urethra [57]. This "conjoined fibrous" tissue acts as a fulcrum for the anterior forces exerted by the rhabdosphincter (compressing the urethra in an anteroposterior direction) and also for the posterior forces exerted by the puboperineal muscles (lifting the membranous urethra in a posteroanterior direction) to maintain urinary continence.

Song [59] reported that the recovery of urinary continence 3 months post RP was related to the thickness of the pelvic diaphragm on sagittal imaging ($p=0.017$), the ratio of the levator ani on the axial image to prostate volume ($p=0.047$), functional urethral length ($p=0.007$) and incontinence before surgery ($p=0.009$). Recovery at 6 months was related to neurovascular bundle sparing ($p=0.013$) and marginally to the pelvic diaphragm on sagittal imaging ($p=0.059$). Pelvic diaphragm thickness and the ratio of levator ani muscle thickness to prostate volume are independent factors predictive of PPI and patients with better developed pelvic floor muscle, especially in relation to the size of the prostate, can be expected to achieve earlier recovery of continence.

In the course of apical and urethral dissection during RP, the pelvic floor musculature can be densely adhered to these important structures and posed considerable challenge to dissect of the membranous urethra. The most distal sphincteric unit consists of rhabdosphincter, paraurethral skeletal musculature and supporting fascia investments. Therefore the integrity of the remaining distal sphincteric unit, of which paraurethral support by the levator ani and its voluntary contractile pressure has the most significant role in the immediate postoperative continence. The Kegel or pelvic floor muscle exercises specifically targets this unit to enhance the pelvic floor musculature and increase resistance on post RP incontinence [60]. Interestingly the benefit of pelvic floor exercises only assists in the earlier recovery of urinary continence with most study participants regaining continence 1 year postoperatively regardless of the pelvic floor exercises.

2.6. Fascia and Supporting Structures

The anatomy of the prostate is complicated by the proximity to other pelvic organs and the narrow male pelvis [45]. The pelvic organs are covered by the pelvic fascias. The parietal component of the pelvic fascia covers the medial aspects of the levator ani muscles and the visceral component covers the pelvic organs such as prostate, bladder and rectum. Some authors refer to the parietal component of the pelvic fascia as endopelvic fascia (EPF) [61], while others consider the entire parietal and visceral pelvic fascia as EPF [62]. Along the pelvic sidewall at the lateral aspect of the prostate and bladder, the parietal and the visceral components of the EPF fused and formed a whitish line, termed fascial tendinous arch of the pelvis. This whitish fascial line stretches from the puboprostatic ligaments to the ischial spine. Some surgeons advocate avoiding incision of the EPF during RP, often in conjunction with an intrafascial nerve sparing approach to improve early urinary continence, but no definite evidence has yet to be established [62, 63]. Incision of the parietal EPF lateral to the fascial tendinous arch exposes levator ani muscle with the LAF adherent to the prostate. In contrast incision of the visceral EPF medial to the fascial tendinous arch results in a dissection plane that leaves the levator ani muscle covered with its fascia without exposure of its muscle fibers [62, 63]. The result is a prostate covered only by prostatic fascia, when present, and not by a layer of LAF [62].

The current literature is littered with various nomenclatures on the fascia covering the outer surface of the prostate gland. Many studies utilized the terms such as lateral pelvic fascia [13, 48]; periprostatic fascia [64]; parapelvic fascia [65]; and prostatic fascia [66] to designate the fascia covering the outer surface of prostate gland. It is important to note that this fascia consisted of several layers, both collagen and adipose tissue elements and can be further subdivided based on anatomical locations. The anterior periprostatic fascia lies on the anterior surface of the prostate and covers the detrusor apron, dorsal vein complex and is fused in the midline with the anterior fibromuscular stroma of the prostate. The lateral periprostatic fascia is encountered lateral to the fascial tendinous arch of the pelvis and medial to levator ani muscle; on the lateral aspect of the prostate gland and covers the prostate capsule. Interestingly, this lateral prostatic fascia is not always adherent to the prostatic capsule and recent anatomical study has demonstrated that 52% of all cases, there was an apparent space between the lateral prostatic fascia and the prostatic capsule is filled with loose connective and adipose tissue [67]. In the remaining 48%, the lateral prostatic fascia was fused with the prostatic capsule with the exception at the posterolateral angle of the prostate and the NVB was identified as a distinct structure. The posterior periprostatic fascia adheres to the posterior aspect of the prostate and fuses with the seminal vesicle fascia to form the DF [68]. In fact some authors consider DF as the fusion of the embryonic peritoneum of the retro-vesical cul-de-sac as it covers the prostate and the seminal vesicle on the dorsal aspect [69]. DF extends distally to the apex of the prostate and the prostatourethral junction, where it has direct continuity to the midline raphe of the central perineal tendon [70]. Therefore the often cited posterior layer of the Denonvilliers' fascia is in fact the fascia proper of the rectum, which is a thin membrane that envelopes the mesorectum and represents a structure independent of the posterior prostatic fascia [67, 69, 71].

The fascial and neural anatomy of the prostate are of special interest in RP, and the fascias in particular represent important surgical dissection planes. The intrafascial dissection of the NVB follows a plane on the prostate capsule, staying medial or internal to the prostatic fascia at the anterolateral and posterolateral aspect of the prostate and anterior to the posterior prostatic fascia [13]. This allows a whole-thickness preservation of the lateral prostatic fascia laterally and therefore presents a complete preservation of the NVB as it remains covered by and lateral to the prostatic fascia. However in doing so, it carries with it the greatest risk of inadvertent iatrogenic capsular penetration [72]. On the other hand, interfascial dissection plane involves the dissection outside or lateral to the prostatic fascia at the anterolateral and posterolateral aspects of the prostate as well as medial to the NVB at the 5 and 7 o'clock positions or the 2 and 10 o'clock positions of the prostate in axial plane. This dissection plane moves the NVB off the prostate so that the posterolateral aspect of the prostate remains covered with fascia but in doing so, it runs the risk of partial resection of the NVB due to possibility of injuring the nerve fibers on the anterolateral surface of the prostate [13, 73]. Lastly, extrafascial dissection involves a dissection plane lateral to the levator ani fascia and posterior to the posterior prostatic fascia. It is associated with the highest risk of post RP ED as the NVB running along the posterolateral aspect of the prostate is completely resected [13].

2.7. Bladder Neck Preservation

The ring-shaped vesical sphincter can be preserved during bladder neck sparing RP. This is not always possible due to anatomic variances of the prostate shape and the surrounding structures. The tissue between the posterior bladder neck and the insertion of seminal vesicles and ampullae of the vasa deferentia is of surgical importance during posterior dissection of the prostate [74]. This tissue layer is believed to contain the anterior layer of the posterior prostatic fascia. The inner tissue lies directly under the bladder mucosa and consists of smooth muscle fibers originating from the outer longitudinal detrusor muscle and inserts into the prostate base. The more posterior layer is found in close contact with the inner layer and composed of fibro-adipose tissue and is in continuity with the bladder adventitia.

Controversy exits in the current literature regarding BN preservation. The reported advantage of earlier return of urinary continence should be balanced against the possibility of an increased positive surgical margin. The preservation of bladder neck during RP is associated with earlier return of urinary continence [13]. On the other hand, a very tight bladder neck reconstruction can lead to bladder neck contracture postoperatively [5]. Stolzenburg [75] found that BN preservation has an impact on early continence immediately after catheter removal and at the 3-month follow up in comparison with those without BN preservation. The positive surgical margin did not differ between the 2 groups. It appeared that BN preservation has an advantage over BN reconstruction approaches in earlier return of urinary continence.

Licht [76] reported that age greater than 65 and occurrence of a bladder neck contracture are adverse predictors for return of urinary continence post RP. Interestingly the study reported that the preservation of the bladder neck did not significantly affect the return of urinary control, instead it was associated with lower risk of bladder neck contracture. Poon [77] found no statistically significant differences in return of urinary continence, bladder neck contracture rates or positive margins between bladder neck preservation, tennis racket reconstruction and anterior bladder tube preservation. In contrast, Selli [78] reported that while bladder neck preservation during RP did not improve long-term results of urinary continence, it contributed substantially to earlier recovery of urinary continence, thus improving the quality of life.

There are several issues to address with BN preservation during RP. The choice of BN preservation needs to be individualized and there are many individual and technical factors to be considered intra-operatively. Cases of larger prostate, prominent middle lobe or poorly defined vesiculoprostatic junction could result in more difficult dissection and less likely for a BN preservation approach. Furthermore, there is no clear consensus on the definition and quantification of BN preservation. Data pertaining to BN preservation and reconstruction can be subjective and could be based on the absence of racket handle repair of the BN and/or direct suturing of the BN on the urethra.

Garg [79] reported a lower incidence of BN (3 in 406 cases) using the intussuscepted vesico-urethral anastomosis, which involves a looped urethral suture that are drawn 'inside-to-out' from staggered points on the urethral stump through the bladder neck opening, and that the urethra is intussuscepted into the bladder neck opening when the sutures are tied down. In contrast, Teber [80] found no difference in the long term continence and stricture rates among the 3 anastomotic techniques in laparoscopic RP. Nontheless intracorporeal continuous anastomotic suture appeared to theoretically reduce the intraoperative time and tension to the anastomosis compared to interrupted suturing.

3. Post-Operative Factors

3.1. Anastomotic Stricture

Anastomotic stricture between the bladder neck and membranous urethra after RP can cause significant voiding dysfunction. The risk factors for anastomotic stricture include excessive intra-operative blood loss, extravasation of urine at the anastomotic site, prior transurethral prostatic operation and history of radiation. Yildrim [81] found that time and the amount of urinary drainage were significantly associated with stricture formation and postulated that might be related to partial disruption of the anastomosis.

Park [82] postulated that the development of anastomotic strictures in some men appears to be related to a generalized hypertrophic wound-healing mechanism. It appeared that men with excessive midline vertical abdominal scar, especially with a maximal scar of greater than 10mm, were eight times more likely to develop strictures than men with smaller post RP scars.

3.2. Post-Micturition Dribble or Urethral Dysfunction

Urinary incontinence post RP is thought mainly due to stress incontinence. However some patients complain of stress-independent urinary leakage following voiding i.e post-micturition dribble, of uncertain origin. Following voiding, a residue of urine becomes trapped and pooled inside the bulbar urethra and begins to drain down the urethra.

Willie [83] confirmed that post-void milk-out of the urethra is often absent in the early postoperative recovery period following RP and that this is associated with post-micturition dribble. There was a statistically significant decrease in the rate of milking and increase in rate of post-micturition dribble from before to after surgery. Urethral dysfunction characterized by the absence of urethral post-void milking, seems to be an additional cause of PPI.

Bader [84] found that the sensory threshold of the membranous urethra increases significantly post RP. In contrast the sensory threshold of the bulbar urethra remained relatively similar pre-and post RP. The change in the sensitivity of the membranous urethra correlates with PPI and post-void dribbling seems to be associated with the loss of urethral milking.

Diagnosis of PPI

The management of PPI differs from that for urge urinary incontinence, which is generally treated with pharmacological agents. Nonetheless it is possible for both conditions to coexist. There are published guidelines for the assessment of men with urinary incontinence occurring with physical activities [85, 86]. A good history provides a good indication that PPI is a result of RP. The initial treatment option for PPI is usually conservative with lifestyle interventions and pelvic floor exercise. However there are controversies surrounding the role of pelvic floor exercise; the different regimen of PFE and combination of PFE with biofeedback [87], and whether preoperative PFE is useful. The timing of continence evaluation is worth mentioning because these anatomical factors were determinants only of early recovery, becoming increasingly insignificant with increasing time after surgery. Nonetheless, many men are debilitated during this time and suffered significant impairment of quality of life.

The clinical workup of a PPI should be methodical with a thorough urinary history with assessment of underlying sphincter function and exclusion of post RP stricture formation, followed by focused physical examination to exclude palpable bladder, a cough/stress test and pad weight/number test. History of recumbent or nocturnal urinary incontinence raises the suspicion of detrusor overactivity; while the ability to interrupt urinary stream during voiding suggests sufficient residual sphincteric function.

Presently, there is no consensus on the severity or grades of urinary incontinence. The number of pads used per day is commonly used to evaluate the degree of urinary incontinence but remains subjective, as there are many reasons that determine how often a patient may change his pad. Some authors advocate the use of 24 hour urinary pad weight to measure daily urine leak while others suggest 1-hour pad weight. The grade of severity can be classified as mild, moderate and severe. Most published literature define mild incontinence as <200ml/day, moderate as 200-500ml/day, and sever as >500ml/day.

Cystoscopic examination should be carried out to exclude urethral stricture, sphincteric defect and anastomotic stricture or bladder neck contracture. Residual sphincter function can be classified normal with sphincter coapts at rest or poor with sphincter remains open. Failure of the urethral sphincter to coapt during active pelvic floor contraction suggests significant sphincter defect and possible periurethral or sphincteric fibrosis [88]. A mid-perineal digital compression in the direction parallel to the membranous urethra during dynamic urethroscopy in a lithotomy position can be utilized to assess urethral mobility and circumferential closure of the urethra [89]. Urodynamics can be carried out to exclude detrusor overactivity, assess sphincteric function with leak point pressures and detrusor function for adequate emptying. This thorough assessment enables confirmation of the diagnosis and evaluate for the various types of anti-incontinence surgery and likely expectations of surgical outcome.

Conclusion

PPI is a complex interplay of many pre-, intra- and postoperative factors. Intra-operative damage to EUS, hypermobility of the sphincteric complex, prolapsed and hypermobility of the membranous urethra and pelvic fascial and musculature dysfunctions have been postulated to contribute to PPI. Despite the advances in surgical techniques and technologies, the increased and earlier detection of prostate cancer with younger men undergoing RP and the proportion of elderly men increasing, greater numbers of men with PPI will likely require treatment. Exciting advances in real-time bioimaging and mathematical modeling of organ function using innovative 3D bioengineering computer platforms could provide much-needed breakthroughs in the evaluation of the pathophysiology of PPI. The clinical workup of PPI should take into account the possible mechanisms of PPI and evaluate the patients for the appropriate treatment options.

References

[1] Kao TC, Cruess DF, Garner D et al. Multicenter patient self-reporting questionnaire on impotence, incontinence and stricture after radical prostatectomy. *J. Urol.* 2000; 163: 858-64.

[2] Kao TC; Bauer RM, Bastian PJ, Gozzi C, Stief CG. Postprostatectomy incontinence: all about diagnosis and management. *Eur. Urol.* 2009; 55: 322-33.

[3] Sanda MG, Dunn RL, Michalski J et al. Quality of life and satisfaction with outcome among prostate-cancer survivors. *N. Engl. J. Med.* 2008; 358: 1250-61.

[4] Fowler Jr FJ, Barry MJ, Lu-Yao G et al. Effect of radical prostatectomy for prostate cancer on patient quality of life: results from a Medicare survey. *Urology* 1995; 45:1007-13.

[5] Sacco E, Prayer-Galetti T, Pinto F et al. Urinary incontinence after radical prostatectomy: Incidence by definition, risk factors and temporal trend in a large series with a long-term follow-up. *BJU Int.* 2006; 97: 1234-41.

[6] Staskin D, Tubaro A, Norton PA, Ashton-Miller JA. Mechanisms of continence and surgical cure in female and male SUI: Surgical research initiatives. *Neurourol. Urodyn.* 2011; 30:704-7.

[7] Flynn BJ, Webster GD. Evaluation and surgical management of intrinsic sphincter deficiency after radical prostatectomy. *Rev. Urol.* 2004; 6: 180-6.

[8] Eastham JA, Kattan MW, Rogers E et al. Risk factors for urinary incontinence after radical prostatectomy. *J. Urol.* 1996; 156:1707-13.

[9] Jhaveri JK, Tan GY, Rao S et al. Impact of total anastomotic reconstruction of the bladder neck in obese men: continence outcomes following robotic prostatectomy. *Urology* 2008; 72(suppl 5):S134.

[10] Ridder DD, Rehder P. The Advance male sling: Anatomic features in relation to mode of action. *Eur. Urol.* 2011: Suppl 10:383-9.

[11] Dorschner W, Stolzenburg JU, Neuhaus J. Structure and function of the bladder neck. *Adv. Anat. Embryol. Cell Biol.* 2011; 159:III-XII, 1-109.

[12] Rehder P, Freiin von Gleissenthall G, Pichler R, Glodny B. The treatment of postprostatectomy incontinence with retroluminal transobturator repositioning sling (AdVance): lessons learnt from accumulative experience. *Arch. Esp. Urol.* 2009; 62: 860-70.

[13] Stolzenburg JU, Schwalenberg T, Horn LC et al. Anatomical landmarks of radical prostatectomy. *Eur. Urol.* 2007; 51:629-39.

[14] Dorscher W, Biesold M, Schmidt F, Stolzenburg JU. The dispute about the external sphincter and the urogenital diaphragm. *J. Urol.* 1999; 162: 1942 5.

[15] Burnett etc; Strasser H, Klima G, Poisel S et al. Anatomy and innervation of the rhabdosphincter of the male urethra. *Prostate* 1996; 28:24-31.

[16] Koyanagi T. Studies on the sphincteric system located distally in the urethra: the external urethral sphincter revisited. *J. Urol.* 1980; 124: 400-6.

[17] Burnett AL, Mostwin JL. In situ anatomical study of the male urethral sphincter complex: relevance to continence preservation following major pelvic surgery. J Urol 1998; 160:1301-6.

[18] Oelrich TM. The urethral sphincter in the male. *Am. J. Anat.* 1980; 158: 229-46.

[19] Dorschner W, Stolzenburg JU, Dieterich F. A new theory of micturition and urinary continence based on histomorphological studies. 2. The musculus sphincter vesicae: continence or sexual function? *Urol. Int.* 1994; 54:154-8.

[20] Sebe P, Schwentner C, Oswald J et al. Fetal development of striated and smooth muscle sphincters of the male urethra from a common primordium and modifications due to the development of the prostate: an anatomic and histologic study. *Prostate* 2005; 62: 388-93.

[21] Tanagho EA, Schmidt RA, de Araujo CG. Urinary striated sphincter: what is its nerve supply? *Urology* 1982;20:415-7.

[22] Strasser H, Bartsch G. Anatomy and innervations of the rhabdosphincter of the male urethra. *Semin. Urol. Oncol.* 2000;18:2-8.

[23] Rocco F, Carmignani L, Acquati P et al. Early continence recovery after open radical prostatectomy with restoration of the posterior aspect of the rhabdosphincter. *Eur. Urol.* 2007; 52:376-83.

[24] Strasser H, Klima G, Poisel S et al. Anatomy and innervation of the rhabdosphincter of the male urethra. *Prostate* 1996;28:24-31.

[25] Rocco F, Carmignani L, Acquati P et al. Restoration of posterior aspect of rhabdosphincter shortens continence time after radical retropubic prostatectomy *J. Urol.* 2006; 175:2201-6.

[26] Rocco B, Rocco F. Re: Assessment of early continence after reconstruction of the periprostatic tissues in patients undergoing computer assisted (robotic) prostatectomy: results of a 2 group parallel randomized controlled trial.

[27] Menon M, Muhletaler F, Campos M, Peabody JO. *J. Urol.* 2008; 180:1018-23; *J. Urol.* 2009; 181:1500-1; author reply 1501.

[28] Myers RP. Detrusor apron, associated vascular plexus, and avascular plane: relevance to radical retropubic prostatectomy- anatomic and surgical commentary. *Urology* 2002; 59:472-9.

[29] Dorschner W, Stolzenburg JU, Neuhaus J. Structure and function of bladder neck. In: *Advances in Anatomy, Embryology and Cell Biology*. Berlin: Spinger-Verlag; 2001. P.31-9.

[30] Steiner MS. The puboprostatic ligament and the male urethral suspensory mechanism: an anatomic study. *Urology* 1994;44:530-4.

[31] Deliveliotis C, Protogerou V, Alargof E, Varkarakis J. Radical prostatectomy: bladder neck preservation and puboprostatic ligament sparing- effects on continence and positive margins. *Urology* 2002; 60:855-8.

[32] Schwalenberg T, Neuhaus J, Dartsch M et al. Functional anatomy of the male urinary continence mechanism. *Urologe A* 2010;49:472-80.

[33] Tewari AK, Bigelow K, Rao S et al. Anatomic restoration technique of continence mechanism and preservation of puboprostatic collar: a novel modification to achieve early urinary continence in men undergoing robotic prostatectomy. *Urology* 2007; 69:726-31.

[34] Lee SE, Byun SS, Lee HJ et al. Impact of variations in prostatic apex shape on early recovery of urinary continence after radical retropubic prostatectomy. *Urology* 2006; 68:137-41.

[35] Paparel P, Akin O, Sandhu JS et al. Recovery of urinary continence after radical prostatectomy: association with urethral length and urethral fibrosis measured by

preoperative and postoperative endorectal magnetic resonance imaging. *Eur. Urol.* 2009; 55(3):629-37.

[36] Schlomm T, Heinzer H, Steuber T et al. Full functional-length urethral sphincter preservation during radical prostatectomy. *Eur. Urol.* 2011; 60(2): 320-9.

[37] Nguyen L, Jhaveri J, Tewari A. Surgical technique to overcome anatomical shortcoming: balancing post-prostatectomy continence outcomes of urethral sphincter lengths on preoperative magnetic resonance imaging. *J. Urol.* 2008;179(5):1907-11.

[38] van Randenborgh H, Raul R, Kubler H et al. Improved urinary continence after radical retropubic prostatectomy with preparation of a long, partially intraprostatic portion of the membranous urethra: an analysis of 1013 consecutive cases. *Prostate Cancer Prostatic. Dis.* 2004; 7:253-7.

[39] Hakimi AA, Faleck DM, Agalliu I et al. Preoperative and intraoperative measurements of urethral length as predictors of continence after robot-assisted radical prostatectomy. *J. Endourol.* 2011;25(6):1025-30.

[40] Gosling JA, Dixon JS, Critchley HO, Thompson SA. A comparative study of the human external sphincter and periurethral levator ani muscles. *Br. J. Urol.* 1981;53:35-41.

[41] Myers RP, Cahill DR, Kay PA et al. Puboperinealis: Muscular boundaries of the male urogenital hiatus in 3D from magnetic resonance imaging. *J. Urol.* 2000;164:1412-15.

[42] Jeong SJ, Chung MS, Kim DS et al. Early recovery of urinary continence after radical prostatectomy: correlation with vesico-urethral anastomosis location in the pelvic cavity measured by postoperative cystography. *Int. J. Urol.* 2011;18(6):444-51.

[43] Tuygun C, Imamoglu A, Keyik B et al. Significance of fibrosis around and/or at external urinary sphincter on pelvic magnetic resonance imaging in patients with postprostatectomy incontinence. *Urology* 2006; 68:1308-12.

[44] Nishida S, Utsunomiya N, Nishiyama H et al. Urethral mobility at catheter removal predicts early recovery of urinary continence after radical prostatectomy. *Int. J. Urol.* 2009; 16(4):375-8.

[45] Baader B, Hermann M. Topography of the pelvic autonomic nervous system and its potential impact on surgical intervention in the pelvis. *Clin. Anat.* 2003;16:119-30.

[46] Lunacek A, Schentner C, Fritsch H et al. Anatomical radical retropubic prostatectomy: 'curtain dissection' of the neurovascular bundle. *BJU Int.* 2005; 95:1226-31.

[47] John H, Hauri D. Seminal vesicle-sparing radical prostatectomy: a novel concept to restore early urinary continence. *Urology* 2000;55:820-4.

[48] Costello AJ, Brooks M, Cole OJ. Anatomical studies of the neurovascular bundle and cavernosal nerves. *BJU Int.* 2004;94:1071-6.

[49] Tewari A, Takenaka A, Mtui E et al. The proximal neurovascular plate and the tri-zonal neural architecture around the prostate gland: importance in the athermal robotic technique of nerve-sparing prostatectomy. *BJU Int.* 2006; 98:314-23.

[50] Narayan P, Konety B, Aslam K et al. Neuroanatomy of the external urethral sphincter: implications for urinary continence preservation during radical prostatectomy. *J. Urol.* 1995; 153-337-41.

[51] Karam I, Droupy S, Abd-Alsamad I et al. The precise location and nature of the nerves to the male human urethral histological and immunohistochemical studies with three-dimensional reconstruction. *Eur. Urol.* 2005;48:858-64.

[52] Takenake A, Murakami G, Soga H et al. Anatomical analysis of the neurovascular bundle supplying penile cavernous tissue to ensure a reliable nerve graft after radical prostatectomy. *J. Urol.* 2004; 172: 1032-5.
[53] Nelson CP, Montie JE, McGuire EJ et al. Intraoperative nerve stimulation with measurement of urethral sphincter pressure changes during radical retropubic prostatectomy: a feasibility study. *J. Urol.* 2003; 169:2225-8.
[54] Bianco FJ Jr, Scardino PT, Eastham JA. Radical prostatectomy: long-term cancer control and recovery of sexual and urinary function ("trifecta"). *Urology* 2005;66 (5 suppl):83-94.
[55] Brooks JD, Chao WM, Kerr J. Male pelvic anatomy reconstructed from the visible human data set. *J. Urol.* 1998;159:868-72.
[56] Porzionato A, Macchi V, Gardi M et al. Histotopographic study of the rectourethralis muscle. *Clin. Anat.* 2005;18:510-7.
[57] Soga H, Takenaka A, Murakami G, Fujisawa M. Topographical relationship between urethral rhabdoshpincter and rectourethralis muscle: a better understanding of the apical dissection and the posterior stitches in radical prostatectomy. *Int. J. Urol.* 2008; 15: 729-32.
[58] Sebe P, Oswald J, Fritsch H et al. An embryological study of fetal development of the rectourethralis muscle- does it really exist? *J. Urol.* 2005; 173:583-6.
[59] Song C, Doo CK, Hong JH et al. Relationship between the integrity of the pelvic floor muscles and early recovery of continence after radical prostatectomy. *J. Urol.* 2007; 178(1): 208-11.
[60] Rarekh AR, Feng MI, Kirages D et al. The role of pelvic floor exercises on post-prostatectomy incontinence. *J. Urol.* 2003;170:130-3.
[61] Wimpissinger TF, Tschabitscher M, Feichtinger H, Stackl W. Surgical anatomy of the puboprostatic complex with special reference to radical perineal prostatectomy. *BJU Int.* 2003;92:681-4.
[62] Takenaka A, Hara R, Soga H et al. A novel technique for approaching the endopelvic fascia in retropubic radical prostatectomy, based on an anatomical study of fixed and fresh cadavers. *BJU Int.* 2005; 95: 766-71.
[63] Stolzenburg JU, Rabenalt R, Do M et al. Intrafascial nerve-sparing endoscopic extraperitoneal radical prostatectomy. *Eur. Urol.* 2008; 53: 931-40.
[64] Tewari A, Peabody JO, Fischer M et al. An operative and anatomic study to help in nerve sparing during laparoscopic and robotic radical prostatectomy. *Eur. Urol.* 2003; 43: 444-54.
[65] Graefen M, Walz J, Open retropubic nerve-sparing radical prostatectomy. *Eur. Urol.* 2006; 49:38-48.
[66] Nielsen ME, Schaeffer EM, Marschke P, Walsh PC. High anterior release of the levator fascia improves sexual function following open radical retropubic prostatectomy. *J. Urol.* 2008;180:2557-64, discussion 2564.
[67] Kiyoshima K, Yokomizo A, Yoshida T et al. Anatomical features of periprostatic tissue and its surroundings: a histological analysis of 79 radical retropubic prostatectomy specimens. Jpn. J. Clin. Oncol. 2004; 34:463-8.
[68] Myers RP. Practical surgical anatomy for radical prostatectomy. *Urol. Clin. North Am.* 2001; 28:473-90.

[69] Lindsey I, Guy RJ, Warren BF, Mortensen NJ. Anatomy of Denonvilliers' fascia and pelvic nerves, impotence, and implications for the colorectal surgeon. *Br. J. Surg.* 2000; 87: 1288-99.

[70] Myers RP, Villers A. Anatomic considerations in radical prostatectomy. In: Kirby RS, Partin AW, Feneley M, Parsons JK, eds. *Prostate cancer: Principles and Practice,* Vol 1. Abingdon, UK: Taylor and Francis; 2006, p. 701-13.

[71] van Ophoven A, Roth S. The anatomy and embryological origins of the fascia of Denonvilliers: a medico-historical debate. *J. Urol.* 1997; 157: 3-9.

[72] Savera AT, Kaul S, Badani K et al.Robotic radical prostatectomy with the "veil of Aphrodite" technique: histologic evidence of enhanced nerve sparing. *Eur. Urol.* 2006; 49:1065-74, discussion 1073-4.

[73] Zorn KC, Gofrit ON, Orvieto MA et al. Robotic-assisted laparoscopic prostatectomy: functional and pathologic outcomes with interfascial nerve preservation. *Eur. Urol.* 2007; 51:755-63, discussion 763.

[74] Secin FP, Karanikolas N, Gopalan A et al. The anterior layer of the Denonvilliers' fascia: ac common misconception in the laparoscopic prostatectomy literature. *J. Urol.* 2007; 177:521-5.

[75] Stolzenburg JU, Kallidonis P, Hicks J et al. Effect of bladder neck preservation during endoscopic extraperitoneal radical prostatectomy on urinary continence. *Urol. Int.* 2010; 85(2):135-8.

[76] Licht MR, Klein EA, Tuason L, Levin H. Impact of bladder neck preservation during radical prostatectomy on continence and cancer control. *Urology* 1994;44(6):883-7.

[77] Poon M, Ruckle H, Bamshad BR et al. Radical retropubic prostatectomy: bladder neck preservation versus recontrsuction. *J. Urol.* 2000; 163(1):194-8.

[78] Selli CM, De Antoni P, Moro U et al. ole of bladder neck preservation in urinary continence following radical retropubic prostatectomy. Scand J *Urol. Nephrol.* 2004; 38(1):32-7.

[79] Garg T, See WA. Bladder neck contracture after radical retropubic prostatectomy using an intussuscepted vesico-urethral anastomosis: incidence with long-term follow-up. *BJU Int.* 2009;104(7):925-8.

[80] Teber D, Erdogru T, Cresswell J et al. Analysis of three different vesicourethral anastomotic techqniues in laparoscopic radical prostatectomy. *World J. Urol.* 2008; 26(6):617-22.

[81] Yildirim A, Basok EK, Ilhan AI et al. The impact of urinary drainage on the development of anastomotic stricture after radical retropubic prostatectomy. *Int. Urol. Nephrol.* 2008;40(3):667-73.

[82] Park R, Martin S, Goldberg JD, Lepor H. Anastomotic strictures following radical prostatectomy: insights into incidence, effectiveness of intervention, effect on continence, and factors predisposing to occurrence. *Urology* 2001;57(4):742-6.

[83] Wille S, Mills RD, Studer UE. Absence of urethral post-void milking: an additional cause for incontinence after radical prostatectomy? *Eur. Urol.* 2000; 37(6):665-9.

[84] Bader P, Hugonnet CL, Burkhard FC, Studer UE. Inefficient urethral milking secondary to urethral dysfunction as an additional risk factor for incontinence after radical prostatectomy. *J. Urol.* 2001;166(6):2247-52.

[85] *EAU guidelines.*

[86] *AUA guidelines.*

[87] Hunter KF, Moore KN, Glazener CMA. Conservative management for postprostatectomy urinary incontinence. *Coch. Datab. Syst. Rev.* 2007. CD001843.

[88] Rehder P, Webster G. The AdVance male sling: patient selection and workup. *Eur. Urol.* 2011;suppl 10:390-4.

[89] Rehder P, Freiin von Gleissenthall G, Pichler R et al. The treatment of post-prostatectomy incontinence with the retroluminal transobturator repositioning sling (AdVance): lessons learnt from accumulative experience. *Arch. Esp. Urol.* 2009; 62: 860-70.

In: Urinary Incontinence
Editor: Eric Chung
ISBN: 978-1-62618-482-4

Chapter 15

Overactive Bladder and Benign Prostatic Hyperplasia: Pathophysiology, Diagnosis and Treatment

Ian McKenzie and Eric Chung
Department of Urology, Princess Alexandra Hospital, Brisbane QLD, Australia

Abstract

Several large population based studies have shown significant overlap between the presence of storage (overactive bladder) and voiding (bladder outlet obstruction) symptoms in men. Long standing bladder outlet obstruction from benign prostatic hyperplasia (BPH) can be associated with detrusor smooth muscle hypertrophy and detrusor overactivty. While the exact pathophysiology for the development of overactive bladder (OAB) in men with BPH has not been fully elucidated, several proposed theories have been put forward and these include progressive denervation of detrusor smooth muscle cells, aberrant sensory feedback mechanism and long-term progressive arterial insufficiency. Behavioural modifications and the use of α-blockers, 5 alpha-reductase inhibitor and anticholinergic drugs either individually or in combination, should be instituted once reversible and/or other sinister causes have been excluded. If medical therapy is unsuccessful, more invasive investigations with urodynamic studies and possibly cystourethroscopy is recommended to guide further treatment.

Bladder overactivity has been described under numerous terminology such as unstable bladder, detrusor instability and detrusor hyperreflexia, over the years. As further work has been done to investigate the potential causes for bladder overactivity it became clear that these descriptions could be classified under a unifying term the Overactive Bladder (OAB). This term was defined in a publication by Abrams and Wein in 1999 following a conference on the subject at the International Continence Society (ICS). The ICS revised the definition in 2002 (revision published in 2003) in their position paper to standardize the terminology in lower urinary tract function [1]. OAB was defined as urgency, with or without urge incontinence, usually with frequency and nocturia. Urgency is the complaint of the sudden compelling desire to void, which is difficult to defer. Urge incontinence is the complaint of involuntary leakage of urine accompanied by or immediately preceded by urgency. Frequency is the complaint by the patient that he or she voids too often by day. Nocturia is the complaint that the individual has to wake at night one or more times to void [1]. All these lower urinary tract symptoms fit under the broad overarching description of storage symptoms.

This definition of overactive bladder is based on symptoms elicited during history taking from the patient. Likewise, history is vitally important in eliciting each patient's symptom complex with respect to the other two broad categories of lower urinary tract symptoms (LUTS), those of voiding and post-micturition. Therefore estimates of the prevalence of these symptoms have mostly been gathered from questionnaire based population studies. Early studies of the prevalence of OAB suffered from varying definitions of the condition. Since the ICS consensus definition in 2002, several large population based studies have been conducted to examine the community prevalence of OAB using this definition. The first large study was the EPIC study, a multinational telephone-based cross-sectional survey. This study assessed LUTS in the general population across five countries. This demonstrated an overall prevalence of OAB of 11.8%. Prevalence was similar in both men and women, and increased in a linear fashion with increasing age. It also showed that there was significant overlap between presence of storage, voiding and post micturition symptoms, with the prevalence of combined storage and voiding LUTS being 17.7% in men and 14.9% in women [2, 3].

The NOBLE study, a telephone-based cross-sectional survey conducted in United States looked specifically at the prevalence of OAB in the general population. This was a smaller study with 5204 participants and demonstrated a prevalence of OAB of 16.5% overall which was higher than that in the larger EPIC study. It however supported the data of EPIC with rates of OAB being similar in men and women, and again prevalence increased with increasing age [4].

The largest population-based study to date, the EpiLUTS study, was an internet based questionnaire conducted across the UK, United States and Sweden, with a total of 30,000 participants, designed to assess both the prevalence of individual LUTS, but also the degree of bother to participants caused by LUTS within the general population. This study used a 5 point scale to assess presence of symptoms. Using the definition of OAB symptoms as 'sometimes present' demonstrated a much higher prevalence of 22.4% for men and 35.7% for women, whereas OAB symptoms present 'often' demonstrated a much lower prevalence of 4.9% for men and 11.1% for women [5]. This survey demonstrates the inherent flaws in questionnaire-based studies with responses strongly influenced by how the question is answered. Regardless, all these population-based studies demonstrate that OAB is common in the general community with a likely prevalence around 11%, with rates similar in both men and women, and increasing in prevalence with increasing age [6].

Pathophysiology

OAB frequently coexists with bladder outlet obstruction (BOO), and can be present in up to 45% of men with BOO [7-9]. It can also however occur in isolation. As shown above,

OAB is present in women at similar rates to men, however BOO is much less common in women than men [10]. There are multiple theories regarding the aetiology of overactive bladder. The majority of these address one of the main underlying causes, detrusor overactivity. The ICS defines detrusor overactivity (DO) as the urodynamic observation characterized by involuntary detrusor contractions during the filling phase which may be spontaneous or provoked [1]. This is because it can be measured objectively using urodynamic studies and therefore is more amenable to scientific research. The subjective nature of urgency symptoms makes them much more difficult to investigate in the laboratory to assess underlying pathophysiology. Previously DO was believed to be the underlying cause of overactive bladder occurring during bladder filling. More recent investigations however demonstrate that urodynamically proven DO does not correlate well with symptomatic urgency and OAB. While DO correlates well with urge incontinence, this is not the case with urgency alone [8]. Not all patients with urgency have DO and not all DO on ambulatory urodynamic studies causes urinary urgency [11]. It is likely that the pathophysiology of OAB is diverse and complex and may differ between patients.

The sensation of bladder fullness travels by the afferent pelvic nerves to the spinal cord with spinal cord efferent nerves stimulating detrusor muscle contraction and bladder neck relaxation. In between are interneurons, which transmit this information to higher centres. The spinal cord micturition reflex is normally under higher centre control from the cortex and brainstem through an intact spinal cord. This reflex can normally be stimulated by both the normal passive bladder distension and active detrusor contraction, but also chemical irritation or thermal stimulation of the bladder mucosa [12, 13]. It is thought that OAB and DO may result from abnormally increased afferent signaling by various methods of sensitization or multiplication of these receptors.

The hypothesis of neurogenic DO can result from any disruption to higher centre control over the micturition reflex, either at the brain or brainstem level, such as with cerebrovascular injury, or damage to the spinal cord decreasing the feedback inhibition [13]. Alternatively sensitization of bladder receptors can lead to inappropriate afferent signaling to stimulate detrusor contraction [14].

A second hypothesis involves changes at the muscle cell level (myogenic hypothesis). This suggests that alterations in smooth muscle cells, by partial denervation, are more prone to spontaneous excitability and contraction. Similarly changes in cell-to cell signaling can lead to more rapid propagation of an abnormal contraction between muscle cells allowing widespread detrusor contraction [10, 14, 15].

The third hypothesis is the integrative hypothesis. This contends that spontaneous localized contractions (micro-motions) of smooth muscle are a normal physiological mechanism to report bladder filling via an interaction between urothelial and interstitial cells. Any alteration in these interactions can cause exaggerated micro-motions resulting in OAB, or excessive propagation resulting in DO [14, 16, 17].

In keeping with these hypotheses, theories to explain the presence of DO with bladder outlet obstruction have been developed and widely investigated. Long-standing BOO leads to bladder smooth muscle hypertrophy. This hypertrophy has been documented to cause a variety of changes, in particular a progressive denervation of muscle cells, which has been demonstrated in both human and animal studies [17, 18]. The larger muscle mass has also been shown to undergo a relative ischaemia with bladder filling and bladder wall distension which also may contribute to denervation of cells. This is due to a greater oxygen demand of the hypertrophied muscle, and decreased oxygen supply in the presence of increased intravesical pressures [10]. This hypertrophy alters the smooth muscle cell-to-cell junctions perhaps by allowing a more rapid propagation of depolarization between these cells. Increased outflow resistance of the bladder has also been shown to change the electrical properties of smooth muscle with re-organisation of the C-fibre-mediated micturition reflex [18, 19]. Whilst this bestows a greater mechanical ability with stronger and faster contractions of muscle cells, it also provides the ability for involuntary activation of cells and propagation of this signal between cells with muscle contraction on a wide front. Another suggested mechanism is that abnormal sensory stimuli from an anatomically altered prostatic urethra can stimulate DO.

One study demonstrated an elimination of DO by local anaesthetic block of the urethra without relieving the outflow obstruction [20]. A similar finding was made in a study of men treated for bladder outlet obstruction with transurethral incision of the prostate. They showed that the majority of men, all with pre-operative urodynamically demonstrated outflow obstruction, had symptomatic improvement regardless of whether outflow obstruction was improved or not [21].

As stated above, not all OAB and DO is related to bladder outlet obstruction. Clearly there are complex changes at the bladder level that can cause OAB symptoms independent of outflow alteration. One possibility that has been investigated is that long-term progressive arterial insufficiency, with associated ischaemia, hypoxia and oxidative stress functionally and structurally alters detrusor smooth muscle leading to DO. A study by Ponholzer assessed the rate of LUTS with vascular risk factors (hypertension, hyperlipidaemia, diabetes and smoking). They found that the incidence of LUTS increased significantly in patients with 2 or more risk factors suggesting an underlying vascular mechanism to their urinary symptoms [22]. This phenomenon has been demonstrated in multiple animal studies. A recent study of rats demonstrated sensitization of afferent nerve signaling mediated by oxidative stress, resulting in DO [18]. This explanation would support the findings of increased prevalence of OAB with increasing age in both sexes, similar to the increased rates of atherosclerotic vascular disease with aging.

Ultimately, while there are many theories, the exact aetiology of overactive bladder has not been fully elucidated. Certainly it is likely that a combination of factors results in both altered sensation of bladder filling and unstable detrusor contractions resulting in a sense of urgency to void. The belief that OAB is solely due to DO has been shown to be inaccurate. The main treatments used focus on cholinergic receptors, implicated in neurogenically mediated DO. Clearly there is an element of heightened sensation of bladder filling unrelated to detrusor activity which may assist in directing treatment for those refractory to initial therapy in the future [7].

Diagnosis

The diagnosis of overactive bladder is, by definition a clinical diagnosis. The important aspect of diagnosing OAB is not just the presence or absence of urinary symptoms, but also the frequency and severity of symptoms, as well as how much these symptoms are affecting the patients quality of life. The presence of urgency, with at least one other symptom is essential for the diagnosis of OAB [1]. Any associated storage, voiding or post-micturition symptoms must also be elucidated. It is also necessary to exclude underlying reversible causes such as urinary infection, endocrine, malignant and neurological conditions. The initial diagnosis therefore involves at least, a full history of symptoms, physical examination and basic investigations such as urinalysis and formal microscopy and culture, and assessment of adequacy of bladder emptying [14].

Pelvic examination must also be performed to assess for pelvic masses, evaluate prostatic enlargement or malignancy. Adequacy of bladder emptying can initially be assessed by abdominal palpation for a distended bladder. A more accurate assessment can be achieved through simple bedside post-void ultrasound scan of the bladder, or with formal urinary tract ultrasound. Urinary tract ultrasound also allows assessment of other causes of urinary symptoms such as abdominal masses and urolithiasis. As OAB symptoms frequently overlap with voiding symptoms, uroflowmetry, simply performed in the clinic, can assess for outflow obstruction at the same time [23, 24]. Another useful assessment tool is a bladder diary. This allows the patient to document, over a period of time, the frequency and volume of voids, any associated urgency or incontinence, and the volume of fluid intake. This can also be useful for more objectively assessing the effect of treatment on a patient's lower urinary tract symptoms [14].

As stated earlier, OAB has been presumed to be partly due to involuntary detrusor contractions. This cannot be objectively measured by symptomatology alone. The best method for this is formal urodynamic studies assessing for unstable detrusor contractions during bladder filling. This however is an invasive, costly and relatively time-consuming test. Furthermore, it is also not 100% sensitive at detecting the presence of DO, which may not be presence during the urodynamic study [8, 11]. For these reasons, it is a common practice is to trial the patient on conservative medical therapy before subjecting the patient to a formal urodynamic study [23].

Also, the drugs used for initial management of OAB are generally safe and efficacious making a trial of therapy prior to invasive testing a valid approach to the management of OAB [14, 24-26]. Indeed the ICS guidelines on the management of urinary incontinence recommends that urodynamic testing for patients with OAB be reserved for those patients that fail initial medical therapy [23].

Management

As discussed in the previous section, it is reasonable to trial initial management of patients with symptom diagnosed OAB. Standard first-line therapy for OAB involves behavioural management [14, 27, 28]. This can include any of:

1. Fluid Management

Teaching the patient to adjust their fluid intake, both in terms of quantity and type of fluid can improve symptoms dramatically. This is where a bladder diary can be extremely useful for assessment of intake, and exacerbating agents such as caffeinated or alcohol containing fluids. If nocturia is especially problematic, decreasing nocturnal fluid intake can be beneficial.

2. Bladder Training

Regular, frequent voiding at fixed time intervals can avoid bladder filling to a volume sufficient to induce a sense of urgency. Having the patient electively void at regular intervals, can improve the distressing urgency and urge incontinence that can occur with bladder distention. Starting at short time intervals, and progressively increasing the time between voids with an aim to reach periods of 2-4 hour intervals. There is however little good evidence of efficacy in the long-term however combination with medical therapy has been shown to produce good efficacy for controlling the symptoms of OAB [29].

Other behavioural modifications such as timed voiding have been used but there is little evidence to support their efficacy in the long term [14].

3. Medical Therapy

The first drug class of choice is usually anticholinergics such as Oxybutynin, Solifenacin, Tolterodine, Darifenacin and Propiverine. All these drugs have been investigated and are effective in the management of overactive bladder symptoms [14, 26]. These drugs block muscarinic receptors on detrusor muscle, inhibiting the action of acetylcholine and effectively decreasing the ability of the bladder to contract [26], thereby improving urinary urgency and increasing the bladder capacity. The exact mechanism for their effect on OAB symptoms remains unclear though they likely act at multiple sites. It is widely accepted that there is no sacral parasympathetic outflow to the bladder during filling [26, 30]. It is believed therefore that their mechanism of action occurs through the inhibition of an acetylcholine-mediated stimulation of detrusor tone, resulting in bladder relaxation and maintenance of low bladder tone during filling. In high doses, anticholinergic can cause urinary retention, and this is a well recognized complication of their use particularly in older patients and those with detrusor hypocontractility [31]. Fortunately the risk of urinary retention is uncommon especially if the pre-treatment bladder residual volume is low [25, 26]. Therefore it is important that post void bladder residual volume be checked prior to the commencement of anticholinergic. These drugs are also not selective for the bladder. They therefore can cause peripheral and to a lesser extent CNS side effects. These can include constipation, dry mouth and tachycardia and loss of accommodation. They are also contraindicated in narrow angle glaucoma [14, 26, 27]. These side effects can be prohibitive for patients therefore decreasing their usefulness clinically.

A Cochrane review of anticholinergic therapy for OAB versus non-drug therapy (in the form of bladder training) was released in 2009. This systematic review of controlled trials demonstrated a benefit for anticholinergic therapy for OAB symptom control. The benefit for anticholinergic therapy combined with bladder training was found to be greater than that of either therapy alone [29]. A further review of randomised controlled trials by Chapple et al. concluded that anticholinergics are safe, efficacious and well-tolerated treatments for overactive bladder symptoms [32]. On this basis, it seems valid to trial a patient on anticholinergic therapy, even before more invasive investigations if a diagnosis of OAB has been made.

There remains therefore the question of the patient with combined OAB and bladder outlet obstruction. As stated, approximately 45% of men with bladder outlet obstruction have concomitant symptoms of OAB. The most common medical therapy for bladder outlet obstruction is α-adrenergic antagonists.

These agents act to relieve with dynamic obstruction associated with increased smooth muscle tone with benign prostatic hypertrophy [26]. In the past, anticholinergic therapy had been avoided in this group of patients due to concerns about aggravating their voiding symptoms or causing urinary retention. More recently, studies have looked at managing patients with both voiding and storage symptoms with α-blockers either alone, or in combination with anticholinergic therapy.

Multiple randomized controlled trials and observational studies have been performed on various anticholinergic drugs used alone, or in combination with alpha (α)-blockers. Meta-analyses of these studies showed that monotherapy with anticholinergic drugs has been overall disappointing [25, 33]. The α-blockers remain the most widely used pharmacologic agents for relief of bladder outlet resistance and are targeted at the dynamic component (increased smooth muscle tone) of BPH. Considering the prevalence and severity of storage symptoms in male patients with increasing age, it is reasonably expected that a combination therapy comprising an α-blocker and an anticholinergic would significantly alleviate OAB and BPH symptoms.

However a more pragmatic approach to real-life practice is to use sequential therapy, where patient is first treated with an α-blocker, and those with continuing OAB symptoms at follow up have an anticholinergic agent added to their therapy. The addition of an anticholinergic agent has been shown to significantly improve symptoms and associated quality of life, with minimal effect on urine flow [25, 32, 33]. For those who fail to adequately respond and have residual symptoms of OAB, an anticholinergic agent can safely be trialled after proper assessment of post-micturition residual volumes [25, 32, 33]. For those patients with elevated residual volumes pre-treatment, there is unfortunately still insufficient data to recommend use of anticholinergic therapy.

The 5-alpha reductase inhibitors (5ARI), such as finasteride and dutasteride, are a class of drug used to treat bladder outlet obstruction and works by reducing the volume of BPH. They have been shown to be safe and effective both used alone, and in combination with α-blockers [27]. An approach to the use of these drugs for OAB associated with bladder outlet obstruction has mirrored that of α-blockers [33]. While there is minimal good quality evidence available, the addition of anticholinergic agents for patients with persistent symptoms of OAB after 6 months of therapy with 5ARIs, has been shown to further improve symptoms and quality of life measures. Similarly, in these studies the incidence of urinary retention was low [33].

More recently the role of phosphodiesterase type 5 (PDE5) inhibitors have been shown to be effective with favorable effect-to-side effect ratio in treatment of BPH/LUTS and the OAB [34]. Immunohistochemical studies revealed the distribution of PDE4 and PDE5 in stromal and glandular areas of the transition zone, and in detrusor muscle fibers and the vascular endothelium.

Therefore the use of PDE5 inhibitors not only alter the blood supply and growth pattern of prostatic stromal and glandular compartments (BPH/LUTS) but also directly on smooth muscle of detrusor to help prevent deleterious alterations of the histological structure of the urinary bladder that may lead to disturbances in urine storage and voiding [34]. This novel approach requires further studies to delineate if PDE inhibitors may gain significance in the treatment of BPH/LUTS, OAB and urge incontinence.

4. Intravesical Therapy

Intravesical therapy has been used with some success for management of OAB and botulinum toxin is perhaps the most promising of these agents. It blocks the release of acetylcholine and other transmitters from pre-synaptic nerve endings. This results in decreased muscle contractility and muscle atrophy at the injection site. This results in a chemical denervation, which reverses with axonal regeneration over 3-6 months. Published literature on intravesical Botulinum toxin A has mostly focused on neurogenic DO with good safety and efficacy, and durable results even with repeat treatments. While there are few studies assessing idiopathic DO, the outcomes have been positive [14, 35]. The ICS position is that intravesical therapy should still be considered second-line therapy at this stage [23].

5. Surgical Treatment

Surgical management of LUTS can be directed at management of either bladder outlet obstruction or DO. Surgical treatment of bladder outlet obstruction is common and usually performed for men whose obstructive symptoms fail to respond to conservative or medical therapy, or for men who have failed to return to spontaneous voiding after catheterization for urinary retention. This is usually in the form of trans-urethral resection of the prostate (TURP) although more recently, laser enucleation and resection of the prostate have become more common. While these treatments are designed to relieve outflow obstruction, studies have shown that they can impact positively on OAB symptoms as well. This seems to be particularly the case in young men, one early study demonstrating that over 60% of men undergoing TURP for lower urinary symptoms, showed improvement in urodynamically demonstrated DO. Symptoms of DO, present in 60% of men pre-operatively, remained in only 25% of men post-operatively. Frequency and nocturia symptoms improved in 60-70% of patients [36]. A more recent study, assessing the long-term efficacy of prostatectomy versus monitoring only, demonstrated a return of DO in the long-term after initial post-operative resolution. In fact, in the long-term follow-up (over 13 years), most men demonstrated DO regardless of treatment [37]. This may mean that long-term bladder outlet obstruction causes irreversible changes to the bladder, which cause persistent increased sensation and overactivity after relief of obstruction. Alternately, it may agree with the theory that changes, possibly age-related occur within the bladder separate to the results of outflow obstruction causing the symptoms of OAB [10]. A study by De Nunzio et al. demonstrated a more significant improvement in DO in men undergoing TURP than medical therapy for bladder outlet obstruction. This occurred despite improvements in flow-pressure measurements in all groups analysed [38].

Surgical management of OAB is reserved for the truly intractable cases. Options include neural stimulation or modulation, detrusor myomyectomy or augmentation cystoplasty [24].

Neural modulation is the least invasive of these therapies. It is believed to work via suppression of inter-neuronal transmission in the micturition reflex pathway. Sacral nerve stimulation has been used for OAB and one randomized prospective study showed significant improvement in frequency, urgency and quality of life measures. Switching off of stimulators at 6 months in this study lead to return to baseline voiding function in these patients. Efficacy of treatment remained up to 24 months post-implantation [39].

Conclusion

OAB is a common, debilitating symptom complex with likely diverse underlying pathophysiology. It is frequently, though not always associated with bladder outlet obstruction. Diagnosis and initial management should be based on thorough history, examination and basic investigations to exclude underlying treatable causes such as infection and malignancy.

Initial therapy with behavioural modification and medical therapy with anticholinergic drugs can then safely be instituted after assessment of bladder emptying. Concomitant bladder outlet obstruction can be managed with medical therapy with α-blockers or 5ARIs alone or in combination.

An anticholinergic agent can be safely and successfully added to treatment for patients whose symptoms fail to respond. While the risk of urinary retention is low in the published literature, these are all conducted on men with low post-void residual volumes. There is still insufficient information to know exactly which patients are suitable for this therapy. It would seem that as long as the post-void residual remains low (<200mL) and urinary flow rate is not significantly impaired, it is then safe to trial this combination. If medical therapy is unsuccessful, further more invasive investigation with urodynamic studies and possibly cystourethroscopy is recommended to guide further treatment such as intravesical therapy and surgery. Further research into the pathophysiology of this very common condition will hopefully guide future developments in management.

References

[1] Abrams, P. et al. The standardisation of terminology in lower urinary tract function: report from the standardisation sub-committee of the International Continence Society. *Urology* 61, 37-49, (2003).

[2] Irwin, D. E. et al. Population-based survey of urinary incontinence, overactive bladder, and other lower urinary tract symptoms in five countries: results of the EPIC study. *Eur. Urol.* 50, 1306-1314; discussion 1314-1305, (2006).

[3] Irwin, D. E. et al. Prevalence, severity, and symptom bother of lower urinary tract symptoms among men in the EPIC study: impact of overactive bladder. *Eur. Urol.* 56, 14-20, (2009).

[4] Stewart, W. F. et al. Prevalence and burden of overactive bladder in the United States. *World J. Urol.* 20, 327-336, (2003).

[5] Coyne, K. S. et al. The prevalence of lower urinary tract symptoms (LUTS) in the USA, the UK and Sweden: results from the Epidemiology of LUTS (EpiLUTS) study. *BJU Int.* 104, 352-360, (2009).
[6] Irwin, D. E., Kopp, Z. S., Agatep, B., Milsom, I. and Abrams, P. Worldwide prevalence estimates of lower urinary tract symptoms, overactive bladder, urinary incontinence and bladder outlet obstruction. *BJU Int.* 108, 1132-1138, (2011).
[7] Chapple, C. R. and Roehrborn, C. G. A shifted paradigm for the further understanding, evaluation, and treatment of lower urinary tract symptoms in men: focus on the bladder. *Eur. Urol.* 49, 651-658, (2006).
[8] Hyman, M. J., Groutz, A. and Blaivas, J. G. Detrusor instability in men: correlation of lower urinary tract symptoms with urodynamic findings. *J. Urol.* 166, 550-552; discussion 553, (2001).
[9] Knutson, T., Edlund, C., Fall, M. and Dahlstrand, C. BPH with coexisting overactive bladder dysfunction--an everyday urological dilemma. *Neurourol. Urodyn.* 20, 237-247, (2001).
[10] Abdel-Aziz, K. F. and Lemack, G. E. Overactive bladder in the male patient: bladder, outlet, or both? *Curr. Urol. Rep.* 3, 445-451 (2002).
[11] Bradshaw, H. D., Radley, S. C., Rosario, D. J. and Chapple, C. R. Towards a better understanding of involuntary detrusor activity. *BJU Int.* 95, 799-803, (2005).
[12] Birder, L. et al. Neural control of the lower urinary tract: peripheral and spinal mechanisms. *Neurourol. Urodyn.* 29, 128-139, (2010).
[13] de Groat, W. C. A neurologic basis for the overactive bladder. *Urology* 50, 36-52; discussion 53-36 (1997).
[14] Foon, R. and Drake, M. J. The Overactive Bladder. *Therapeutic Advances in Urology* 2, 147-155 (2010).
[15] Brading, A. F. A myogenic basis for the overactive bladder. *Urology* 50, 57-67; discussion 68-73 (1997).
[16] Drake, M. J., Mills, I. W. and Gillespie, J. I. Model of peripheral autonomous modules and a myovesical plexus in normal and overactive bladder function. *Lancet* 358, 401-403, (2001).
[17] Andersson, K. E. Storage and voiding symptoms: pathophysiologic aspects. *Urology* 62, 3-10, (2003).
[18] Yamaguchi, O., Aikawa, K., Shishido, K. and Nomiya, M. Place of overactive bladder in male lower urinary tract symptoms. *World J. Urol.* 27, 723-728, (2009).
[19] Steers, W. D. Pathophysiology of overactive bladder and urge urinary incontinence. *Rev. Urol.* 4 Suppl 4, S7-S18 (2002).
[20] Yokoyama, O., Nagano, K., Kawaguchi, K., Ueki, O. and Ohkawa, M. The influence of prostatic urethral anesthesia in overactive detrusor in patients with benign prostatic hyperplasia. *J. Urol.*151,1554-1556(1994).
[21] Sirls, L. T. et al. Transurethral incision of the prostate: an objective and subjective evaluation of long-term efficacy. *J. Urol.* 150, 1615-1621 (1993).
[22] Ponholzer, A., Temml, C., Wehrberger, C., Marszalek, M. and Madersbacher, S. The association between vascular risk factors and lower urinary tract symptoms in both sexes. *Eur. Urol.* 50, 581-586, (2006).
[23] Abrams, P. et al. Fourth International Consultation on Incontinence Recommendations of the International Scientific Committee: Evaluation and treatment of urinary

incontinence, pelvic organ prolapse, and fecal incontinence. *Neurourol. Urodyn.* 29, 213-240, (2010).

[24] Abrams and Drake. in *Campbell-Walsh Urology* Vol. 3 eds Wein AJ et al. Ch. 61, 2079-2090 (Saunders Elsevier, 2007).

[25] Chapple, C. Antimuscarinics in men with lower urinary tract symptoms suggestive of bladder outlet obstruction due to benign prostatic hyperplasia. *Curr. Opin. Urol.* 20, 43-48, (2010).

[26] Andersson, K. E. et al. Pharmacological treatment of overactive bladder: report from the International Consultation on Incontinence. *Curr. Opin. Urol.* 19, 380-394, (2009).

[27] Woo, H. H., Gillman, M. P., Gardiner, R., Marshall, V. and Lynch, W. J. A practical approach to the management of lower urinary tract symptoms among men. *Med. J. Aust.* 195, 34-39, (2011).

[28] Payne. in *Campbell-Walsh Urology* Vol. 3 eds Wein AJ et al. Ch. 63, 2125-2146 (Saunders Elsevier, 2007).

[29] Alhasso, A. A., McKinlay, J., Patrick, K. and Stewart, L. Anticholinergic drugs versus non-drug active therapies for overactive bladder syndrome in adults. *Cochrane Database Syst. Rev.*, CD003193, (2006).

[30] Athanasopoulos, A. Antimuscarinics and bladder outlet obstruction: From a contraindication to an indication? *Neurourol. Urodyn.* 29 Suppl 1, S46-50, (2010).

[31] Andersson, K. E. Antimuscarinics for treatment of overactive bladder. *Lancet Neurol.* 3, 46-53, (2004).

[32] Chapple, C. R. et al. The effects of antimuscarinic treatments in overactive bladder: an update of a systematic review and meta-analysis. *Eur. Urol.* 54, 543-562, (2008).

[33] Athanasopoulos, A. et al. The role of antimuscarinics in the management of men with symptoms of overactive bladder associated with concomitant bladder outlet obstruction: an update. *Eur. Urol.* 60, 94-105, (2011).

[34] Uckert S and Oelke M. Phosphodiesterase (PDE) inhibitors in the treatment of lower urinary tract dysfunction. *Br. J. Clin. Pharmacol.* 72(2), 197-204 (2011)

[35] Duthie, J. B., Vincent, M., Herbison, G. P., Wilson, D. I. and Wilson, D. Botulinum toxin injections for adults with overactive bladder syndrome. Cochrane *Database Syst. Rev.* 12, CD005493, (2011).

[36] Abrams, P. H., Farrar, D. J., Turner-Warwick, R. T., Whiteside, C. G. and Feneley, R. C. The results of prostatectomy: a symptomatic and urodynamic analysis of 152 patients. *J. Urol.* 121, 640-642 (1979).

[37] Thomas, A. W. and Abrams, P. Lower urinary tract symptoms, benign prostatic obstruction and the overactive bladder. *BJU Int.* 85 Suppl 3, 57-68; discussion 70-51 (2000).

[38] de Nunzio, C. et al. The evolution of detrusor overactivity after watchful waiting, medical therapy and surgery in patients with bladder outlet obstruction. *J. Urol.* 169, 535-539, (2003).

[39] Hassouna, M. M. et al. Sacral neuromodulation in the treatment of urgency-frequency symptoms: a multicenter study on efficacy and safety. *J. Urol.* 163, 1849-1854 (2000).

In: Urinary Incontinence
Editor: Eric Chung
ISBN: 978-1-62618-482-4

Chapter 16

Surgical Treatment for Male Stress Urinary Incontinence

Eric Chung*
Department of Urology, Princess Alexandra Hospital, Brisbane QLD, Australia

Abstract

While research has shown that urinary incontinence (UI) affects women about twice as common as men, one in twenty men suffer from UI and this figure is higher in older men. Men with chronic illness, depression, pelvic trauma and prostatic diseases especially prostate cancer, are associated with higher risk of stress urinary incontinence (SUI). In the past, the options for the treatment of male SUI following failure of conservative measures were limited. Men are offered bulking agents if the SUI is mild or received artificial urinary sphincter (AUS) in severe cases. Over the last decade, the introduction of various synthetic male slings and other surgical urinary continent devices has expanded the armamentarium in the surgical treatment of male SUI. This chapter evaluates the current surgical options and clinical outcomes following the surgical treatment of male SUI.

Introduction

Stress urinary incontinence (SUI) is defined as involuntary leakage of urine on effort or exertion, or on sneezing or coughing [1]. The incidence and prevalence of female SUI far outnumber that of male SUI. However, male SUI is an increasingly common condition particularly following surgery for prostate cancer and can occur in upwards of 60% of men in the initial months post radical prostatectomy [2]. Due to the substantial numbers of radical prostatectomy performed following the advent of prostate specific antigen testing and greater public awareness for prostate cancer, there is an increasing number post-prostatectomy SUI.

* Corresponding author: Dr Eric Chung, Department of Urology, Princess Alexandra Hospital, Ipswich Rd, Brisbane QLD 4103, Australia. (T): +617-33242468, (F):+617-33242546, ericchg@hotmail.com.

The incidence of post-prostatectomy urinary incontinence (PPI) depends on the definition of urinary incontinence and the length of follow up [3]. Although most cases of PPI resolve within months using conservative treatment option such as pelvic floor physiotherapy and trial of pharmacotherapy, some 5-10% of men continue to experience PPI at 12 months post-prostatectomy [4]. In these men, PPI remains a debilitating disorder that markedly impairs the quality of life and is associated with significant social stigmata and economic burden [5].

In patients with persistent PPI, surgical treatment is recommended [6]. Presently, there are no guidelines concerning the timing of surgical treatment in the postoperative setting. Furthermore there is no accepted formal definition of the degree of SUI and the choice of various surgical treatments although most experts agree that men with mild to moderate SUI should receive male slings while men with severe SUI need artificial urinary sphincter (AUS) implant [7]. In recent years, a plethora of minimal invasive treatment options for male SUI have become commercially available [7]. While these synthetic male slings are effective in men with SUI, the AUS has shown excellent clinical success rate and to date remains the gold standard of male SUI treatment [8]. Nonetheless, when given the choice, most men with post-prostatectomy SUI opt for less invasive treatment options over the AUS [9]. The following chapter evaluate the contemporary management of post-prostatectomy SUI.

1. Urethral Bulking Agents

Urethral bulking agents work by adding bulk to the urethral wall to improve urinary continence by increasing bladder neck and sphincter coaptation. It remains the most minimally invasive treatment for PPI after conservative measures. Several agents have been used including bovine collagen (Contigen; Bard, Covington, Georgia, USA), and silicone macroparticles (Macroplastique; Uroplasty, Minnetonka, Minnesota, USA). The success rates for PPI range from 36%-69%, with 4-20% of patients reported to be dry [10-12]. Several main issues pertaining to urethral bulking injections are low cure rate, the need for multiple injections, and deterioration of effect over time. Collagen injection success rate diminishes in patients who receive radiotherapy, high grade SUI, low abdominal leak point pressure and significantly scarred or stricture urethra [13].

More recently, Mitterbeger [14] reported the first human trial of injecting myoblasts and fibroblast around the rhabdosphincter. While the initial reported cure rate was impressive at 65%, a later retraction of similar data from the authors cast doubt on the validity of this trial.

2. Male Slings (See Table 1)

In the last ten years, synthetic slings for PPI have gained popularity because of cost and its non-mechanical action. Most experts agree that proper patient selection is paramount for urinary sling to be effective [15]. The ideal candidate should have mild to moderate degree of SUI with adequate residual sphincter function and is able to generate strong detrusor contraction to overcome the fixed resistance of the sling in order to void. Although Berry [16] was the first to describe the male sling, it was Kaufman [17] who popularised one of the earlier external compressive devices of the bulbous urethra for the treatment of PPI.

Table 1. Surgical treatment of PPI

Device	Maker	Description	Mode of action	References
Invance	American Medical Systems	Bone-anchored silicon rectangular sling	Compresses bulbar urethra	[22-27]
Argus	Promedon	Adjustable sling with silicone foam and conical elements/washers	Compresses bulbar urethra	[29-31]
Remeex	Neomedic	Adjustable sling with mesh and mechanical regulator	Compresses bulbar urethra	[32-34]
AdVance	American Medical Systems	Polypropylene mesh sling; 2 arms	Relocates bulbar urethra	[35-45]
Virtue	Coloplast	Polypropylene mesh sling; 4 arms	Compresses and relocates bulbar urethra	[47-50]
AMS 800	American Medical Systems	3 pieces; 3 parts - Urethral cuff - Pressure regulating balloon - Control pump	Occluding cuff	[51-58]
Flowsecure	?	1 piece; 4 parts - Regulator balloon - Stress release balloon - Urethral cuff - Control pump	Occluding cuff	[61-65]
Zephyr ZSI375	Mayor group	1 piece; 2 parts - Urethral cuff - Pressure regulating tank	Occluding cuff	[66]
Pro-ACT	Uromedia	2 piece; 2 parts -Silicone balloon with titanium ports X2	Occluding 'cuff'	[67-71]
Periconstrictor device	Silimed	2 piece; 2 parts - Urethral cuff - Self sealing port	Occluding cuff	[72-73]

Nonetheless Kaufman's urinary device was associated with low success rates and high complication rates resulting in these slings fell out of favour [18].

Since then various male sling procedures have been developed for the treatment of male SUI. Furthermore it was shown that more than 90% of men with moderate degree of PPI will choose a male sling over artificial urinary sphincter, when given a choice [9]. There are several reasons why male slings present an attractive alternative to AUS. From the patient perspective, there is no postoperative waiting period for healing to occur prior to activation of the device. The patient can void without any device manipulation and is able to achieve an instantaneous significant improvement in their continence rates following removal of the catheter. With regards to the device design, the male sling is not a circumferential occluding device therefore the risk of urethral atrophy and erosion is minimal and uncommon [9].

2.1. InVance Sling

The InVance sling (American Medical Systems, Minnetonka, MN, USA) was first introduced in 2000 [19] and later popularised by Comiter [20, 21]. This non-adjustable male sling consists of a silicon-coated polyester rectangle sling which is positioned under the bulbar urethra through a perineal incision to achieve urethral compression. The sling compresses the bulbar urethra with the aids of 3 titanium screws attached to the anteromedial aspects of the descending pubic rami bilaterally.

As one of the earliest male sling introduced for the treatment of male SUI, it has the longest follow up study [22]. The published pad-free rates range from 36% to 65% in patients with mild to severe SUI [22-27]. Postoperative perineal pain occurs in up to 76% of the patients but usually resolves after 3 months. Other reported complications include the increased residual urine (up to 12%), the need for explantation due to infection (up to 15%), and bone-anchor dislodgement (up to 5%).

The severity of preoperative incontinence correlated with the outcome of the operation. There is higher failure rate (up to 85%) in slings for men who have undergone pelvic radiotherapy [22, 25]. Importantly salvage surgery for failed bone-anchor sling remains effective [28]. Unlike the AUS, urethral atrophy with loss of coaptation has not been reported and the efficacy is maintained with a low risk of late failure [22].

2.2. Argus Sling

The Argus (Promedon, Cordoba, Argentina) system was first popularised in 2006 [29]. It consists of a silicone foam pad for compression of the bulbar urethra and two silicone columns of multiple conical elements and silicone washers that allow for regulation of the desired tension on the bulbar urethra. The recommended maximum intra-operative leak point pressure is 45 cm H_20. The Argus sling can be implanted via a retropubic approach and more recently the Argus-T was introduced as a transobturator re-adjustable sling. In the event of suboptimal intra- or post-operative tension, sling tightening may be accomplished through a minimally invasive "readjustment" technique.

The published dry rate among men with mild to moderate SUI was up to 65% [29,30]. Recent study on the outcome of Argus sling in moderate to severe SUIT demonstrated a dry rate of 79% and adjustment of the sling was required in 39% of the cases [31]. Most postoperative complications for Argus sling relate to the large silicone burden and that include transient perineal pain (up to 15%), sling explantation from sling infection (6%) and/or erosion (13%) into the urethra, bladder and through the abdominal wall. However salvage surgery with AUS following failed Argus sling was quite favourable [31].

2.3. Remeex Sling

The Remeex sling (Neomedic, Barcelona, Spain) is another adjustable sling located under the bulbar urethra and was first introduced in 2004 [32]. A mesh is connected via two monofilament traction threads to a suprapubic mechanical regulator which is implanted subcutaneously over the abdominal rectum fascia 2 cm above the pubis. Further adjustment of the sling is performed though an external manipulator.

The reported dry rates in patients with mild to moderate SUI are comparable to the Argus sling with results of up to 65% [33, 34]. Up to 90% of patients require at least 2 adjustments to achieve urinary continence. The reported complications include intra-operative bladder injuries (up to 11%) and explantation of device (up to 12%) due to device infection and/or urethral erosion. Postoperative perineal pain is a common postoperative complaint.

2.4. AdVance Sling

In contrast to the current male slings, the AdVance sling is not compressive in nature. The trans-obturator Advance sling repositions the bulbo-membranous urethra and the lax undescended supporting structures of the posterior urethra and sphincteric structure towards the bladder neck and works by displacing the proximal urethra from a vertical to horizontal plane underneath the membranous urethra; where the force is applied parallel to the urethral lumen [35]. Critical success factors for AdVance surgery include good mobility of the sphincter region and a good residual function of the sphincter with a coaptive zone of > 1 cm [36].

The reported dry rates of AdVance sling surgery are 51.4% to 73.7% [37-39], and this number increased further to 90% in men wearing 1 to 2 pads [40]. Radiotherapy, bulking agents, failed stem cell therapy and previous AUS placement and urethral fibrosis are all compromising factors. In patients who have received radiation therapy, the success rates decreased to 25% to 35% [41, 42]. Major postoperative complications include transient urinary retention requiring temporary re-catheterization, local wound infection and perineal pain. The risk of explantation for AdVance sling is low [43].

In patients with failed AdVance sling, the implantation of a second AdVance sling has demonstrated good results with more than a third of patient requiring no pad [44]. Failure of AdVance sling can also be salvaged with AUS or prostate adjustable continence therapy [45]. Similarly, men who suffer from recurrent urinary incontinence secondary to cuff compression atrophy can be made continent by the placement of a male sling and by not revising the AUS device [46]. The advantages of using AdVance to salvage recurrent SUI in AUS patients are the lower risk of postoperative infection due to non-violation of AUS pseudo-capsule and the potential that patient may not need to rely upon the use of his AUS to maintain continence.

2.5. Virtue Sling

The Virtue sling (Coloplast, Humlebaek, Denmark) was introduced by Dr Comiter in early 2009.

This quadratic ventral elevation urethral sling consists of monofilament polypropylene mesh with four mesh arms, 2 (inside-out) transobturator arms and 2 (outside-in) prepubic arm [47, 48]. The proposed mechanisms of action include ventral urethral elevation from the transobturator arms and distal urethral compression from the prepubic arms. It was shown that this (VUE + Levera) sling, provided sufficient urethral compression against the perineal membrane using a pre-pubic approach and ventral elevation and compression of the bulbar urethral using the transobturator approach in the cadaveric study [49]. The same article also reported that the 2 men who were enrolled in this early study found improvement in their urinary incontinence. The reported success rate showed that 54% of men had >50% reduction in pad weight at 6 months but 10% of men reported worse urinary incontinence [50]. The potential adverse events include bladder perforation, wound infection, perineal pain and urinary retention requiring catheterisation. The author has had some experience with Virtue sling and found that while patients reported excellent immediate urinary continence, more than 50% of patients experienced recurrent of SUI at 6 months.

3. Artificial Urinary Sphincter-Like Device

While synthetic male slings have a niche in the treatment of mild to moderate PPI, they are not effective in the moderate to severe PPI and in high risk groups such as men with past history of radiotherapy, urethral bulking agents, sling infection/erosion, transurethral prostate surgery or urethral fibrosis. A urinary cuff provides a circumferential occlusion to the urethral lumen and therefore ensures complete mucosal coaptation. Furthermore, the transmission of fluid from a reservoir increases the pressure in the occluding cuff to simulate more physiological sphincter.

3.1. AMS 800

The first AUS-like device was first developed in 1973 and has evolved into the current AMS 800 device (American Medical Systems, Minnetonka, MN, USA). Currently, it remains the treatment of choice for persistent moderate and severe PPI and is still regarded as the gold treatment for male SUI.

This device consisted of an inflatable occluding cuff, pressure regulating balloon and control pump. The AUS has the longest tract record in the treatment of PPI and published literature has supported the AMS 800 device as a highly durable, effective and safe treatment option for SUI. The reported success rate is up to 90% and is associated with high patient satisfaction rate [51-57].

While AMS 800 is a safe, durable and effective treatment for SUI, this device has several limitations. Revision and explantation rates are due to mechanical failure, urethral atrophy, infection, and erosion vary considerably among published studies. The reported reoperation rate for AUS is 17-35%, with about 50% of these cases caused by mechanical complications and 50% by non-mechanical complications [54, 55, 57].

The use of the double-cuff system was introduced to reduce the urethral atrophy and increase continence rate. However, men with double-cuff systems have a higher risk of complications [58].

Revisions include replacement of the malfunctioning part, cuff replacement, repositioning or downsizing due to urethral atrophy, and a second tandem cuff or transcorporal cuff placement [59, 60]. There appears to be no difference in continence outcomes but a higher revision rate in patients undergoing double-cuff implant versus single-cuff after longer follow up [58].

3.2. FlowSecure Device

The FlowSecure™ AUS device (London, UK) was designed by Dr Craggs and associates [61,62]. This new AUS device attempts to address two major weakness of the AMS 800 namely the inability to protect patients against incontinence secondary to sudden increases in intra-abdominal pressure, suggesting that the PRB is not always efficient; and to alter the cuff pressure and correct for cuff atrophy without further surgery. The FlowSecure device is implanted as a single unit, thus eliminating the need for tubing connections. This one-piece silicone device is prefilled with 30 ml of 0.9% saline and comprises of four parts connected together by silicone connecting tubes - a regulator balloon, a stress release balloon, a circular occluding urethral cuff and a control pump.

The stress relief balloon is placed extraperitoneally and transmits transient intra-abdominal pressure changes to the urethral cuff to increase occlusion pressure during periods of stress (conditional occlusion). The pressure-regulating balloon establishes a basal occlusive pressure and is identical to the stress relief balloon.

The regulating pressure is adjusted in the range of 0-80 cmH_2O and can be altered by the injection or removal of fluid (on the basis of continence status) from the device in situ. Device pressure can therefore be titrated against continence for each individual patient, removing the need to select a specific pressure range before operation. Pressurization of the device occurs after scrotal swelling resides, typically after 2-4 weeks post-operatively.

The cuff features a pre-moulded and adjustable rounded internal surface for homogenous pressure transmission to reduce the risk of potential cuff stress fracture. Although it is specifically designed for a male urethra, urethral circumference of up to 7cm may be supported, large enough to accommodate female bladder neck [63]. One of the earlier concerns with the FlowSecure design was the risk of cuff perforation during pressurization but this appeared to have been rectified with the new control pump that features a resistance valve [64].

While a preliminary report on the outcomes of the FlowSecure device in nine male patients followed for a minimum period of 12 months were encouraging with a ten-fold decrease in mean daily leakage volume (770.6ml to 55.1ml) and an overall improvement in the Continence Index from 54% to 97% [14], recent followed study on 100 patients with FlowSecure device highlighted 6% mechanical failure, 5% risk of infection and 9% risk of pump assembly perforation with repeated puncture of the self-sealing port [65].

3.3. Zephyr ZSI 375

The Zephyr ZSI 375™ (Mayor group, Villeurbanne, France) is a one piece, silicone elastomer urinary continence device manufactured in France [66]. Unlike the AMS 800 and FlowSecure devices, it comprises of two components, a circular urethral cuff and a pressure regulating tank placed in the scrotum. The cuff consists of a moulded curved silicone rubber and comes in a range of different diameters from 3.75cm to 5cm and three different pressure ranges – 60-70 cmH_2O, 70-80 cmH_2O and 90-100 cmH_2O. The pressure regulating tank consists of an activation button, hydraulic circuit and a compensation pouch, and sits in the patient's scrotum. At rest, a piston mechanism, under spring loaded tension, exerts pressure on the fluid in the hydraulic chamber. When the activation button is pressed, the piston descends forcing fluid from the cuff into the hydraulic circuit and the compensation chamber. Auto-inflation of the cuff occurs within 2-3 minutes.

The theoretical advantages of Zephyr device over the AMS 800 product are that it is possible to adjust the pressure of the device by injecting or removal fluid from the compensating pouch, and the lack of a third component to be placed in the retropubic space thereby decreasing the risk of bladder injury and device migration. However, to date, there is no peer-reviewed publication or follow up studies on this new continence device.

3.4. Adjustable Continence Therapy (Pro-ACT)

Pro-ACT device™ (Uromedia Inc, MN, USA) is an adjustable continence device that consists of two silicone balloons on the proximal end and a titanium port in the distal end. The two balloons are placed trans-perineally under fluoroscopy or trans-rectal ultrasound guided to the level of the urethra-vesical anastomosis bilaterally, and can be inflated or deflated to compress the urethral lumen and provide outlet resistance [67, 68]. The proposed advantages of ProACT device include technical ease of insertion, low morbidity, relatively low cost, the lack of circumferential urethral compression and the ability to adjust the degree of mechanical compression with a titratable volume injected into the titanium port.

Earlier published literature on ProACT device [67] showed that there was a substantial improvement in patient continence rate following an average of three balloon volume adjustments. Despite the initial high cure rate, more than third of patients were unsatisfied with the surgical outcome in the long term. Early series on ProACT device reported relatively high complications rates such as device infection and revision [69, 70] but recent studies have shown that ProACT device is effective and safe therapeutic option in a select group of patients with moderate degree of SUI [71].

3.5. Periurethral Constrictor

The periurethral constrictor continence device (Silimed, Rio de Janeiro, Brazil) was developed by Dr Fabio Vilar specifically to treat paediatric patients with deficient bladder sphincter function [72]. It consists of a constrictor cuff linked by a tube to a hydraulically activated self-sealing valve. The cuff is made of a silicone membrane shaped like an open and inflatable ring, with a polyurethrane-foam coat on the internal surface and a polyester tissue reinforcement band on the external surface. The external band contains two pairs of buttons and four pairs of holes along its length to allow for adjustment of the device around the bladder neck or the bulbar urethra. The two sections of silicone tubes (200 and 500 mm long) are joined by a plastic connector linking the valve to the constrictor cuff and allow for adjustment of the distance between the valve and the cuff. The system works in a hydraulic fashion through the injection of sterile saline into the self-sealing port. In order to minimize tissue ischemia and subsequent cuff erosion, Vilar [72] advocated that the pressure should be relieved for about two months each year. The initial report demonstrated satisfactory outcomes in men with post-prostate UI and that 73.3% of the patients had functional devices and were socially continent at a mean follow up of 42.1 months [73]. Nonetheless, the periurethral constrictor device is plagued by high complication rates such as the need for additional fluid in the port to increase the occlusive static pressure of the cuff (7 patients), urethral erosion (4 patients), device infection (3 patients) and device malfunction from leakage of saline solution (4 patients) [73]. It is postulated that the leakage was inadvertently caused by needle perforations at the edge of the valve (where the silicone is thin) during the activation of the device.

Unlike AMS 800™ device, this compressive urinary device is relatively inexpensive and patient avoids the need to manipulate a pump to void. However patients are required to void against resistance created by the device and the long-term effects of this mechanical compression on the urethra and upper urinary tract are unknown. While the preliminary outcomes on this periurethral constrictor device are encouraging, larger patient participation and longer term follow-up need to be conducted to address the long-term effectiveness and safety of this urinary device.

Conclusion

Male SUI especially PPI is not uncommon. At present the AMS 800 AUS device remains the gold standard of PPI treatment with the longest efficacy and safety records. Male slings are an attractive alternative for patients who wish to avoid mechanical handling for urinary void and with intermediate data supporting their safety and efficacy in men with moderate degrees of PPI. Other AUS-like devices are designed to address the current AMS 800 limitations. Newer experimental AUS models are innovative and ambitious with the goal of producing a device implant that closely simulates a healthy human sphincter and is driven by different external and internal stimuli. Until the emergence of a better engineered AUS device, and/or further successes in stem cell or tissue engineering, significant challenges remain in the research for an ideal urinary sphincter device.

References

[1] Abrams P, Cardozo L, Fall M et al. the standardization of terminology of lower urinary tract function: report from the Standardisation Sub-committee of the International Continence Society. *Neurourol. Urodyn.* 2002;21:167-78.

[2] Kao TC, Cruess DF, Garner D, et al. Multicenter patient self-reporting questionnaire on impotence, incontinence and stricture after radical prostatectomy. *J. Urol.* 2000;163:858-64.
[3] Krupski TL, Saigal CS, Litwin MS. Variation in continence and potency by definition. *J. Urol.* 2003;170:1291-4.
[4] Peyromaure M, Ravery V, Boccon-Gibod L. Management of stress urinary incontinence after radical prostatectomy. *BJUI Int.* 2002;90:155-61.
[5] Sandhu JS. Treatment options for male stress urinary incontinence. *Nat. Rev. Urol.* 2010;7:222-8.
[6] Herschorn S, Thuroff J, Bruschini H et al. Surgical treatment of urinary incontinence in men. In: Abrams P, Cardozo L, Khoury AE, Wein A, editors. Incontinence: Third international consultation. Paris: Health Publications Ltd; 2005. P. 1241-96.
[7] Bauer RM, Bastian PJ, Gozzi C et al. Post-prostatectomy incontinence: All about diagnosis and management. *Eur. Urol.* 2009; 55(2):322-33.
[8] Herschorn S. The artificial urinary sphincter is the treatment of choice for post-radical prostatectomy. *Can. Urol. Assoc. J.* 2008;2:536-9.
[9] Kumar A, Litt ER, Ballert KN, Nitti VW. Artificial urinary sphincter versus male sling for post-prostatectomy incontinence-what do patients choose? *J. Urol.* 2009;181: 1231-5.
[10] Aboseif SR, O'Connell HE, Usui A et al. Collagen injection for intrinsic sphincter deficiency in men. *J. Urol.* 1996;155:10-3.
[11] Cespedes RD, Leng WW, McGuire EJ. Collagen injection therapy for postprostatectomy incontinence. *Urology* 1999;54:597-602.
[12] Klutke JJ, Subir C, Andriole G et al. Long-term results after antegrade collagen injection for stress urinary incontinence following radical retropubic prostatectomy. *Urology* 1999;53:974-7.
[13] Smith DN, Appell RA, Rackley RR et al. Collagen injection therapy for post-prostatectomy incontinence. J Urol 1998;160:364-7; Klutke et al. *Urology* 1999.
[14] Mitterberger M, Marksteiner R, Margreiter E et al. Myoblast and fibroblast therapy for postprostatectomy urinary incontinence: 1-year follow up of 63 patients. *J. Urol.* 2008;179:226-31.
[15] Bauer RM, Gozzi C, Hubner W et al. Contemporary management of postprostatectomy incontinence. *Eur. Urol.* 2011;59:985-96.
[16] Berry J. New procedure for correction of urinary incontinence: a preliminary report. *J. Urol.* 1961;85:771-5.
[17] Kaufmann JJ. Urethral compression operations for the treatment of post-prostatectomy incontinence. *J. Urol.* 1973;110:93-6.
[18] Durrani AF, Rosenbaum TP, Shaw PJ et al. Does the Kaufman prosthesis still have a place? Review of thirteen years' experience. *Urology* 1991; 38: 328-31.
[19] Madjar S, Jacoby K, Giberti C et al. Bone anchored sling for the treatment of post-prostatectomy incontinence. *J. Urol.* 2001; 165:72-6.
[20] Onur R, Rajpurkar A, Singla A. New perineal bone-anchored male sling: lessons learned. *Urology* 2004; 64:58-61.
[21] Comiter C. The male perineal sling: intermediate-term results. *Neurourol. Urodyn.* 2005; 24:648-51.

[22] Guimaraes M, Oliveira R, Pinto R et al. Intermediate-term results, up to 4 years, of a bone-anchored male perienal sling for treating male stress urinary incontinence after prostate surgery. *BJU Int.* 2009;103:500-4.
[23] Fassi-Fehri H, Badet L, Cheras A et al. Efficacy of InVance male sling in men with stress urinary incontinence. *Eur. Urol.* 2007;51:498-503.
[24] Giberti C, Gallo F, Schenone M, Cortese P. The bone-anchor suburethral sling for the treatment of iatrogenic male incontinence: subjective and objective assessment after 41 months of mean follow-up. *World J. Urol.* 2008;26:173-8.
[25] Giberti C, Gallo F, Schenone M, Cortese P, Nonotta G. The bone anchor suburethral synthetic sling for iatrogenic male incontinence: critical evaluation at a mean 3-year followup. *J. Urol.* 2009;181:2204-8.
[26] Carmel M, Hage B, Hanna S et al. Long-term efficacy of the bone-anchored male sling for moderate and severe stress urinary incontinence. *BJU Int.* 2010;106;1012-6.
[27] Athanasopoulos A, Konstantinopoulos A, McGuire E. Efficacy of the InVance male sling in treating stress urinary incontinence: a three-year experience from a single centre. *Urol. Int.* 2010;85(4):436-42.
[28] Fisher MB, Aggarwal N, Vuruskan H, Singla AK. efficacy of artificial urinary sphincter implantation after failed bone-anchored male sling for postprostatectomy incontinence. *Urology* 2007;70:942-4.
[29] Romano SV, Metrebian SE, Vaz F et al. An adjustable male sling for treating urinary incontinence after prostatectomy: a phase III multicentre trial. BJUI 2006; 97:533-9.
[30] Romano SV, Metrebian SE, Vaz F et al. Long-term results of a phase III multicentre trial of the adjustable male sling for treating urinary incontinence after prostatectomy: minimum 3 years [in Spanish]. *Actas. Urol. Esp.* 2009;33(3):309-14.
[31] Hubner WA, Gallistl H, Rutkowski M, Huber ER. Adjustable bulbourethral sling: experience after 101 cases of moderate-to-severe male stress urinary incontinence. *BJU Int.* 2011;107:777-82.
[32] Sousa-Escandon A, Rodriguez Gomez JI, Uribarri Gonzalez C, Margues-Queimadelos A. Externally readjustable sling for treatment of male stress urinary incontinence: points of technique and preliminary results. *J. Endourol.* 2004;18:113-8.
[33] Campos-Fernandes JL, Timsit MO, Paparel P et al. REMEEX: A possible treatment option in selected cases of sphincter incompetence [in French]. *Prog. Urol.* 2006;16:184-91.
[34] Sousa-Escandon A, Cabrera J, Mantovani F et al. Adjustable suburethral sling (male Remeex system) in the treatment of male stress urinary incontinence: a multicentric European study. *Eur. Urol.* 2007;52:1473-80.
[35] Rehder P and Gozzi C. Transobturator sling suspension for male urinary incontinence including post-radical prostatectomy. *Eur. Urol.* 2007; 52:860-7.
[36] Rehder P, Freiin von Gleissenthall G et al. The treatment of postprostatectomy incontinence with retroluminal transobturator repositioning sling (Advance): lessons learnt from accumulative experience. *Arch. Esp. Urol.* 2009;62:860-70.
[37] Bauer RM, Mayer ME, Gratzke C et al. Prospective evaluation of the functional sling suspension for male postprostatectomy stress urinary incontinence: Results after 1 year. *Eur. Urol.* 2009;56:928-33.

[38] Cornu JN, Sebe P, Ciofu C et al. The AdVance transobturator male sling for postprostatectomy incontinence: Clinical results of a prospective evaluation after a minimum of 6 months. *Eur. Urol.* 2009;56:923-7.
[39] Rehder P, Mitterberger MJ, Pichler R et al. The 1 year outcome of the transobturator retroluminal repositioning sling in the treatment of male stress urinary incontinence. *BJU Int.* 2010;106;1668-72.
[40] Gozzi C, Becker AJ, Bauer RM et al. Early results of transobturator sling suspension for male urinary incontinence following radical prostatectomy. *Eur. Urol.* 2008; 54:960-1.
[41] Cornu JN, Sebe P, Ciofu C et al. Mid-term evaluation of the transobturator male sling for post-prostatectomy incontinence: focus on prognostic factors. BJU Int. In press, DOI:10.1111/j.1464-410X.2010.09766.x.
[42] Bauer RM, Soljanik I, Fullhase C et al. Results of AdVance transobturator male sling after radical prostatectomy abd adjuvant radiotherapy. *Urology* 2011;77:474-9.
[43] Bauer RM, Mayer ME, May F et al. Complications of the AdVance transobturator male sling in the treatment of male stress urinary incontinence. *Urology* 2010;75:1494-8.
[44] Soljanik I, Becker AJ, Stief CG et al. Repeat retrourethral transobturator sling in the management of recurrent postprostatectomy stress urinary incontinence after failed first male sling. *Eur. Urol.* 2010;58:767-72.
[45] Al-Najar A, Kaufmann S, Boy s et al. Management of recurrent post-prostatectomy incontinence after failed previous failed retrourethral male slings. *Can. Urol. Assoc. J.* 2011;5(2):107-11.
[46] Christine B, Knoll LD. Treatment of recurrent urinary incontinence after artificial urinary sphincter placement using the AdVance male sling. *Urology* 2010;76(6): 1321-4.
[47] http://www.straighttalk.net/wp-content/uploads/70001950_rev_b.pdf.
[48] http://www.coloplast.com.au/About/news/Pages/VirtueincontinenceslinglaunchedinUS. aspx.
[49] Comiter CV, Rhee EY. The “ventral urethral elevation plus’ sling: a novel approach to treating stress urinary incontinence in men. *BJU Int.* 2008;101(2):187-91.
[50] http://joachimfocking.files.wordpress.com/2011/03/drrheeeau-2011final-21.pdf.
[51] Elliot DS, Barrett DM. Mayo Clinic long-term analysis of the functional durability of the AMS 800 artificial urinary sphincter: a review of 323 cases. *J. Urol.* 1998;159(4):1206-8.
[52] Grousse AE, Madjar S, Lambert MM, Fishman IJ. Artificial urinary sphincter for post-radical prostatectomy urinary incontinence: long-term subjective results. *J. Urol.* 2001;166:1755-8.
[53] Madjar S, Grousse AE, Lambert MM et al. Artificial urinary sphincter implantation for radical prostatectomy urinary incontinence: Which factors influence patient satisfaction? *BJU Int.* 2000;86:121-XX.
[54] Kim SP, Sarmast Z, Daignault S et al. Long-term durability and functional outcomes among patients with artificial urinary sphincters: a 10-year retrospective review from the University of Michigan. *J. Urol.* 2008;179:1912-6.
[55] Lai HH, Hsu EI, The BS et al. 13 years of experience with artificial urinary sphincter implantation at Baylor College of Medicine. *J. Urol.* 2007;177:1021-5.

[56] Haab F, Trockman BA, Zimmern PE, Leach GE. Quality of life and continence assessment of the artificial urinary sphincter in men with minimum 3.5 years of follow up. *J. Urol.* 1997;158:435-9.
[57] Venn SN, Greenwell TJ, Mundy AR. The long-term outcome of artificial urinary sphincters. *J. Urol.* 2000;164:702-6, discussion 706-7.
[58] O'Connor RC, Lyon MB, Guralnick ML, Bales GT. Long-term follow-up of single versus double artificial urinary sphincter insertion for the treatment of severe prostatectomy stress urinary incontinence. *Urology* 2008;71:90-3.
[59] DiMarco DS, Elliot DS. Tandem cuff artificial urinary sphincter as a salvage procedure following failed primary sphincter placement for the treatment of post-prostatectomy incontinence. *J. Urol.* 2003;170:1252-4.
[60] Guralnick ML, Miller E, Toh KL et al. Transcorporal artificial urinary sphincter cuff placement in cases requiring revision for erosion and urethral atrophy. J. Urol. 2002;167:2075-8, discussion 2079.
[61] Craggs MD, inventor. Prosthetic sphincter device. UK patent [135308]. 1992.
[62] Knight SL, Susser J, Greenwell T, Mundy AR, Craggs MD. A new artificial urinary sphincter with conditional occlusion for stress urinary incontinence: preliminary clinical results. *Eur. Urol.* 2006;50:574-80.
[63] Garcia-Montes F, Vicens-Vicens A, Ozonas-Moragues M, Oleza-Simo J, Mora-Salva A. Surgical implantation of the new Flow Secure artificial urinary sphincter in the female bladder neck. *Urol. Int.* 2007;79(2):105-10.
[64] Garcia-Montes F. FlowSecure artificial urinary sphincter for the treatment of stress urinary incontinence after radical prostatectomy. *Ach. Esp. Urol.* 2009;62(10):845-50
[65] Alonso Rodriguez D, Fes Ascanio E, Fernandez Barranco L, Vicens Vicens A. One Hundred FlowSecure Artificial Urinary Sphincters (Abstract). Vienna : EAU Annual Congress 2011.
[66] http://zephyr-si.com/.
[67] Hubner WA. Schlarp OM. Treatment of incontinence after prostatectomy using a new minimally invasive device: adjustable continence therapy. *BJU Int.* 2005;96:587-94
[68] Gregori A, Romano AL, Scieri F, Pietrantuono F, Incarbone P, Salvaggio A, Granata A, Gaboardi F. Transrectal ultrasound-guided implantation of Adjustable Continence Therapy (ProACT): surgical technique and clinical results after a mean follow-up of 2 years. *Eur. Urol.* 2010;57(3):430-6.
[69] Lebret T, Cour F, Bencherit J, Grise P, Bernstein J, Delaporte V, Chartier-Katler E, Botto H, Costa P. Treatment of postprostatectomy stress urinary incontinence using a minimally invasive adjustable continence balloon device, ProACT: results of a preliminary, multicenter, pilot study. *Urology* 2008;71(2):256-60.
[70] Gilling PJ, Bell DF, Wilson LC, Westernberg AM, Reuther R, Fraundorfer MR. An adjustable continence therapy for treating incontinence after prostatectomy: a minimum 2-year follow up. *BJU Int.* 2008;102(10):1426-30, discussion 1430-1.
[71] Gregori et al; Aboseif SR, Sassani P, Franke EI, Nash SD, Slutsky JN, Baum NH, Le Tu M, Galloway NT, Pommerville PJ, Sutherland SE. Treatment of moderate to severe female stress urinary incontinence with the adjustable continence therapy (ACT) device after failed surgical repair. *WJU* 2011; 29:249-253.
[72] Vilar FO, Araujo LAP, Lima SVC. Periurethral constrictor in paediatric urology: long-term follow-up. *J. Urol.* 2004;171:2626-8.

[73] Schiavini JL, Damiao R, Dutra JA et al. Treatment of post-operative surgery urinary incontinence with the periurethral constrictor: A retrospective analysis. *J. Urol.* 2009;75(6):1488-92.

In: Urinary Incontinence
Editor: Eric Chung
ISBN: 978-1-62618-482-4

Chapter 17

Dual Prostheses Implantation for the Treatment of Male Urinary Incontinence and Erectile Dysfunction

Eric Chung*
Department of Urology, Princess Alexandra Hospital,
Brisbane QLD, Australia

Abstract

Despite technical and technological advances, radical prostatectomy is associated with substantial morbidity and post operative complications such as post prostatectomy urinary incontinence (PPI) and erectile dysfunction (ED) continue to persist and pose management issues. Patients that failed conservative therapy will require the implantation of prosthetic devices. The purpose of this article is to review the existing literature pertaining to dual implantation of artificial urinary sphincter (AUS) and penile prosthesis (PP). Improvements in mechanical properties and functional capabilities of these devices as well as innovative surgical techniques have shown that dual implantation of urinary and penile prostheses is feasible and safe provided that strict adherence to prosthetic surgical protocols are adhered to and, has been shown to be cost effective and highly efficacious to treat men with PPI and ED.

Introduction

The introduction of prostate-specific antigen testing has resulted in increased incidence of prostate cancer diagnosis worldwide. The American Cancer Society estimates that more than 200 000 new cases of prostate cancer have been diagnosed each year in United States alone and the number of radical prostatectomies has increased dramatically [1]. While technical and

* Corresponding author: Dr Eric Chung; Department of Urology, Princess Alexandra Hospital, Ipswich Rd, Brisbane; QLD 4103; Australia.; (T): +617-33242468; (F):+617-33242546; ericchg@hotmail.com.

technological advances have been made such as minimally invasive robotic laparosopic-assisted radical prostatectomy, radical prostatectomy is associated with substantial morbidity [2], with major quality of life issues such as postoperative erectile dysfunction and urinary incontinence continue to persist and pose management issues.

The incidence of post radical prostatectomy urinary incontinence (PPI) varies from 0.4 to 80% and up to 10% of men reported significant impact on quality of life due to the ongoing urinary incontinence [2]. The most likely cause of PPI is due to the deficiency and/or damage of the external urethral sphincter following surgery. However other factors such as dysfunction of the bladder neck, shortened urethral length and changes in the urethral axis as well as intra-operative damage to both nerve and pelvic floor musculature all play a causative role [3]. While synthetic male slings have been shown to be an effective treatment option in the mild PPI cases, artificial urinary sphincter (AUS) remains the gold standard management in men with PPI and has been shown to have a durable and effective continence rate of over 90% [4].

Erectile dysfunction (ED) continues to occur relatively frequent despite nerve sparing radical prostatectomy. Systematic review of prognostic factors following radical prostatectomy revealed the mean potency rate after radical prostatectomy in the general urologic practice is only 19%, regardless of the surgical technique used [5]. The advent of phospho-diesterase type-5 (PDE5) inhibitors has assisted many impotent men following nerve sparing radical prostatectomy but it is not without its own limitations. Second line treatment for ED such as intracavernosal vasoactive agent injection is associated with significant dropout rate, and many men will require the implantation of penile prosthesis to treat their ED following radical prostatectomy.

In a significant number of men, both PPI and ED co-exist, understandably contributing to a significant decline in quality of life. Recent publication by Wille [6] showed a statistically significant higher rate of urinary incontinence among men who had poor erectile function both before and after surgery.

This raised the possibility that injury to the neurovascular bundle and potential higher tumour burden could be common etiologic factors in both PPI and ED. Penile prosthesis (PP) and artificial urinary sphincter (AUS) implantation are therefore the logical surgical option in men with severe PPI and refractory ED.

Historical Perspective

The modern versions of both the AUS and PP were popularised by Scott and colleagues in the early 1970s [7, 8]. The current AUS (AMS 800; American Medical Systems, Minnetonka, MN) is the latest of a series of modification of an earlier model, the AMS 721. AMS 800 consisted of a cuff that surrounds the urethra or bladder neck, a scrotal pump that regulates flow of fluid into or out of the cuff, and the pressure-regulating balloon (PRB) that maintains the pressure within the cuff and acts as a reservoir for the fluid. Over the years, several technological advances have been made to the AMS 800 device such as the introduction of narrow-backed silicone gel coated cuff, kink-resistant tubing, quick connectors, poppet valve in the sphincter pump and InhibiZone® antibiotic coating, and current AMS 800 is a very effective and durable urinary device for the treatment of PPI. The

AUS implant can be performed through either a perineal or trans-scrotal approach. The former approach is more common and allows for direct and more proximal placement of the sphincter cuff at the bulbar urethra.

A second incision is required in the infrapubic region for placement of the PRB in the perivesical space and the tubing from the cuff and scrotal pump are routed to the infrapubic wound for connection. In contrast, trans-scrotal placement of AUS has the advantage of all components of the AUS positioned through a single incision.

Penile prosthesis (PP) implant can be either inflatable, with two or three-piece devices, or semi-rigid, which include the malleable and mechanical types. The three-piece inflatable PP best mimics a normal erect penis, and it consists of a paired cylinder, placed in each corpus cavernosal body, a scrotal pump and a fluid reservoir, usually placed in the perivesical space. Improvements in PP designs such as the introduction of parylene coating, rear tip extenders, quick connectors and InhibiZone® impregnated device have greatly improved the longevity and satisfaction associated with this device.

There are 2 approaches to penile prosthesis implant namely trans-scrotal or infrapubic approach. While both approaches allow for placement of all components through a single incision, the trans-scrotal placement is more common due to the lower risk of penile neurovascular injury.

Dual Implantation

Most men with PPI generally reported improvement of their urinary symptoms after 1 year post-operative. Men with severe urinary incontinence are usually not sexually active due to significant urine leak and the high incidence of climaturia.

While nerve sparing radical prostatectomy aims to preserve the underlying erectile function, neuropraxia and other intraoperative complications could potentially delay the return of erection. The use of drugs such as PDE5 inhibitors in penile rehabilitation program and the availability of alternative therapies for ED have made it more likely that the AUS placement will predate the PP implant. In a patient who develops both PPI and ED, it may become necessary to place both prostheses, either synchronously or sequentially. Candidates for dual implant are usually patients who have failed conservative management for both conditions.

In the vast majority of patients, dual implantation of AUS and PP effectively relieve both urinary incontinence and erectile dysfunction. However synchronous prostheses implant is not common and popular due to theoretical concerns of patient confusion and the difficulty of manipulating the two scrotal pumping devices. The risk of urethral or corporal injury could preclude the consideration of a simultaneous dual implant. Furthermore, the duration and extent of dissection required to insert and place the components, potentially increase the risks of infection and mechanical failure.

On the other hand, a 2-stage procedure requires more attentive surgery in order to avoid damaging the components of the existing implant and possibly operating in less well defined tissue planes.

In either situation, patients need to be counselled on the pros and cons of dual vs. staged implants and technical considerations for the device placement will vary depending on the sequence of device implant and the surgeon preferences.

Assessment of Patient

A comprehensive evaluation of all patients should be undertaken to identify the underlying etiology of ED and PPI. All patients should be trialled on conservative measures such as PDE5 inhibitors and/or vasoactive agents for their ED, with pelvic floor exercise and anti-muscurinic agents for men with PPI prior to consideration for implant surgery. Video urodynamics is required to evaluate sphincter incompetence and underlying detrusor overactivity, while cystoscopic examination of the urethra and bladder neck regions should be performed to exclude stricture disease. The cause of ED in post prostatectomy patient is usually obvious but if there is any doubt as to the diagnosis of ED, a full ED work-up should be performed, including hormonal and penile colour Doppler studies where appropriate.

All patients should be instructed on the use of these mechanical devices and advised on potential complications. The patient should possess good intellectual capacity and manual dexterity to allow them to use the devices correctly. Any stricture disease should be treated and stabilised first prior to the AUS implant. Careful preoperative preparation of patient is critical to reduce the incidence of infection during implant. It is important to exclude urinary tract infection and care should be taken to ensure that the genital and perineal skin is clear of irritation and signs of cellulitis. Some surgeons even recommend that the patients use a chlorhexidine-based anti-staphylococcal wash 24 hours prior to surgery to reduce the overall bacterial load on the skin.

Intra-Operative Care and Positioning

Since the introduction of trans-scrotal placement of AUS by Wilson [9], dual implantation of urinary and penile prostheses has been shown to constitute a safe and efficient method to treat both conditions through a single incision. For the purpose of this article, we described the trans-scrotal approach for placement of these prostheses.

Following induction of anaesthesia, the patient is placed in a modified leg-frogged position i.e supine with the legs slighted abducted. The patient genital region is shaved and a 5-10 minute surgical scrub with povidine iodine is performed to minimise intra-operative bacterial colonisation. All patients receive preoperative intravenous antibiotic, usually broad-spectrum antibiotics that cover both aerobic and anaerobic organisms (the author uses 500g vancomycin and 240mg gentamicin). They should be continued in this fashion for 24 hours, after which they may be given orally, usually for 1-2 weeks. A 14 Foley urinary catheter is placed in the urethra to facilitate the identification urethra during surgery.

Surgical Technique

A single transverse or vertical scrotal incision is made followed by dissection and exposure of the bulbar urethra and corporal bodies. Once adequate exposure is obtained, the choice is to place either the sphincter cuff or prosthesis cylinder first. Most surgeons advocate the dissection and mobilisation of the proximal bulbar first as inadvertent urethral injury would require abandoning or modifying the procedure without discarding any of the prostheses.

The AUS cuff placement requires adequate mobilisation of the urethra with dissection at the level of the corporal bodies and the bulbocavernosus to expose the entire bulbous urethra. To access the proximal bulb, the bulbospongiosus muscle must be retracted ventrally while continuing to divide the midline attachment to the raphe and dissection should continued until the perineal body is encountered and divided sharply.

It is important to ensure that the dissection is performed outside of the muscle and avoid denuding the spongiosus muscle bulb to minimise the risk of urethra injury and subsequent cuff erosion. Circumferential dissection of the urethra is then performed to allow for placement of a 2.0 cuff width. The urinary catheter is removed and the correct AUS cuff is then determined using the measuring device and the appropriate sized cuff is placed.

Once the cuff has been placed, bilateral vertical corporotomies can be made and corporal bodies are dilated and sized for the cylinders. Corporal dilatation must proceed cautiously in the proximal part of corporal near the cuff. Single-step dilatation may be a better option than sequential dilatation to avoid injuring the urethra. At the level of the bulbar urethra, the corporal bodies have already diverged and therefore the likelihood of injuring the cuff or urethra is lower. Once the appropriate cylinders are in place, the corporotomies are sutured watertight to avoid further bleeding from the corporotomy and later hematoma formation.

The bladder is then emptied and the reservoirs are then placed on either side in the perivesical space by puncturing the transversalis fascia lateral to the external inguinal ring. Care is taken to avoid the spermatic cord laterally and the bladder medially. The pump for each device is placed in the ipsilateral hemi-scrotum.

During the placement, the tubing must exit straight toward their pump without crossing-over or entangling. Similarly, the tubing to the respective reservoir and PRB must not cross-over and each must be placed on the ipsilateral side. Both reservoir and PRB are filled to the correct amount and the tubing is then connected using the quick-connectors.

The AUS is then cycled and left in a deactivated state while the PP is left partially inflated overnight to minimise bleeding risk. The scrotal wound is checked for any bleeding sites and the fascial layers are closed with continuous absorbable suture with the tubing quarantined in separate tissue compartments. Meticulous care not to damage any prosthetic material and avoidance of hematoma infection are important manoeuvres to minimise post-operative infection and pain. Application of "Henry mummy wrap" to the scrotum [10] and ice packs to the scrotal and perineal region are to reduce post-operative edema and assist with pain control. If the implants are not placed synchronously, the AUS is usually placed first followed by penile prosthesis for the reasons cited above. In sequential device implant, the greatest concern is accidental damage to the pre-existing device and its tubing. Great care needs to be taken to avoid damaging the AUS cuff when subsequently placing the penile cylinders. Some authors proposed that malleable penile prosthesis is utilised in sequential implant because of lesser components required and that the implant could be performed more distally on the corporal bodies and hence avoid encountering the AUS device.

While it is expected that all implants should have ipsilateral tubing and reservoir placement, surgeons should exercise precaution such as reviewing previous surgical records or organising pre-operative imaging study to avoid intra-operative surprise and the placement of the second implant can be planned for the pump and reservoir at the contralateral side. The incision should be performed away from the existing device, with meticulous dissection and the use of cutting currents to avoid damage to any components of the first device.

Post-Operative Care

Patients can usually be discharged within 24 hours of surgery on oral antibiotics. The inflatable PP can be recycled as early as week 2 if the patient is comfortable and there is minimal bruising and swelling to the scrotum. If there is marked penile fibrosis and scrotal discomfort post-operatively, the device cycling can commence at week 6 when the AUS can also be activated at the same time. It is important to advice patients to avoid any significant physical activities during the first 4 weeks and to seek medical attention if there is on-going significant pain, scrotal swelling and redness.

Current Literature on Dual Implantation of Urinary and Penile Prostheses

At present very few centres routinely perform simultaneous dual implant. Although much has been written about the excellent outcomes of AUS and PP implant alone, there is very minimal quality data published on the outcomes of synchronous insertion of AUS and PP. One of the earliest reports on dual implant of AUS and PP was disappointing and Graham [11] reported almost 100% failure rate in patients who received Kaufman urinary prosthesis and penile implant. However with newer devices, Parulkar [12] showed that 90% of patients reported good social continence following AUS implant and 98% of patients had functional penile prosthesis. More importantly, the authors did not detect any increase risk of surgical or mechanical problems between the synchronous implant and sequential implants groups. Another dual-incision approach was described by Bhalchandra [13] who found excellent urinary continence and PP function among the 40 patients of whom had implants performed simultaneously. Although this study did not distinguished those patients who had synchronous insertion of AUS and PP to sequential implants group, the overall erosion/infection rate was reported at 11%.

Prior to the year 2000, synchronous dual implants were performed using a dual-incision approach. Since the publication of trans-scrotal insertion of AUS implant [9, 14], synchronous dual implants are now performed mostly through a single incision. Wilson [14] first reported that synchronous dual implants is technically feasible and safe with a single incision, and that it is possible to preserve one device when the other infected device was removed. Bryan [15] showed that even infected dual implants may be amenable to salvage procedures. Three patients who had simultaneous dual implant had their device successfully salvage and one patient underwent two dual salvage procedures.

In a multi-institutional study on dual implant, Kendirci [16] reported no prosthetic infection postoperatively among the 22 men over a mean follow up of 17 months following a single upper transverse scrotal approach. The overall revision rate was 14%, mostly due to complications associated with the AUS device such as cuff erosion. Sellers [17] showed significant benefits in operative time and greater cost savings with dual implantation in a single staged procedure. The authors reported that dual implantation was associated with approximately a $7000 cost savings compared with individual procedures. Furthermore over the 16 months of follow up, there was no report of infective complications or device erosion. Mancini [18] also reported encouraging outcomes in patient satisfaction, ease of use and functionality in the dual implantation group that are similar to those observed in individual prosthesis group. In fact the majority of patients (94%) stated that they would recommend dual implantation procedure to others and have the procedure done again.

The literature on patients who received radiotherapy and the results of combination therapy with AUS and PP is limited. Kendirci [16] reported that the only erosions following synchronous insertion of AUS and PP occurred in the irradiated patients post radical prostatectomy.

The higher AUS revision rates in patients who received previous radiation were also confirmed by Martins [19]. The poorer surgical outcomes in post irradiated population is likely attributed to several factors such poorer quality of urethral tissue, difficult surgical dissection and unrecognised injury to the urethra during dissection as well as improper sizing and higher rates of cuff atrophy. Nonetheless the limited published literature on the incidence and risks of prosthesis erosion and infection in the irradiated population with an AUS is inconsistent [19-21]. On the other hand, there does not appear to be increased risk of erosion or infection on the use of PP in the context of the irradiated patients but the literature is very scarce. Dubocq [22] reported only a 7% malfunction rate with no incidences of prosthesis infection or erosion in men who received PP implant following radiotherapy after a mean follow up of 40 months.

Prosthetic infection is the most dreaded complication and generally occurs due to inadvertent introduction of skin organisms at the time of surgery and early postoperative bacteremia. Shortening the operative time would seem a logical way of decreasing this incidence but published literature on synchronous and sequential dual implants has not revealed any higher incidence of prosthetic infection, probably due to the low incidence of prosthesis infection of 1-3%. Given up to 40% of patients with previous prosthetic implant might have asymptomatic colonization of device [23], reoperation in the same area could potentially predispose to a clinical infection from these existing organisms and indeed, prosthetic infection rate in patients undergoing a redo surgery are higher than those in primary implant [24].

In the event of an infection, the concern is that it will spread to all components necessitating their removal and making revision surgery more technically challenging. While device erosion without infection may make salvaging one of the devices possible, in the context of device infection, it is often difficult to ascertain which device is affected and therefore it would be safer to remove both devices. However Bhalchandra [13] argues that in this situation, provided that the infected device is identified early, and if one acts early to locate the components affected, it is possible to salvage the components of the unaffected device. Indeed there are several pertinent points to consider before performing a dual implant [25, 26]. The patients should be adequately counselled on the procedure and potential complications, and have sufficient manual dexterity to recycle either pump as required. In a carefully selected group of patients, there is no doubt that most patients are satisfied with the outcomes and highly appreciative of the improvements in their quality of life. From the surgeon point of view, dual implant of urinary and penile devices is technically challenging and the surgeon should be competent at placing either device independently before contemplating a dual implantation. Dual implantation of urinary and penile prostheses is feasible and safe provided that strict adherence to prosthetic surgical protocols are adhered to and, has been shown to be cost effective and highly efficacious to treat men with PPI and ED.

Conclusion

Dual implantation of AUS and penile prosthesis is feasible, safe, efficient and cost-effective for the surgical treatment of PPI and ED. Implanting these two devices through a single surgical procedure provides encouraging outcomes in patient satisfaction, functionality and is highly rewarding, and should be considered and offered to patients who require both devices.

References

[1] Jemal A, Siegel R, Xu J, Ward E. Cancer statistics, 2010. *CA Cancer J. Clin.* 2010;60:277-300.

[2] Sanda MG, Dunn RL, Michalski J et al. Quality of life and satisfaction with outcome among prostate-cancer survivors. *N Engl. J. Med.* 2008;358:1250-61.

[3] Porena M, Mearini E, Mearini L et al. Voiding dysfunction after radical retropubic prostatectomy: more than external urethral sphincter deficiency. *Eur. Urol.* 2007; 52:38-45.

[4] Montague DK, Angermeier KW. Postprostatectomy urinary incontinence: the case for artificial urinary sphincter implantation. *Urology* 2000;55:2-4.

[5] Dubbelman YD, Dohle GR, Schroder FH. Sexual function before and after radical retropubic prostatectomy: a systematic review of prognostic indicators for a successful outcome. *Eur. Urol.* 2006;50:711-8.

[6] Wille S, Hendenreich A, Hofmann R, Engelmann U. Preoperative erectile function is one predictor for post prostatectomy incontinence. *Neurourol. Urodyn.* 2007;26:140-3.

[7] Scott FB, Bradley WE, Timm GW. Treatment of urinary incontinence by an implantable prosthetic sphincter. *Urology* 1973;1:252-9.

[8] Scott FB, Bradley WE, Timm GW. Management of erectile impotence: use of implantable inflatable prosthesis. *Urology* 1973;2:80-2.

[9] Wilson SK, Delk JR. A new approach for implantation of artificial urinary sphincter: upper transverse scrotal incision. *J. Urol.* 2001;165:256.

[10] Henry GD. The Henry mummy wrap and the Henry finger sweep surgical techniques. *J. sex Med.* 2009;6(3):619-22.

[11] Graham SD Jr, Carson CC 3rd, Anderson EE. Long term results with the Kaufman prosthesis. *J. Urol.* 1982;128:328-30.

[12] Parulkar BG, Barrett DM. Combined implantation of artificial sphincter and penile prosthesis. *J. Urol.* 1989;142:732-5.

[13] Bhalchandra G, Barrett P, Barrett DM. Combined implantation of artificial sphincter and penile prosthesis. *J. Urol.* 1989;142:732-5.

[14] Wilson SK, Delk JR II, Henry JR et al. New surgical technique for sphincter urinary control system using upper transverse scrotal incision. *J. Urol.* 2003;69:261-4.

[15] Bryan DE, Mulchahy JJ, Simmons GR. Salvage procedure for infected noneroded artificial urinary sphincters. *J. Urol.* 2002;168:2464-6.

[16] Kendirci M, Gupta S, Shaw L, Morey A, Jones L, Hakim L, Hellstrom WJ. Synchronous prosthetic implantation through a transscrotal incision: an outcome analysis. *J. Urol.* 2006;175:2218-22.

[17] Sellers CL, Morey AF, Jones LA. Cost and time benefits of dual implantation of inflatable penile and artificial urinary sphincter prosthetics by single incision. *Urol.* 2005;65(5):852-3.

[18] Mancini JG, Kizer WS, Jones LA, Mora RV, Morey AF. Patient satisfaction after dual implantation of inflatable penile and artificial urinary sphincter prostheses. *Urol.* 2008;71(5):893-6.

[19] Martins FE, Boyd SD. Artificial urinary sphincter in patients following major pelvic surgery and/or radiotherapy: are they less favourable candidates. *J. Urol.* 1995;153:1188-93.

[20] Gomha MA, Boone TB. Artificial urinary sphincter for post-prostatectomy incontinence in men who had prior radiotherapy; a risk and outcome analysis. *J. Urol.* 2002;167 (2 Pt 1):591-6.

[21] Perez LM, Webster GD. Successful outcome of artificial urinary sphincters in men with post prostatectomy urinary incontinence despite adverse implantation features. *J. Urol.* 1992;148:1166-70.

[22] Dubocq Jr FM, Bianco FJ, Maralani SJ, Foreman JD, Dhabuwala CB. Outcomes analysis of penile implant surgery after external beam radiation for prostate cancer. *J. Urol.* 1997;158:1787-90.

[23] Licht MR, Montague DK, Angermeier KW, Lakin MM. Cultures from genitourinary prostheses at reoperation: questioning the role of Staphylococcus epidermidis in periprosthetic infection. *J. Urol.* 1995;154:387-90.

[24] Wilson SK, Delk JR. Inflatable penile implant infection: predisposing factors and treatment suggestions. *J. Urol.* 1995;153:659-61.

[25] Zafirakis H, Wang R, Westney OL. Combination therapy for male erectile dysfunction and urinary incontinence. *Asian J. Androl.* 2008;10(1):149-54.

[26] Kumar R, Nehra A. Dual implantation of penile and sphincter implants in the post-prostatectomy patient. *Curr. Urol. Rep.* 2007;8(6):477-81.

Special Section: Other Types of Urinary Incontinence

In: Urinary Incontinence
Editor: Eric Chung
ISBN: 978-1-62618-482-4

Chapter 18

Urinary Incontinence in the Paediatric Population: Congenital Bladder Outlet Obstruction and Urinary Incontinence in Boys

Hideo Nakai
Children's Medical Center Tochigi, Jichi Medical University, Japan

Abstract

In order to document mild congenital bladder outlet obstruction as a cause of refractory daytime incontinence and/or nocturnal enuresis, indications for VCUG and its diagnostic criteria, urethroscopic diagnostic criteria, surgical procedure for endoscopic incision, and evaluation of the results of endoscopic incision were standardized. Outcome analysis revealed that posterior urethral valves (type 1 and/or type 3), although they are near at its mildest spectrum, might well cause high pressure voiding resulting in refractory daytime incontinence and/or nocturnal enuresis. In addition, dyssynergic voiding pattern was sometimes concomitant with these mild form of posterior urethral valves, resulting in ineffectiveness of endoscopic treatment. Conclusively, urologists should not hesitate to indicate VCUG (1~2 frame per second in voiding phase) for boys with refractory incontinence and should sophisticate the methodology of endoscopic incision to these mild posterior urethral valves.

Introduction

Congenital bladder outlet obstruction (BOO) in boys is well known as an underlying disorder resulting in dysuria that causes successive urinary tract infections and kidney failure in infancy, and a degree of consensus has been achieved with regard to the diagnostic and treatment methods for conditions such as posterior urethral valve. However, despite the fact that even mild congenital BOO can underlie urinary incontinence and nocturnal enuresis from early childhood and school age, sufficient consensus on the diagnosis and treatment of minor organic lesions has yet to be achieved [1, 2].

In Japan, congenital bulbar urethral ring stenosis (urethral ring) [3] has been well known since the 1980s, and the effectiveness of endoscopic optic urethrotomy for improving vesicoureteral reflex (VUR) and urinary incontinence is accepted by many urological surgeons. Unfortunately, however, "urethral ring" is not globally accepted as a form of congenital BOO. Although a range of other conditions has been reported, including mini-valve, Cobb's collar (1968), [4] Moorman's ring (1972), [5] and congenital obstructive posterior urethral membrane (1992), [6] specialist opinion is also divided on the differences between these disease concepts. This is the first problem.

Next, although endoscopic treatment for mild congenital BOO, including urethral ring, is comparatively effective for improving diurnal urinary incontinence, it is generally regarded as not very effective for nocturnal enuresis. The diagnostic criteria for mild BOO are still ambiguous, however, and because endoscopic incision for individual suspected obstructions is of low invasiveness, there is a general attitude of "try cutting and see if it works." Thus, the second problem is that the level of evidence-based medicine is still low.

This paper summarizes the knowledge that has been obtained to date and reports the progress of our own clinical research, with the aim of improving the evidence level for medical care in this field.

Embryology and Morphology of Congenital Posterior Urethral Valve

We will start by looking at the embryology of posterior urethral valve (Figure 1). According to Stephens' description, [7] the typical posterior urethral valve (Type 1) develops as an abnormality of the position of the opening of the mesonephric duct into the genitourinary sinus. That is, the mesonephric duct, which would normally open into the distal posterior wall of the genitourinary sinus, opens proximally, close to the midline of the anterior wall to the extent that it forms a severe urethral valve. During subsequent development, the opening migrates to the cranial side while gradually moving around the lateral wall, finally rising to the site of formation of the verumontanum, while hypertrophy of the urethral wall occurs after the migrating opening has passed through the urethral wall. In other words, a valvular or membranous structure persists on a line diagonal to the long axis of the urethra after the positional migration of the abnormal opening.

The morphology of posterior urethral valve was first described and categorized in 1919 by Young, and it was later expanded by Stephens on the basis of endoscopic findings [7, 8] (Table 1). Type 1 presents a valvular morphology in an *oblique* positional relationship with the long axis of the urethra and is continuous with the verumontanum on the posterior wall midline when traced back cranially. In this case, the verumontanum is large (compared with Type 3, described below), and the morphology of the inferior crest (a ridge line continuous with the verumontanum in the 6 o'clock direction on the posterior wall) is thick and fin-shaped. Type 2 is regarded as an over-classification by Young and is now considered to represent over-evaluation of protrusions into the lumen proximal to the verumontanum as BOO. Type 3 is formed when the border of the genitourinary diaphragm persists in the form of a ring during the process of development when this diaphragm ruptures and the urethra passes through, and it has a membranous or septal morphology, with its positional relationship being transverse to the long axis of the urethra. The verumontanum is small, and there is no continuity between this lesion and the verumontanum. There is no obvious inferior crest, and only fine membranous ruffles are visible. Type 4 is regarded as an original category introduced by Stephens, and its details are omitted here.

Understanding the development and morphology of posterior urethral valve, as described above, is very important for elucidating the actual nature of BOO in the posterior, membranous, and bulbar urethra in boys, including posterior urethral valve.

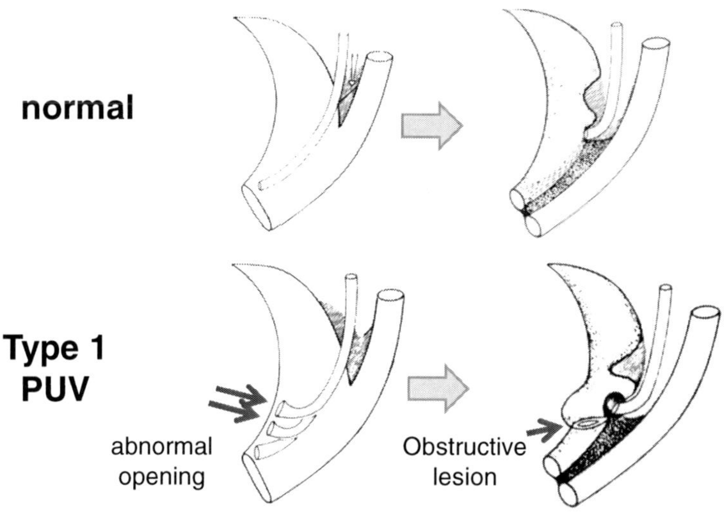

Figure 1. Embryology of PUV Congenital anomalies of the urinary and genital tracts. (Isis Medical Media Ltd.1996, modified).

Table 1. Stephens' description of PUV morphlogy in his textbook 1996

	embryology	shape	Orientation to urethral axis	continuity to veru.	veru	inferior crest
type 1	originate from abnormally located wollfian duct orifices	Valvular	oblique	continuous	big	thick fin like
type 2	overestimation or overclassification					
type 3	originate from persistent urogenital membrane	Membrane or diaphragm	transverse	no	small	very fine
type 4	?	deep Infold of anterior and anterolateral walls	transverse	no		

Changes and Confusion in the Concept of BOO

In 1919, Young's classification of posterior BOO in boys was created on the basis of findings observed when the urethra was opened in the 12 o'clock direction during dissection. Today, it has been pointed out that findings observed with a 12 o'clock incision actually bias these morphological descriptions. That is, if the urethral wall is opened in the 12 o'clock direction, in Type 1 lesions the obstruction on the anterior wall is divided bilaterally, making it appear as if there are structures with venous valve-like morphology on each of the lateral walls of the opened urethra. Type 1 lesions were named "valves" for this reason, but as subsequent studies have shown, most lesions do not comprise the double-valve structures shaped like the sails of a yacht that would be inferred from an analogy with venous valves.

In 1992, Dewan pointed out that the name "valve" does not objectively indicate the actual nature of posterior BOO in boys, which comprises a spectrum ranging from severe to mild, and proposed that Type 1 posterior urethral valve be renamed "congenital obstructive posterior urethral membrane" (COPUM).[6)] He understood the lesion causing the obstruction to consist of a membrane and pointed out that this membrane possesses a posterior defect, that is, a foraminal defect close to the posterior urethral wall, projecting not only from the left and right, but also from the anterior wall, to cause BOO (Figure 2). This analysis was regarded as extremely useful, and it served as an important warning call that the diagnosis and treatment of this disorder based on the name "valve" could be misleading for inexperienced urological surgeons (particularly in terms of not emphasizing endoscopic incision in the 12-o'clock direction). Nevertheless, it remains unclear whether COPUM as a concept is applicable not only to severe posterior urethral valve but also to the sort of mild BOO discovered in 7-10-year-old boys with urinary incontinence.

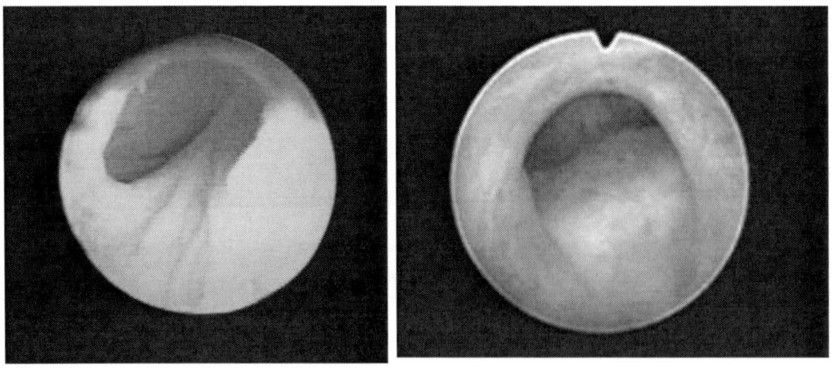

a b

a. looks like bilateral valve formation.
b. looks like membrane structure with posterior foraminal defect

Figure 2. Concept of valve or membrane.

In addition to morphological diagnosis of the lesion, localization is also important, but there has been no consistency among previous reports on this point. Although there have been numerous reports in Japan of the discovery of mild BOO as a result of urinary incontinence in

5- and 6-year-olds [9, 10, 11] (Table 2), a comparison of these reports shows that the percentage of bulbar BOO is extremely high, while others describe a high rate of posterior BOO. [12, 13].

Table 2. Urethral anomalies seen in enuretic patients. Difference in location and incidence among articles

author	year	Total number of patients	Posterior Urethral Valve	Bulbar Urethral Stenosis
Shima	**1998**	**170**	**3**	**42**
Yamanishi 2000		**157**	**3**	**26**
Sugimoto 2005		15	0	15
Yeung	**1999**	**33**	**4**	**3**
Kihara 2008		**37**	**5**	**4**

A regional diagnosis of whether the obstruction is proximal or distal to the membranous urethra can be determined overall based on findings from voiding cystourethrography (VCUG) and endoscopic observation, but there has been no clear description to date concerning the location or extent of the obstruction in terms of its positional relationship with the membranous urethra.

As described above, in 1989, Mori et al. collated 226 cases of congenital bulbar urethral stenosis (urethral ring) and described the efficacy (improved VUR and nocturnal enuresis) of endoscopic incision (cold incision at 12 o'clock or 6 o'clock), in a report that broke new ground in raising awareness within Japan of the importance of the diagnosis and treatment of mild BOO. [3] Their concept of this condition comprised a congenital stenosis that develops at the junction of the endodermal urethra and ectodermal urethra in boys, visible endoscopically as a ring morphology immediately outside the external urinary sphincter, and comprising a different condition from posterior urethral valve or anterior urethral valve.

According to Stephens, Cobb's collar (1968) [4] and Moormann's ring (1972) [5] are congenital BOOs seen at the bulbomembranous junction. There is now a consensus view that these constitute the same condition as the Type 3 posterior urethral valve described above. Nonomura et al. collated 74 cases of Cobb's collar and reported the effectiveness of endoscopic incision (cold incision) in improving VUR and urinary incontinence, but as with mild Type 1 posterior urethral valve, some experts also hold a negative opinion with regard to the clinical significance of these lesions [14]

In Japan, great attention has been paid to the clinical significance of congenital bulbar urethral stenosis (urethral ring), and to date it has been diagnosed and treated with no new scrutiny as to how it differs from posterior urethral valve. Before this, however, we believe that it is necessary to elucidate how this differs from the standard view of posterior urethral valve (Types 1 and 3) worldwide, in order to pursue the association between mild BOO and urinary incontinence and nocturnal enuresis in greater depth.

The reason we have placed such emphasis above on the morphological and positional diagnosis of obstructions is that these are directly related to treatment procedures. The actual nature of the obstruction must be determined in order to elucidate where, to what extent, and how deep to make the incision. It can easily be conceived that the extent of the obstruction is different in Cobb's collar and Type 1 posterior urethral valve, and there may be more than one lesion. An explanation must include the issue of which name most universally describes these lesions: valve, membrane, collar, ring, or something else.

Strategies for the Scientific Study of Pediatric BOO

Although the problems described above involve a range of different factors, chief among them is the fact that there is no global agreement with regard to evaluation methods at any of the various stages of the diagnosis of obstructions, their treatment, and evaluation of outcomes, meaning that standardization of the various evaluation criteria is required (Figure 3). We are engaged in a clinical study incorporating high-resolution video recording of endoscopic findings and voiding urodynamics with the aim of standardizing the diagnosis and treatment of this condition, and our findings to date are described below. These studies have been approved by the Ethics Committee of Jichi Medical University.

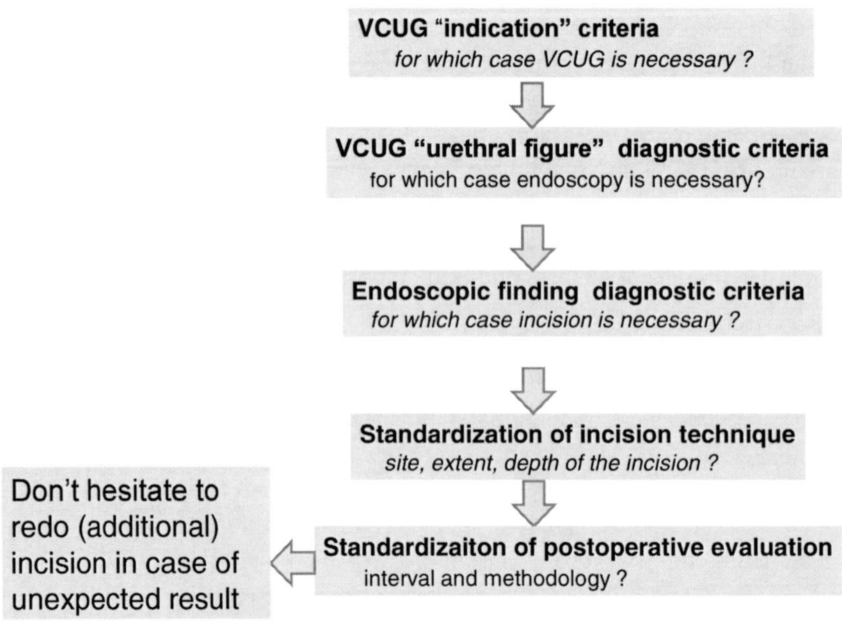

Figure 3. Our strategy for scientific evaluation of BOO in children (5 steps for standardization).

(1) Indications for VCUG and Diagnostic Criteria

There are no clear worldwide criteria for the diagnosis of obstruction in boys by means of VCUG, particularly for mild lesions. In a European clinical study in which four clinicians (two pediatric urological surgeons and two pediatric radiologists) evaluated the results of VCUG in 72 boys, although the diagnostic concordance rate for VUR and bladder diverticulum was 80%, that for posterior BOO was only 30%, indicating a tendency for diagnosis to be dependent on the evaluator [1] To resolve this problem, we routinely use imaging at two continuous frames per second in order to improve the accuracy of VCUG in cases where an obstruction is suspected. We have described the details of this method in another report [15]

As is already widely known, the indication for endoscopy is findings of segmental stenosis with differences in diameter before and after the stenosis, but the routine use of continuous frame imaging frequently shows that this finding is not continuously present during urination, but rather it makes an extremely transient appearance. Typically, this finding only comes to light around the time of maximum urinary flow. In practice, it should really be described as circumferential dilatation or posterior flexure of the posterior urethra (Figure 4), and the causes of such transient urethral dilatation or deformation may be related to the mobility of the posterior urethra in boys before puberty or urinary flow rate-dependent obstruction (secondary urethral flexion generated at the lesion site). In 1997, Hoebeke et al. reported that stenotic lesions from the membranous to the bulbar urethra produced ballooning of the posterior urethra by the same mechanism involved in dose-dependent hydronephrosis in uteropelvic junction stenosis, causing obstruction, and this is probably the same phenomenon that we have identified [16] Endoscopy is also indicated in this case.

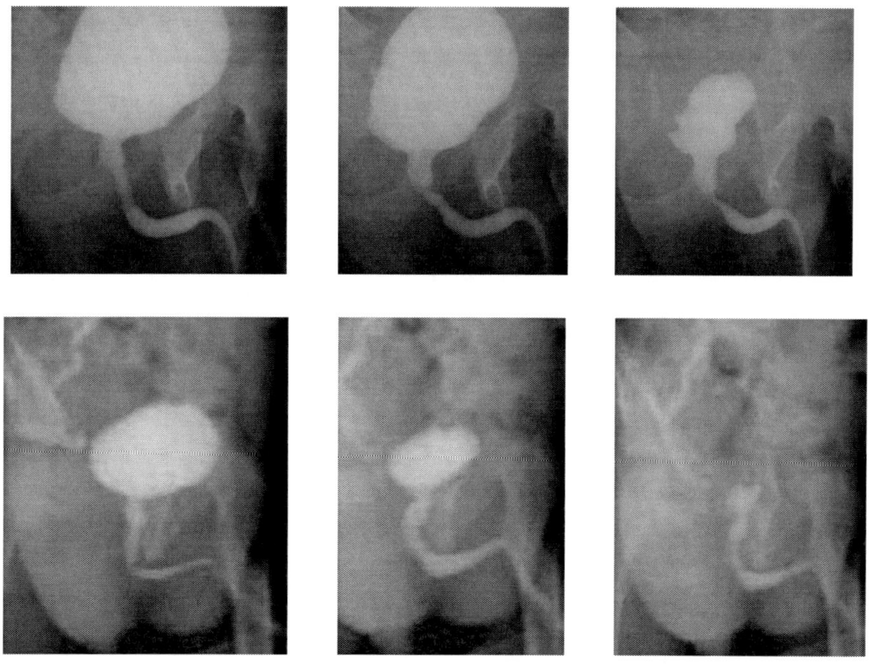

Figure 4. "Transient"deformity of urethra in VCUG for evaluation of boys with refractory nocturnal enuresis and daytime incontinence.

Finally, in two reports, lesions were suspected among 46% (17/37) and 51% (22/43), respectively, of boys with urinary incontinence (aged ≥6 years) and nocturnal enuresis (aged ≥8 years) with ≥1 year of resistance to conservative therapy [12, 15]. In addition, endoscopy confirmed the presence of lesions in 91% (20/22). It is impossible to tell at this point whether this high detection rate is the result of over-diagnosis of BOO or if it is actually genuine, and we are evaluating this in conjunction with the further standardization of clinical findings described in the following sections.

(2) Urethroscopic Diagnostic Criteria

When 25 European pediatric urological surgeons were shown endoscopic video recordings of the urethras of 17 boys, including healthy urethras and a range of mild to severe cases of posterior urethral valve in 2008, there was complete diagnostic concordance (100%) for only one video recording, with moderate concordance (≥80%) for 11 and low concordance (50–75%) for five. [2] This also demonstrates that, even when endoscopy is performed, this does not result in uniform diagnosis of congenital BOO, and global standards have yet to be established.

We started by using pediatric endoscopes from 8.5 Fr to 11.5 Fr as observation endoscopes to observe lesions. If a lesion was suspected, the observation endoscope was exchanged for a resectoscope fitted with a sickle-type cold knife, and an incision was made. Dilatation of the lower urinary tract by water pressure reveals the morphology of the obstruction more clearly, and therefore we basically performed observations and incisions with the bladder and lower urinary tract somewhat dilated, while being careful to avoid excessive dilation to nonphysiological levels. We considered that this test procedure could be carried out with almost no discrepancy among specialist pediatric urological clinics.

Endoscopic diagnosis and classification of BOO were based on the reports of Stephens (Table 1) and Lu. [7, 17] The concept of COPUM, that is, the view that has the universal structure of a membrane possessing a foraminal defect close to the posterior urethral wall, with the border of the membrane being continuous with the verumontanum, was extremely useful in the identification of this condition. We made an endoscopic diagnosis of latent BOO in the anterior wall direction if a comparatively large verumontanum was present with an inferior crest continuous with this on the posterior wall that branched in the direction of the lateral walls the further distally it continued, extending to the anterior wall, regardless of whether the membrane was clearly visible (Figure 5). If these findings were not evident, the obstruction was diagnosed as constriction by the external urinary sphincter rather than as an anterior wall lesion (Figure 6).

Cobb's collar (Type 3 posterior urethral valve) was diagnosed if a membranous or septal morphology was present in either the membranous or bulbar urethra with a transverse positional relationship to the long axis of the urethra. We confirmed that the verumontanum was small and discontinuous with the lesion (Figure 7).

Ultimately, BOO could be classified into two aggregate types, Type 1 posterior urethral valve and Cobb's collar, and among the 22 subjects, Type 1 posterior urethral valve was present in 11 patients, Cobb's collar (Type 3 posterior urethral valve) was present in 2, and both were present in 7. A retrospective investigation found that it was difficult to predict these categories and the degree of obstruction from VCUG findings.

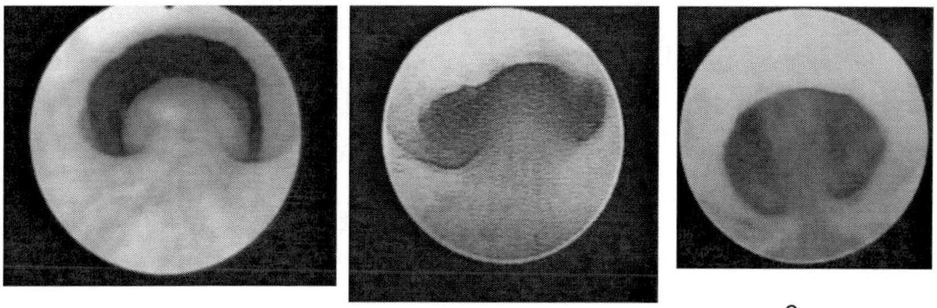

a b c

a. The location of the most distal part of the lesion looks consistent with the sphincter level.
b. The location of the most distal part of the lesion looks just distal to the sphincter level.
c. The location of the most distal part of the lesion looks far distal to the sphincter level.

Figure 5. Variety of posterior wall findings suggestive of latent BOO.

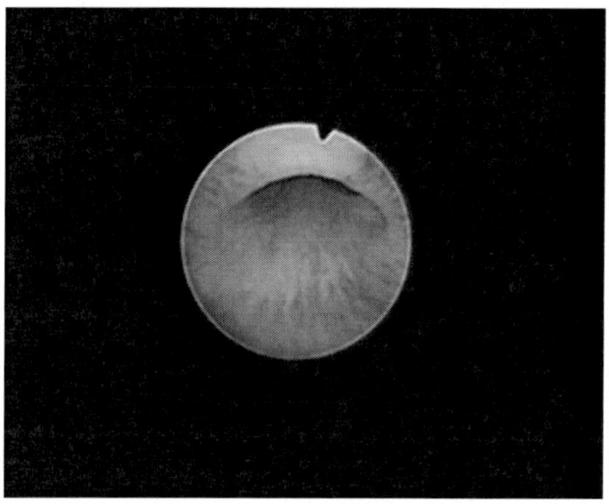

Without BOO the margin of the constriction of the sphincter looks like having no continuity to the verumontanum and inferior crest.

Figure 6. Constriction at the sphincter level in normal case.

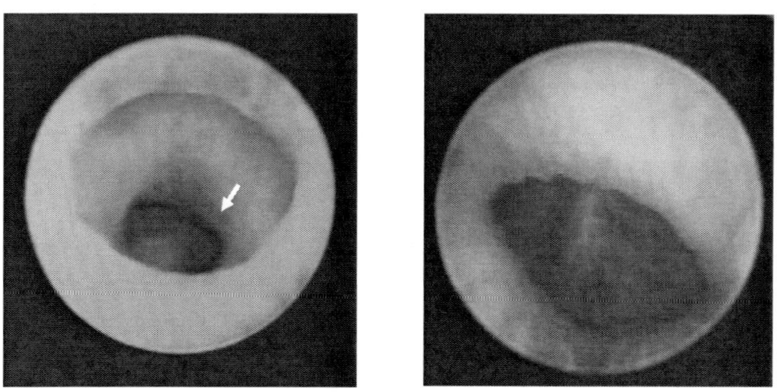

a b

a. The location of the lesion is distal to the sphincter level. (The arrow indicates sphincter.)
b. The location of the lesion is consistent with the sphincter level. (overlapping the sphincter) There is no continuity between the lesion and the verumontanum.

Figure 7. Cobb's collar (type 3 PUV).

Type 1 posterior urethral valve anterior wall lesions may extend past the external urinary sphincter to its distal side, which Dewan termed "prolapse of the obstructive lesion." [18] Rather than terming this phenomenon "prolapse," which implies a secondary meaning, we regard such lesions as being originally present in that location. Although a differential diagnosis was rendered difficult by proximity to the location of Cobb's collar, even in such cases, observation of the posterior wall of the urethra enabled these conditions to be differentiated by checking structural continuity between the lesion and the verumontanum (Figures 5c, 7b). It is important to recognize that the location of the lesion by itself is insufficient to distinguish between posterior urethral valve and Cobb's collar.

Previously, Mori et al. stated that, with respect to the morphology of congenital bulbar urethral stenosis (urethral ring), "although typically the foraminal defect is evident in the center, as its name suggests, it may sometimes approach the posterior wall." [3] By analogy with the results from our own patients, it is conceivable that most of the lesions diagnosed as urethral ring in Japan could be classified as distally extended Type 1 posterior urethral valves, with a minority being Cobb's collars.

Based on the criteria above, if the presence of BOO could not be determined, a policy was adopted of actively performing an incision in the 12 o'clock direction at the suspected location. Even in this case, however, it was important to clarify intraoperative findings specific to BOO, and we were careful to use a consistent method for making the incision, as described in the following section.

(3) Standardization of the Surgical Procedure for Endoscopic Incision

We fitted a sickle-type cold knife to an 8.5-Fr or 11.5-Fr resectoscope and made an incision in the 12 o'clock direction in cases of both Type 1 posterior urethral valve and Cobb's collar. In terms of extent and depth, we endeavored to make an incision until the stratum containing fibers running in an annular direction was visible and the anterior urethral wall became flat. As a result, 12 o'clock incisions for Type 1 posterior urethral rings usually required at least 20 strokes. Even when there was a possibility that the anterior wall lesion overlapped the external urinary sphincter, we attempted to make an incision in all cases, as long as the site of the suspected lesion consisted of firm tissue with poor circulation. As a result, in mild Type 1 posterior urethral valve, we came to focus not on lesions represented by lateral "valves" or circular "membranes," but on comparatively thick, protruding structures formed on the anterior wall that could be compared to "dikes" or banks" (Figure 8). It has been suggested that lesions with these characteristics not only cause direct urinary resistance, but they may also generate the sort of urinary flow rate-dependent obstruction reported by Hoebeke et al. as a result of insufficient local distensibility of the urethral wall [16]. If an adequate 12 o'clock incision was initially performed, the valvular structures on both lateral walls frequently disappeared. If lesions nevertheless persisted on the lateral walls (sufficient to snag the sickle-type cold knife), these were excised.

At present, there is no consistent approach for posterior urethral valve incisions, which are generally made by using one of two types of device, either by electrocauterization using a resection loop or by sharp incision using a cold knife. However, we believe that incision using a sickle-type cold knife should become standard. The first reason for this is that incision using a sickle-type cold knife enables the surgeon to control the extent and depth of incision almost completely, whereas these are more difficult to control with electrocauterization, and there is thus particularly greater risk of sphincter damage and perforation, which increases with incision depth. Secondly, using a sickle-type cold knife enables confirmation that the incision site consists of a lesion with poor blood circulation while the incision is in progress, a factor that is useful in differentiating between the obstructive lesion and the external urinary sphincter during surgery.

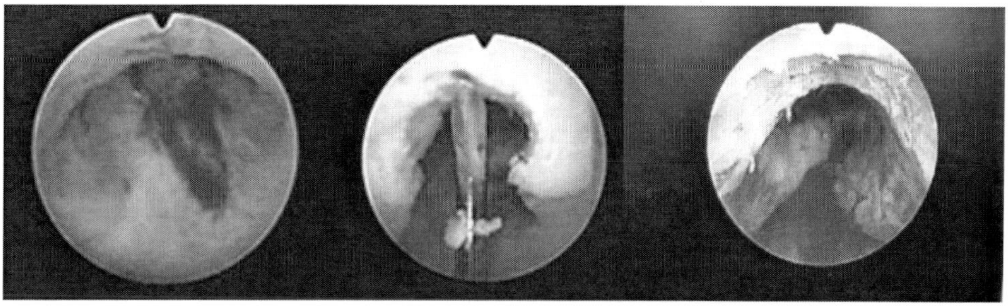

a b c

a. before endoscopic incision. The obstructive lesion is suspected to be located just on sphincter level.
b. endoscopic incision with sickle type knife. Bilateral cut-edges fall down and cut-surface shows vascular poor tissue.
c. after endoscopic incision. The extension and depth of the incision are rather long and deep.

Figure 8. Intraoperative findings of anterior wall lesion with PUV type 1 suggestive of latent BOO.

There were no cases in which incision had to be abandoned midway due to hemorrhage or other problems, nor in which electrocoagulation had to be used after incision to provide additional hemostasis. There were also no cases of postoperative increased urinary incontinence that would suggest the possibility of damage to the external urinary sphincter.

VCUG performed 3–4 months after endoscopic resection using this technique found that persistent lesions requiring repeated incision were present comparatively early on in the series, with a frequency of 20% (4/20). Generally, reported rates of repeated incision range from 18% to 47%. [14, 19] In our case, we made video recordings of endoscopic incision and viewed them repeatedly, gradually becoming better able to make immediate decisions and recognize the presence or absence of obstructive lesions, as well as the correct extent and depth of incisions. In other words, there was a learning curve for the techniques of diagnosis and incision of anterior wall lesions.

(4) Standardization of the Evaluation of the Results of Endoscopic Incision

To judge whether or not the theory and practice of endoscopic incision provides the correct level of treatment, further improvements in the scientific level of methods of evaluating its efficacy are also required. Until now, evaluation of endoscopic incision efficacy in terms of voiding function has only involved a comparison of urethrography findings and changes in the frequency of diurnal urinary incontinence and nocturnal enuresis before and after surgery, rather than routine urodynamic testing [9, 10, 11] The evaluation period has been inconsistent between reports, with evaluation sometimes taking place after more than a year has passed since surgery. The possibility that indirect effects due to growth may also be present must be eliminated as far as possible.

In order to standardize the evaluation of efficacy, we adopted the International Children's Continence Society (ICCS) evaluation criteria for urinary incontinence and nocturnal enuresis and evaluated lower urinary tract symptoms at set periods of 3–4 months and 6 months postoperatively [15]. We also performed VCUG and urodynamic tests 3–4 months postoperatively under the same conditions as preoperative testing. Urodynamic tests included uroflowmetry following fluid intake (repeated three times), cystometry using an 18-gauge central venous double-lumen catheter, and a voiding pressure flow study. (In patients who required repeated endoscopic incision, these were performed after the second operation.) As in adults, voiding urodynamics are also important in pediatric lower urinary tract obstructive disorders, and to enable this to be performed in school-aged children, we used a fine 18-G pliable central venous double-lumen catheter. We attempted to create a friendly testing environment for children with consistent voiding conditions (not making them wait, but allowing them to urinate at will).

Yamanishi et al. performed endoscopic incision on a total of 34 patients (29 boys, 5 girls) in whom BOO was discovered as a result of intractable nocturnal enuresis, and they reported that the frequency of nocturnal urination improved by ≥90% in 72% of boys, and that voiding dynamics, performed in from one-third to one-half of all subjects, also showed significant improvements in detrusor pressure at peak flow rate (PdetQmax), cystometric bladder capacity, and maximum flow rate [10]

In our study, diurnal urinary incontinence and nocturnal enuresis at 3–4 months postoperatively improved by 50% and 35%, respectively (full response and partial response according to the ICCS evaluation criteria), while at 6 months postoperatively, they had both improved by 50% (Table 3). This improvement rate of around half meant that we were unable to arrive at any conclusion concerning the validity of our endoscopic treatment (the possibility of over-indication and over-treatment could not be ruled out). We therefore compared voiding urodynamic parameters before and after surgery in all cases to investigate its validity [15]

Table 3. Symptomatic response of TUI after 3 to 4 months postoperatively

	Synergic n=13	Dyssynergic n=7	Total, n=20
Daytime incontinence (n=14)			
FR	7/8 (87.5%)	0/6 (0%)	7/14 (50%)
PR	0/8 (0%)	0/6 (0%)	0/14 (0%)
Nocturnal enuresis (n=20)			
FR	5/13 (38.5%)	0/7 (0%)	5/20 (25%)
PR	2/13 (15.4%)	0/7 (0%)	2/20 (10%)

We first concluded that two types of preoperative voiding urodynamics were present: one in which maximum detrusor pressure occurred after the onset of voiding (appearance of urine), and another in which maximum detrusor pressure occurred immediately before the onset of voiding. We named these types “synergic” and “dyssynergic” (Figure 9).

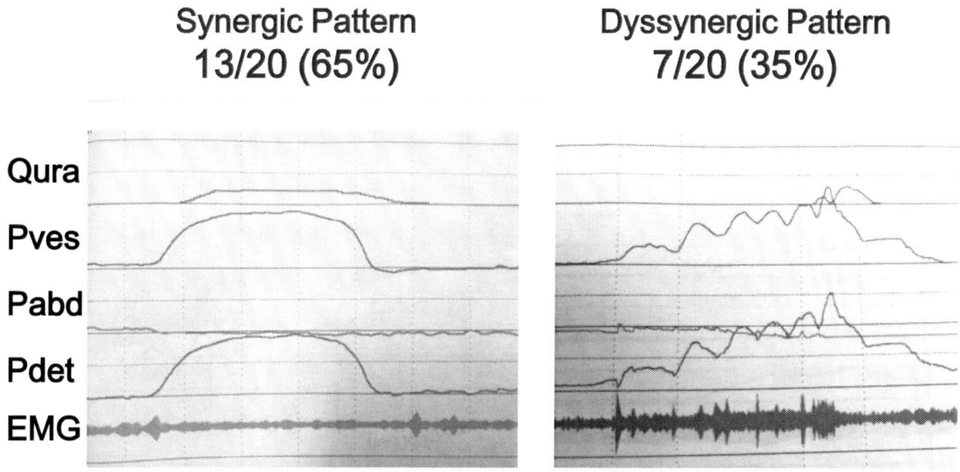

Figure 9. Two patterns of voiding urodynamics for boys with congenital urethral obstructive lesion.

They were present at frequencies of 65% (12/20) and 35% (7/20), respectively. Postoperative voiding urodynamics showed no change in these patterns. Secondly, a comparison of the rates of improvement in diurnal urinary incontinence and nocturnal enuresis in terms of these two types found that, for the synergic types, these improved by 87.5% and 53.9%, respectively (at 3–4 months postoperatively), whereas for the dyssynergic type, the rates were both 0%, a dramatic difference (Table 3). This difference was even more pronounced at 6 months postoperatively (Table 4). The dyssynergic type was conjectured to reflect sphincter dysfunction, suggesting the possibility of latent functional abnormality caused by the presence of organic BOO. Endoscopic incision may thus not have any efficacy if a functional abnormality is also present, but it may have a marked effect in cases of BOO alone.

Table 4. Symptomatic response of TUI after 6 months postoperatively

	Synergic n=13	Dyssynergic n=7	Total, n=20
Daytime incontinence (n=14)			
FR	7/8 (87.5%)	0/6 (0%)	7/14 (50%)
PR	0/8 (0%)	0/6 (0%)	0/14 (0%)
Nocturnal enuresis (n=20)			
FR	6/13 (46.2%)	0/7 (0%)	6/20 (30%)
PR	4/13 (30.8%)	0/7 (0%)	4/20 (20%)

Table 5. Parameter change of voiding urodynamics

Synergic Pattern (n=13)	bofore TUI	3 ~ 4 months after TUI	P value*
Pdet at maximum flow rate (Q_{max}; cm H_2O)	83.2 ± 26.9	45.8 ± 17.3	0.0004
Maximum bladder capacity (mL)	198.2 ± 103.3	260.4 ± 82.4	0.036
Post-voiding residual urine volume (mL)	25.7 ± 20.4	35.0 ± 43.7	0.467
Q_{max} (mL/s)	17.8 ± 4.8	21.8 ± 6.4	0.169
Dyssynergic Pattern (n=7)			
Pdet at maximum flow rate (Q_{max}; cm H_2O)	54.3± 8.34	52.1 ± 7.0	0.677
Maximum bladder capacity (mL)	147.0 ± 37.7	121.9 ± 36.5	0.252
Post-voiding residual urine volume (mL)	19.4 ± 18.4	9.0 ± 16.0	0.422
Q_{max} (mL/s)	20.3 ± 4.7	20.1 ± 5.7	0.959

A comparison of preoperative and postoperative voiding urodynamic parameters for the synergic pattern alone showed a significant decrease in PdetQmax and a significant increase in cystometric bladder capacity (maximum voiding volume when uroflowmetry was performed three times after fluid intake and waiting to urinate at maximum desire to void.) (Table 5). From these findings, improvements in diurnal urinary incontinence and nocturnal enuresis can be brought about by reducing detrusor pressure and increasing bladder capacity by means of the endoscopic incision of organic lesions, provided that there are no functional abnormalities, indicating the validity of our diagnostic criteria, treatment indications, and treatment method. Conversely, additional treatments must be developed for cases including functional abnormalities.

Summary

Although it must be noted that our hospital specializes in pediatric urological surgery, imaging diagnosis showed suspected lesions in around 50% of school –aged boys with intractable urinary incontinence and nocturnal enuresis, and among these, stenosis was diagnosed endoscopically in 90%. Excluding the one-third of these patients with functional abnormalities, endoscopic treatment for this stenosis improved diurnal urinary incontinence in around 90% and nocturnal enuresis in around 80% of cases at 6 months postoperatively, reducing their frequency to less than half. A rough calculation shows that congenital BOO was present at the high frequency of one in four of school –aged boys with urinary incontinence and nocturnal enuresis for whom lifestyle guidance and conservative treatment were ineffective, suggesting that this condition may be more prevalent than is generally thought. Further clinical epidemiological studies including a larger number of patients will be required to verify this, and greater consistency of diagnostic criteria (VCUG and endoscopic findings) and treatment procedures may also be necessary.

At this point, VCUG offers the most reliable form of screening, and not only is further effort required to improve its diagnostic accuracy, but the development of less invasive testing techniques is also desirable. To find out how bladder ultrasound and uroflowmetry can be effectively used for screening, it will first be important to investigate the sensitivity and specificity of bladder wall thickness and abnormalities seen on urethrography. The future identification of biochemical substances in urine that can detect lower BOO with high sensitivity is also anticipated.

Conclusions

(1) Congenital obstruction of the posterior and membranous urethra in boys can be generally divided into Type 1 posterior urethral valve and Cobb's collar, and both may be present simultaneously.
(2) Severe Type 1 posterior urethral valve is characterized by lesions consisting of valves or a membrane adjoining the verumontanum, but mild Type 1 posterior urethral valve is characterized by thick lesions located more distally on the anterior wall while maintaining continuity with the verumontanum.
(3) Severe Type 1 posterior urethral valve causes direct urinary resistance due to valves or a membrane, but mild Type 1 posterior urethral valve causes kinking at the site of the lesion due to ballooning of the posterior urethra, resulting in secondary urinary resistance.
(4) BOO suppresses the spontaneous resolution of diurnal urinary incontinence and nocturnal enuresis by increasing detrusor pressure and reducing bladder capacity.
(5) Functional obstructions of the urethra are also present in around one in three cases of BOO, and endoscopic incision is ineffective for urinary incontinence and nocturnal enuresis in these patients

References

[1] de Kort LM, Uiterwaal CS, Beek EJ, Jan Nievelstein RA, Klijn AJ, de Jong TP. Reliability of voiding cystourethrography to detect urethral obstruction in boys. *Urology*, 2004 May; 63(5):967-71; discussion 971-2.

[2] de Jong TP, Radmayr C, Dik P, Chrzan R, Klijn AJ, de Kort L; Pediatric Urology Club Meeting, Stans, Austria, January 2007. Posterior urethral valves: search for a diagnostic reference standard. *Urology*, 2008 Nov:72(5):1022-5. Epub 2008 Jun 30.

[3] Mori Y, Matsui T, Ogino T, Hosokawa S, Ihara H, Terakawa T, Shima H, Arima M, Ikoma F. *Treatment Of Congenital Urethral Stenosis* (Urethral Ring) In Children: O*ptic Internal Urethrotomy in the Congenital Bulbar Urethral Stenosis in Boys.* Nihon Hinyokika Gakkai Zasshi. 1989 May;80(5):704-10..

[4] Cobb B, Wolf JJ, Ansell J. Congenital stricture of the proximal urethral bulb. *J Urol.* 1968 May: 99:629-31.

[5] Moormann J. Congenital bulbar urethral stenosis as a cause of diseases of the urogenital junction. *Urologe* A. 1972 May: 11:157-60.

[6] Dewan P, Zappala S, Ransley P, Duffy P. Endoscopic reappraisal of the morphology of congenital obstruction of the posterior urethra. *Br. J. Urol.* 1992 Oct: 70:439-44.

[7] F Douglas Stephens, E Durham Smith, and John M Hutson, *Congenital anomalies of the urinary and genital tracts*. (Isis Medical Media Ltd.1996) 91-112.

[8] Young H, Frontz W, Baldwin J. Congenital obstruction of the posterior urethra. *J Urol.* 1919:3: 289-355.

[9] Shima H, Mori Y, Nojima M, Miyamoto I, Chokyu H, Ikoma F. Lower urinary tract problems in patients with enuresis. *Eur Urol.* 1998: 33 Suppl 3:37-40.

[10] Yamanishi Urethral Obstruction in Patients with Nighttime Wetting: Urodynamic Evaluation and Surgical Incision, 2000.

[11] Sugimoto M, Kakehi Y, Yamashita M, Matsuki T, Inui M, Taketa S. Ten cases of congenital urethral stricture in childhood with enuresis. *Int J Urol.* 2005 Jun: 12: 558-62.

[12] Kihara T, Nakai H, Mori K, Sato R, Kitahara S, Yasuda K. Variety of congenital urethral lesions in boys with lower urinary tract symptoms and the results of endoscopic treatment. *Int. J. Urol.* 2008 Mar: 15:235-40.

[13] Yeung CK, Chiu HN, Sit FK. Bladder dysfunction in children with refractory monoxymptomatic primary nocturnal enuresis. *J. Urol.* 1999 Sep;162(3Pt2):1049-54;discussion 1054-5.

[14] Nonomura K, Kanno T, Kakizaki H, Koyama T, Yamashita T, Koyanagi T. Impact of congenital narrowing of the bulbar urethra (Cobb's collar) and its transurethral incision in children. *Eur. Urol.* 1999 Aug: 36:144-8; discussion 9.

[15] Nakamura S, Kawai S, Kubo T, Kihara T, Mori K, Nakai H. Transurethral incision of congenital obstructive lesions in the posterior urethral in boys and its effect on urinary incontinence and urodynamic study. *BJU Int.* 2010 Aug 27, Epub ahead of pring.

[16] Hoebeke PB, Van Laecke E, Raes A, Vande Walle J, Oosterlinck W. Membrano-bulbo-urethral junction stenosis. Posterior urethra obstruction due to extreme caliber disproportion in the male urethra. *Eur. Urol.* 1997;32(4):480-4.

[17] Lu Y, Dewan P. Congenital urethral obstruction: the video-endoscopic perspective. *BJU Int.* 2006 Nov: 98:953-9.

[18] Dewan P, Keenan R, Morris L, Le Quesne G. Congenital urethral obstruction: Cobb's collar or prolapsed congenital obstructive posterior urethral membrane (COPUM). *Br. J. Urol.* 1994 Jan: 73:91-5.

[19] Imaji R, Dewan PA. Congenital posterior urethral obstruction: re-do fulguration. *Pediatr. Surg. Int.* 2002 Sep;18(5-6):444-6.

In: Urinary Incontinence
Editor: Eric Chung
ISBN: 978-1-62618-482-4

Chapter 19

Voiding Dysfunction and the Elderly: Pathophysiology, Types and Management

Chasta Bacsu and Lewis Chan
Department of Urology,
Concord Repatriation General Hospital,
University of Sydney, Australia

Abstract

Voiding dysfunction and urinary incontinence are common in the elderly often overlooked as a normal part of ageing or due to embarrassment. Lower urinary tract (LUTS) and urinary incontinence can contribute to substantial morbidity and reduced quality of life.

Age-related changes of the genitourinary, neurologic and endocrine systems as well as an increased propensity to have multiple medical co-morbidities contribute to the increased prevalence of voiding dysfunction in the elderly.

Causes of LUTS and urinary incontinence in the elderly are often multi-factorial. Baseline evaluation of the elderly should include at thorough history, physical examination and urinalysis. Other investigations such as voiding diaries, validated questionnaires, serum and urine studies, imaging, and urodynamics can be considered depending on the clinical scenario.

Management strategies for common types of voiding dysfunction affecting the elderly (e.g. detrusor overactivity, detrusor hyperactivity impaired contractility, stress urinary incontinence, and bladder outlet obstruction) are reviewed. Symptoms of geriatric voiding dysfunction and incontinence are not always reflective of the underlying pathology that if not recognized, may result in treatments with limited therapeutic benefit and unpleasant adverse effects.

The impact of voiding dysfunction and urinary incontinence can depend on the severity, functional status, comorbidities, coping strategies, treatment goals and expectations which are unique to each patient and need to be thoroughly discussed to optimize patient satisfaction.

Introduction and Epidemiology

Voiding dysfunction and urinary incontinence are common in the elderly. Over age 60, 41-74% of men and 46-74.5% of women experience at least one urinary storage symptom, and 37% men and 25% of women experience at least one urinary voiding symptom [1].

Women are at least twice as likely than men to have urinary incontinence [2, 3, 4]. Prevalence of urinary incontinence of elderly living in the community are 12.2-48% in women and 10.4-31% in men [1, 4, 5-13]. Prevalence of urinary incontinence in nursing homes is 44-77% [14]. Discrepancy in prevalence rates of voiding dysfunction and urinary incontinence has been attributed to variance in inclusion criteria and poor adherence to ICS definitions [9, 15].

Age is a well-known risk factor for voiding dysfunction and urinary incontinence [2, 4, 15, 16]. With the ageing population, it is anticipated that the prevalence of voiding dysfunction and urinary incontinence will also increase [17].

In the elderly, urinary incontinence and lower urinary tract symptoms (LUTS) are often overlooked as a normal part of aging or can be too embarrassing to seek medical attention [10, 18]. LUTS and urinary incontinence have been associated with worsening quality of life (QOL) [9]. Urinary incontinence affects both physical and mental aspects of QOL [9, 19]. In one study, urinary incontinence had greater impact on patient-perceived QOL than did diabetes, cancer and arthritis [19].

Morbidity of urinary incontinence includes increased risk of falls, urinary tract infections (UTIs), urinary retention, renal deterioration and skin irritation [10, 20, 21, 22]. Urinary incontinence also contributes to a substantial economic burden for both society and the sufferer. In Australia, the overall cost of incontinence in 2010 was estimated to be $66.7 billion or $14,014 per person with urinary incontinence [16].

Physiology of Geriatric Voiding Dysfunction

Ageing affects the lower urinary tract and is a well-known risk factor associated with both voiding dysfunction and urinary incontinence. Ageing and its associated medical conditions have considerable impact on bladder storage and emptying [22]. Causes of voiding dysfunction are often multifactorial [22]. Mobility, manual dexterity, accessibility to toileting, mental capacity, general health and medication use are important factors in urinary continence [22]. For example, diabetes causes polyuria and neurologic impairment of urinary control [22]. Neurological conditions such as cerebral vascular accidents (CVA) and Parkinson's disease affect bladder storage and emptying. A detailed discussion regarding these conditions, medical co-morbidities and effects of medication are beyond the scope of this discussion.

In females, estrogen levels decline with menopause. Decreased estrogen levels are associated with atrophy of the epithelium and the supporting tissue of the urethra and vagina consequently increasing the risk of pelvic floor hypermobility, intrinsic sphincter deficiency (ISD) and pelvic organ prolapse (POP) [23]. Cadaveric studies have demonstrated reduced striated and circular smooth muscle densities in the urethra of elderly women, most notably in the posterior urethra [24, 25, 26]. These factors likely contribute to the reduction of urethral closure pressures and functional urethral length often seen in ageing women [17].

Ageing in men is typically associated with prostate enlargement. Observational cohort studies have found median prostate growth rates of 1.9-2.5% [27, 28]. Increased prostatic volume may cause bladder outlet obstruction which can result in long term changes to the bladder including detrusor hypertrophy, bladder trabeculation and fibrosis, detrusor overactivity, decreased bladder compliance or atonic distended bladder.

Bladder capacity, bladder sensation, detrusor contractility, ability to postpone urination are reduced in elderly [10, 29]. Urinary flow rates also decrease with ageing but it is more profound in males associated with benign prostatic hyperplasia (BPH) [10]. Ageing is associated with increased prevalence of involuntary detrusor contractions and post-void residual [10, 15, 29, 30]. Structural and histopathological changes associated with ageing have been investigated using electron microscopy of endoscopic detrusor biopsies and cadaveric studies [31]. The ageing detrusor typically has a dense-band pattern characterized by decreased caveolae with elongation of sarcolemma dense bands and widening between muscle cells with some collagen fibrils and diminished elastic fibers [31].

Nocturnal urine production and frequency of nocturnal urination also increases with age. Causes may include altered anti-diuretic hormone (ADH) secretion, congestive heart failure, fluid redistribution with aging, medications such as diuretics, high fluid intake, diabetes, sleep disturbance or anxiety conditions and decreased bladder capacity [15, 23].

Neurologic changes related to ageing affect lower urinary tract functioning. Positron emission tomography (PET) and functional magnetic resonance imaging (fMRI) studies reveal alterations in activation and deactivation of cortical pathways involved in normal bladder control in elderly compared to younger subjects [32]. Decreased activation of non-frontal cortical regions such as the right and left insula have been demonstrated in response to bladder filling in the elderly groups which may correlate to the decline in bladder sensation seen with ageing [32]. Decreased activation may be related to cerebral changes of ageing, impaired bladder afferent input from peripheral nerves or unrecognized brain pathology [32]. Detrusor overactivity and impaired bladder sensation in the elderly has been associated with cortical hypoperfusion on single photon emission computed tomography (SPECT) [31, 33].

Assessment of Voiding Dysfunction in the Elderly

As geriatric voiding dysfunction is often multifactorial, comprehensive history and physical examination are essential [34]. Assessment should be individualized to the patient's clinical situation, needs and goals. Although history should be obtained from the patient, medical records and caregivers can provide supplemental information. History attained over a series of visits may be helpful in gaining a better appreciation of the patient's overall health, expectations and psychosocial influences. History should address both storage and voiding LUTS. Storage symptoms include frequency, urgency, nocturia and incontinence [35, 36]. Voiding symptoms include slow stream, hesitancy, intermittency, terminal dribble, splitting of the stream, incomplete emptying, need to immediately re-void, urinary retention and dysuria [35, 36]. Duration, severity and progression of LUTS, as well as degree of bother should be assessed. Haematuria should be ruled out as it could signify serious pathology. Past urologic history such as UTIs, urosepsis, urologic malignancy, BPH, urolithiasis, incontinence should be elicited along with previous investigations, medical and surgical interventions [34]. Other risk factors for voiding dysfunction such as obstetrical history, trauma or radiation are important to elicit [37]. Fluid intake and caffeine habits may contribute to LUTS.

History should include medical co-morbidities and a detailed assessment of medications [18, 34, 37]. Transient causes of urinary incontinence should be ruled out [18, 37]. Transient causes of incontinence have been included in the mnemonic DIAPPERS: delirium, infection atrophic vaginitis, pharmaceuticals, psychological factors, excess urine production, restricted mobility and stool impaction [10, 38]. It is estimated at nearly 40% of patients over 65 take more than 5 different medications [18]. Many medications can affect urine production, bladder storage and emptying or can interact with the pharmacologic agents used for voiding dysfunction [34, 37].

Functional assessments should include performance of both basic activities of daily living and instrumental activities of daily living [34, 37]. The Folstein mini-mental is often helpful in assessing cognitive impairment [34]. Environment factors such as accessible toileting are also important [34].

A thorough physical exam is helpful in assessing occult causes of voiding dysfunction. General appearance, hygiene, cognition, mobility and functional status help provide clues for diagnosis. Exam should include cardiovascular, respiratory and neurological systems [34]. Abdominal exam should document prior incisions, any tenderness, constipation and palpable bladder [18, 37]. Genital and pelvic exam are useful to assess for atrophic vaginitis, POP, pelvic floor strength and signs of skin irritation or breakdown [10, 36, 37]. Rectal examination should be performed as it evaluates prostate size and consistency, presence of prostatic or rectal masses, sphincter tone and constipation [37].

Urinalysis should be performed in all patients presenting with voiding dysfunction [34]. Urine culture and sensitivity should be performed if symptoms suggest UTI or abnormal urinalysis [20, 34]. Serum electrolytes, creatinine, calcium and glucose are useful especially in patients with confusion or suspected renal impairment [18, 37]. Results of these investigations help tailor further investigations [20].

Voiding diaries performed for 2 or 3 days may be helpful in further characterizing voiding dysfunction [10, 18, 34, 37]. Voiding diaries should include timing of urination and incontinence; volumes of intake and output can be helpful but is more time consuming [10, 34, 37]. Validated questionnaires such as the International Prostate Symptom Score (IPSS) or International Consultation on Incontinence Questionnaire-Urinary Incontinence Short Form (ICIQ-UI SF) may be used to further assess the degree of bother or impact to quality of life.

Measurement of post void residual (PVR) should be performed following intentional voiding to rule out urinary retention [10, 37]. In possible stress urinary incontinence (SUI), urinary leakage can be assessed by a urinary stress test with a full bladder in a relaxed environment and provoking maneuvers like cough or valsalva.

Urodynamics are useful to evaluate LUT function, especially in complex patients. In the elderly, LUTS do not always correlate of the urodynamic diagnosis [10, 17]. A study of urodynamics performed on elderly women with LUTS resulted in a complete change in management in 43% of the patients following urodynamics and may avoid empirically prescribing medications with adverse effects [17]. In this study, patients with pure storage symptoms had the most discrepancy with their urodynamic findings having only 29% positive predictive value of detrusor overactivity [17]. There are no specific guidelines for urodynamics in the elderly. Urodynamic studies would be most helpful in patients with significant LUTS, neurologic disease, prior urologic/pelvic surgery, high post-void residuals or when urologic surgery for the complaint is considered [10]. Urodynamics are generally well tolerated in geriatric patients providing adequate cognition and mobility [10, 17]. Risk of UTI following urodynamics is approximately 6% [17]. Antibiotic prophylaxis may be helpful in this population to reduce this risk [10, 38]. Other complications include gross haematuria and urinary retention [10]. Although urodynamics can be very helpful, risks and benefits of the study should be weighed for each patient [10, 37].

Types of Voiding Dysfunction and Management Strategies

Detrusor Overactivity

The constellation of urinary frequency, urgency and nocturia in the absence of infection or pathology is typically referred to as overactive bladder (OAB) syndrome [36]. The EPIC study demonstrated a prevalence of OAB in 13.9% of respondents over 40, which increased with age in both sexes [15]. OAB was more common in women < 60 years but more common in men over 60 years [15]. Patient perceived OAB does not correspond to rates physician perceived OAB [39]. Patient perceived OAB rates were 22.4% compared to 9.5% perceived by their primary care physicians [39]. The discrepancy was even higher in patients over 70 with patient perceived prevalence at 29.7% [39]. The differential diagnosis of OAB symptoms include detrusor overactivity, UTIs, bladder cancer and carcinoma in situ (CIS), bladder calculi, medications, fluid intake, habit or misperception of normal voiding.

Detrusor overactivity is a urodynamic diagnosis of involuntary detrusor contractions on filling cystometry [36]. Detrusor overactivity is the most common cause of incontinence in both elderly men and women. Neurogenic detrusor overactivity occurs in the presence of a neurological condition or lesion such as CVA or Parkinson's disease while idiopathic detrusor overactivity occurs in the absence of a neurological cause [36].

Lifestyle modification including avoidance of caffeine and bladder irritants, adjustments to fluid intake and bladder retraining should be initial management [18, 34]. Prompted voiding is useful strategy in those with cognitive impairment [18, 34]. Some male patients find it is useful to have a bedside commode [18]. Adjustments to timing of medications may also be helpful if urinary frequency.

Pharmacologic treatment of detrusor overactivity typically includes anticholinergics. Dry mouth is the most common side effect. Other side effects include confusion, constipation, visual disturbances, GORD, tachycardia and urinary retention [40]. Contraindications for anticholinergic include narrow-angle glaucoma and urinary retention [40]. Anticholinergics may aggravate co-existing medical conditions and have many interactions with other medications so detailed medical history, pharmacologic review and close monitoring throughout treatment is essential [18, 40]. Oxybutinin and tolterodine are the original formulations and have been used safely in the elderly by starting at lowest dose and gradually increasing the dose to minimize side effects. Newer anticholinergic agents include darifenacin, solifenacin and trospium. These medications are thought to have a reduced side effect profile but there are a limited number of studies in the geriatric population.

Refractory urgency incontinence may be managed by intravesical botulinum toxin A injection. One study of non-neurogenic refractory urgency incontinence patients over 75 years of age treated with intravesical botox had 76% response rate and no treatment related complications [41]. Mean treatment effect was 7.1 months (range 5-11 months) [41]. Potential side effects include haematuria, UTI, urinary retention and weakness.

Sacral neuromodulation has also been reported as a safe and effective management approach in refractory non-neurogenic detrusor overactivity in a limited number of studies [42, 43, 44]. Elderly patients are more likely to have contraindications for sacral neuromodulation that include cognitive impairment, sacral anatomic abnormalities, conditions requiring possible MRI or cardiac pacemakers [42]. In two small studies, age over 55 years was associated with lower success rates 17-37% compared to younger cohorts with success rates of 40-65% [42, 43, 44]. Morbidity of sacral neuromodulation was not increased in these elderly patients [42, 43, 44].

Patients refractory, unfit or opposed to pharmacologic and surgical intervention can be managed with protective absorbents pads and continence products. Urinary catheters should be used as last resort as catheters can worsen detrusor overactivity and cause bypassing around the catheter.

Detrusor Hyperactivity with Impaired Contractility (DHIC)

Detrusor hyperactivity with impaired contractility (DHIC) is a condition increasingly recognized in the elderly [45]. It was first described by Yarra et al. in 1987 [45]. It is thought to be a paradoxical voiding disorder as there is detrusor overactivity with ineffective voiding [45]. On urodynamics, DHIC is characterized by low-pressure involuntary detrusor contractions associated with reflexic urethral relaxation and reduced bladder emptying [33]. Pathophysiology is poorly understood [33, 45]. Misdiagnosis is common often being mistaken as bladder outlet obstruction (BOO) or ISD [33, 40]. Misdiagnosis may result in unnecessary surgery [33]. Currently there is a paucity of data on the clinical management of DHIC. Management strategies are formulated on the basis of symptomatic complaints, urodynamic findings and patient tolerability. If symptoms of DHIC are minimally bothersome, it can be managed conservatively with adjustments to fluid intake, bladder retraining and pelvic floor exercises [33]. If the symptoms are predominantly related to detrusor overactivity, a trial of low dose anticholinergic agents can be initiated. Careful follow-up to monitor cognitive status, post-void residuals and related side effects should be coordinated throughout treatment [33]. If symptoms are more related to impaired bladder emptying, alpha-blockers may be considered to decrease the outlet resistance or added in combination with a low dose anticholinergics. In select patients, TURP can be considered. Clean intermittent catheterization and indwelling catheters can also be a suitable way to manage elevated post void residuals associated with DHIC [33]. Fifty-six males with urodynamic proven DHIC were reviewed from 2005 to 2009 with mean follow up of 16.2 months [46]. Mean age was 76 years [46]. Mean post-void residual was 102 ml [46]. Approximately 52% of patients noted improvement following intervention, 46% reported no change and 2% deteriorated [46]. In this series, only 1 patient developed acute urinary retention [46]. The study demonstrated that anticholinergics and alpha-blockers could safely be used in DHIC [46]. Prompted voiding programs have been effective in up to 50% of nursing home populations [47]. Patients failing prompted voiding can be alternatively managed with protective incontinence devices and catheters.

Nocturia

Nocturia occurs more often in the elderly. Nocturia can cause daytime fatigue, impaired cognitive functioning and increased fall risk [18]. Medical conditions should be ruled out and treated if they are an underlying cause of nocturia. Lifestyle modification is also helpful. Afternoon ambulation may also help in promote diuresis prior to sleeping. Low dose anticholinergics can be considered if conservative measures fail. Desmopressin should not be used in the elderly as it causes significant hyponatremia.

Stress Urinary Incontinence

Stress urinary incontinence (SUI) is defined as "involuntary urinary loss associated with effort or physical exertion, sneezing or coughing" [36]. It is a common cause of incontinence in elderly women. Most often it is due to pelvic floor hypermobility. Ageing leads to urethral atrophy and impaired urethral closure pressures which may contribute to reduced sphincteric function adding an ISD component [17, 23, 24, 25, 26]. Severe ISD is rare and usually associated with operative trauma and long-term indwelling catheterization. In women, conservative management of SUI includes weight loss, smoking cessation, and bladder retraining [37].

Biofeedback and pelvic floor exercises can reduce the severity of SUI. Pessaries may be an option for patients with POP, unfit or reluctant to have surgery. Topical estrogens are often used in combination with pessaries to reduce erosion risk [37]. On failure of lifestyle modification, surgery can be considered. Surgical options for female SUI include periurethral bulking agents, mesh suburethral slings, autologous suburethral slings and open abdominal bladder suspensions such as the Burch procedure.

Suburethral slings are less invasive than the traditional open procedures such as the Burch [48, 49]. Success rates, safety profiles and more rapid recovery make mesh suburethral slings acceptable for patients regardless of age providing they are suitable surgical candidates [18, 48, 49]. Success rates for suburethral slings in the elderly are highly variable, ranging from 45-96% [48, 49, 50, 51, 52, 53, 54, 55, 56]. This discrepancy is likely due to study design, definitions and assessment of success, age, parity, obesity, duration of follow-up and concomitant procedures [50].

Morbidity of suburethral slings is not significantly higher in the elderly compared to younger cohorts [48-56]. Rates of de novo urgency, urinary retention and UTIs were variable and not consistently associated with increased risk in the older patients [48-56]. Even if success rates are reduced compared to younger patients, a multicentre, prospective randomized trial performed in women over age 70 demonstrated significant improvement in quality of life, patient satisfaction and urinary symptoms compared to non-treated women awaiting the procedure [57].

SUI in men most often iatrogenic in the setting of prior prostatectomy and related sphincteric damage. Radiation and trauma may also be a contributor to male SUI. Management options include weight loss, smoking cessation, behavior modification, pelvic floor exercises, penile clamp, periurethral bulking agents, male urethral sling or artificial sphincter.

Bladder Outlet Obstruction (BOO)

Benign prostatic hypertrophy (BPH) is a common cause of BOO in men. BPH is often associated with progressive LUTS [58, 59, 60]. The clinical dilemma is in differentiating whether LUTS are due to OAB, BOO, detrusor underactivity or DHIC. Urodynamics can be especially helpful in diagnosis and treatment planning as symptoms may poorly correspond to urodynamic findings. BPH can present with recurrent UTIs, bladder calculi, gross haematuria, upper tract deterioration with renal impairment, overflow incontinence, acute urinary retention, detrusor overactivity and bladder decompensation [59, 60, 61]. Chronic bladder obstruction has been associated with structural changes of trabeculation, fibrosis, and reduced bladder compliance [62].

International Prostate Symptom Score (IPSS) can be used to assess bother and help guide management. For minimal bother, patients may be offered conservative lifestyle modification and observation. Lifestyle modification could include restriction of late day fluid intake, avoidance of caffeine, adjustments in medications like diuretics, pelvic floor exercises, prevention of constipation, and bladder retraining. For moderate to severe bother, options include observation, medical management, minimally invasive therapy and surgical therapy. Alpha-blockers work by relaxing prostatic smooth muscle. Alpha-blocking agent traditionally used include tamsulosin, doxazosin, alfuzosin, and terazosin. Typical side effects from alpha-blockers included postural hypotension, rhinitis, retrograde ejaculation, and asthenia [61]. Tamsulosin and alfuzosin have improved tolerability with less postural hypotension compared to doxazosin and terazosin [63]. Alpha-blockers especially tamsulosin have been associated with increased complications following cataract surgery [64]. Increased risk of cardiac failure was seen in elderly men treated with doxazosin as an antihypertensive in the ALLHAT trial [65]. In the elderly, drug interactions and baseline blood pressure should be assessed prior to initiating alpha-blockers as they may increase the patient's fall risk. 5-alpha reductase inhibitors (5ARIs) include finasteride and dutasteride studied in MTOPS and CombAT respectively [59, 60, 61]. Typical side effects from 5ARIs include erectile dysfunction, ejaculatory disturbances, decreased libido, gynecomastia, and hair growth [59, 60, 61]. In patients suffering BPH and concomitant detrusor overactivity, addition of an anticholinergic to alpha-blocker therapy may be considered if low PVR.

Surgical indications for BPH include renal failure due to BOO, refractory urinary retention, recurrent UTIs, bladder calculi, persistent prostatic bleeding, and failure of medical therapy. Surgery for BPH include transurethral incision of prostate (TUIP) for small prostates, transurethral resection of prostate (TURP), laser vaporization of prostate, holium laser enucleation of the prostate and open prostatectomy. Early complications of TURP include TURP syndrome, bleeding requiring transfusion, clot retention, bladder injury, urosepsis, urinary retention, and death [63]. Anesthetic and peri-operative risks also includes myocardial infarction, pulmonary emboli, deep vein thrombosis, CVA or transient ischemic attack but are relatively rare. Long-term complications associated with TURP include bladder neck contracture, urethral strictures, urinary retention, retrograde ejaculation, urinary incontinence, erectile dysfunction, persistence of LUTS or need for repeat surgery [63]. Complications post-TURP, particularly need for transfusion, are higher in the elderly. TURP is well tolerated if patients are appropriately selected [67].

Laser vaporization of the prostate appears to reduce bleeding complications and need for transfusion in patients on anticoagulants or anti-platelet agents [66]. Laser and bipolar technology to perform prostatic resection using saline avoids risk of TURP syndrome for which the elderly are at increased risk [67]. Age has is a risk factor for increased mortality post TURP [67, 68]. TURP mortality has been reported 0-3.2% in patients over 80 years [67, 68].

Increased age has also been associated with increased resection volumes and preoperative bacteriuria [68]. Rates of voiding dysfunction increase 5.3% for each year older, where patients greater than 70 years had twice the chance of incontinence post procedure [69]. Minimal invasive treatments for BPH include transurethral microwave therapy (TUMT) and transurethral needle ablation (TUNA) may be performed in an ambulatory setting but have reduced long-term efficacy compared to TURP. In select patients unfit for surgery, prostatic stents may be considered surgical but otherwise not recommended. Long-term indwelling catheter or clean intermittent catheterization is necessary in patients with acute urinary retention, surgically unfit or persistent postoperative urinary retention.

BOO is uncommon in women. It could occur with severe atrophic vaginitis, POP, urethral stricture, post-anti-incontinence procedures or pelvic malignancy [70].

Detrusor Underactivity

Detrusor contractility declines with age [10, 29, 71]. Detrusor underactivity is the preferred ICS term to describe "detrusor contraction of reduced strength and/or durations, resulting in prolonged bladder emptying and/or failure to achieve complete bladder emptying within a normal time span" [36]. Detrusor underactivity is likely under-diagnosed and frequently mistaken for BOO. In a study of nearly 200 community dwelling patients over 70 with urinary symptoms, detrusor underactivity was found in 48% of men and 12% of women on urodynamics [72]. Debate exists regarding its pathophysiological mechanism whether it's a result of myogenic failure or bladder wall ischemia [31, 32, 73]. Detrusor underactivity may be idiopathic, caused by medication, neurologic disease, end stage BOO or radical pelvic surgery [73, 74]. History of catheterization and retention are predictive of detrusor underactivity [72]. Presence of diabetes and neurologic disease did not predict detrusor underactivity [72]. Urodynamics are essential to confirm diagnosis of bladder underactivity and help guide treatment [72]. Urodynamics has been criticized as it does not indicate severity of detrusor underactivity and can miss co-existent BOO [75]. Bladder contractility index (BCI) has been used to help diagnose detrusor underactivity [76]. BCI=pdet@Qmax + 5Qmax; where BCI < 100 indicates underactivity [76]. Initial management for detrusor underactivity is lifestyle modification to help optimize voiding with treatment of constipation, pharmacologic review and increased mobilization. Parasympathomimetic medications such as bethanecol for detrusor underactivity are generally ineffective and place the patient at risk for increased side effects [73, 77, 78]. The role of TURP in detrusor underactivity is controversial with conflicting results [75, 79]. A prospective study of patients with detrusor underactivity demonstrated improved IPSS and QOL scares, mean Q max, Pdet Max and reduced PVR at 12 months [75]. Another study had 60% patient satisfaction with surgical outcomes and urinary symptoms [78]. Informing the patients that success rates of TURP are lower than in patients without detrusor underactivity can be helpful to ensure that patients have realistic expectations. Improvement following TURP may be due to reduce outflow resistance or undiagnosed BOO [75]. Further research efforts in detrusor underactivity are necessary given its increasing prevalence and limited management options [80].

References

[1] Irwin DE, Milsom I, Steinar H, Reilly, Kopp Z, Herschorn S, Coyne K, Kelleher C, Hampel C, Artibani, Abrams. Population-based survey of urinary incontinence, overactive bladder, and other lower urinary tract symptoms in five countries: Results of the EPIC study. *Eur. Urol.* 2006; 50: 1306-1315.

[2] Landefel CS. Bowers BJ, Feld AD, Hartmann KE, Hoffman E, Ingber MJ, King JT, McDougal WS, Nelson H, Orav EJ, Pignone M, Richardson LH, Rohrbaugh RM, Siebens HC, Trock BJ. National Institutes of Health State-of-the-Science conference statement: prevention of fecal and urinary incontinence in adults. *Ann. Intern. Med.* 2008; 148:449-458.

[3] Moore KN, Gray M. Urinary incontinence in men: current status and future directions. *Nurs. Res.* 2004; 53: S36-41.

[4] Tennstedt SL, Link CL, Steers WD, McKinlay JB. Prevalence of and risk factors for urine leakage in a racially and ethnically diverse population of adults: The Boston Area Community Health (BACH) Survey. *Am. J. Epidemiol.* 2008; 167: 390-399.

[5] Hawthorne G. Measuring Incontinence in Australia. A report from the Commonwealth of Australia. 2006: 1-104.

[6] Dooley Y, Kenton K, Cao G, Luke A, Durazo-Arvizu R, Kramer H, Brubaker L. Urinary incontinence prevalence: Results from the National Health and Nutrition Examination Survey. *J. Urol.* 2008; 179: 656-661.

[7] Anger JT, Saigal CS, Litwin MS, and the Urologic Diseases of America Project. The prevalence of urinary incontinence among community dwelling adult women: Results from the National Health and Nutrition Examination Survey. *J. Urol.* 2006; 175: 601-604.

[8] Temml C, Haidinger G, Schmidbauer J. Schatzl G, Maderbacher S. Urinary incontinence in both sexes: Prevalence rates and impact on quality of life and sexual life. *Neurourol. Urodyn.* 2000; 19: 259-271.

[9] Kwong PW, Cumming RG, Chan L, Seibel MJ, Naganathan V, Creasey H, Le Couteur D, Waite LM, Sambrook PN, Handelsman D. Urinary incontinence and quality of life among older community-dwelling Australian men: the CHAMP study. *Age Ageing.* 2010; 39: 349-359.

[10] Gomes CM, Arap S, Trigo-Rocha FE. Voiding dysfunction and urodynamic abnormalities in elderly patients. *Rev. Hosp. Clin. Fac. Med.* S Paulo. 2004; 59: 206-215.

[11] McGrother C. Epidemiology and etiology of urinary incontinence in the elderly. *World J. Urol.* 1998; 16; S3-9.

[12] Anger JT, Saigal CS, Stothers L, Thom DH, Rodriguez LV, Litwin MS and the Urologic disease of America Project. The prevalence of urinary incontinence among community dwelling men: Results from the National Health and Nutrition Examination Survey. *J. Urol.* 2006; 276: 2103-2108.

[13] Markland AD, Goode PS, Redden DT, Borrud LG, Burgio KL. Prevalence of urinary incontinence in Men: Results from the National Health and Nutrition Examination Survey. *J. Urol.* 2010; 184: 1022-1027.

[14] Offermans MP, Du Moulin MF, Hamer JP, Dassan T, Halfens RJ. Prevalence of urinary incontinence and associated risk factors in nursing home resident: a systematic review. *Neurourol. Urodyn.* 2009; 28: 288-294.

[15] Milsom I, Irwin DE. A cross-sectional, population based, multinational study of the prevalence of overactive bladder and lower urinary tract symptoms: Results from the Epic study. *Eur. Urol. Supp.* 2007; 6: 4-9.

[16] Deloitte Access Economics. The economic impact of incontinence in Australia. Continence Foundation of Australia. 2011: 1-60.

[17] Bromage SJ, Dorkin TJ, Chan L, Tse V. Urodynamics in the octogenarian female: is it worthwhile? *Int. Urogynecol. J.* 2010; 21: 117-1121.

[18] Guzzo TJ, Drach GW. Major urologic problems in geriatrics: Assessment and management. *Med. Clin. N Am.* 2011; 253-264.

[19] Hawkins, K, Pernarelli J, Ozminkowski RJ, Bai M, Gaston SJ, Hommer C, Migliori RJ, Yeh CS. The prevalence of urinary incontinence and its burden on the quality of life among older adults with medicare supplement insurance. *Qual. Life Res.* 2011; 20: 723-732.

[20] Gammack JK. Lower urinary tract symptoms. *Geriatr Clin.* 2010; 26: 249-260.

[21] Morris V, Wagg A. Lower urinary tract symptoms, incontinence and falls in elderly people: time for an intervention study. *Int J Clin Pract.* 2007; 61: 320-3.

[22] Kevorkian R. Physiology of incontinence. *Clin. Geriatr. Med.* 2004; 20: 409-425.

[23] Ouslander JG. Aging and the lower urinary tract. *Am. J. Med. Sci.* 1997; 314: 214-218.

[24] Clobes AM, De Lancey JOL, Morgan DM. Urethral circular smooth muscle in young and old women. *Am. J. Obstet. Gynecol.* 2008; 198: 587.e1-587e.5.

[25] Carlile A, Davies I, Rigby A Brocklehurst JC. Age changes in the human female urethra: A morphometric study. *J. Urol.* 1988; 139: 532-535.

[26] Perucchini D, De Lancey JO, Ashton-Miller JA, Peachers U, Kataria T. Age effects on urethral striated muscle. I. Changes in number and diameter of striated muscle fibers in the ventral urethra. *Am. J. Obstet. Gynecol.* 2002; 186: 351-355.

[27] Loeb S, KettermannA, Carter HB, Ferrucci L, Metter EG, Walsh PC. Prostate volume changes over time: results from the Baltimore Longitudinal Study of Aging. *J. Urol.* 2009; 182: 1458-1462.

[28] Fitzpatrik JM. The natural history of benign prostatic hyperplasia. *BJU Int.* 2006; 97 Supp 2: 3-6.

[29] Madersbacher S, Pycha A, Schatzi G, Mian C, Klinger CH, Marbey M. The aging lower urinary tract: A comparative urodynamic study of men and women. *Urology.* 1998; 51: 206-212.

[30] Homma Y, Imajo C Taskahashi S, Kawabe K, Aso Y. Urinary symptoms and urodynamics in a normal elderly population. *Scand. J. Urol. Nephrol.* 1994; 157: S27-30.
[31] Elbadawi A, Yalla AV, Resnick NM. Structural basis of geriatric voiding dysfunction. II. Aging detrusor normal versus impaired contractility. *J. Urol.* 1993; 150: 1657-67.
[32] Griffiths D, Tadic SD, Schaerfer W, Resnick NM. Cerebral control of the lower urinary tract: How age-related changes might predispose to urge incontinence. *Neuroimage.* 2009; 47: 981-986.
[33] Yalla SV, Sullivan MP, Resnick NM. Update on detrusor hyperactivity with impaired contractility. *Curr. Bladder. Dysfunct. Rep.* 2007; 2: 191-196.
[34] DuBeau CE. The aging lower urinary tract. J Urol. 2006; 175: S11-S15.
[35] Abrams P, Cardozo L, Fall M, Griffiths D, Rosier P, Ulmsten U, van Kerrebroeck P, Victor A, Wein A; Standarisation Sub-Committee of the International Continence Society. The standardisation of terminology of lower urinary tract function: report from the Standardisation Sub-Committee of International Continence Society. *Neurourol. Urodyn.* 2002; 21: 167-178.
[36] Haylen BT, de Riddle D, Freeman RM, Swift SE, Berghmans B, Lee J, Monga A, Petri E, Rizk, Sand PK, Schaer GN. An International Urogynecological Association (IUGA)/ International Continence Society (ICS) joint report on the terminology for female pelvic floor dysfunction. *Neurourol. Urodyn.* 2010; 29: 4-20.
[37] Griebling TL. Urinary incontinence in the elderly. *Clin Geriatr Med.* 2009; 25: 445-457.
[38] Wolf JS. Bennett CJ, Dmochowski RR, Holenbeck BK, Pearle MS, Schaffer AJ et al. Best Practice Policy Statement on Urologic Surgery Antimicrobial Prophylaxis. *American Urological Association.* 2008.
[39] Yoshida M, Inadome A, Matsumoto K, Otani M, Masunaga K, Yono M . Overactive bladder in female patients with chronic diseases visiting primary care doctors: eVect of age on prevalence and bothersomeness. *LUTS.* 2009; 1:45–50.
[40] Good PS, Burgio KL. Pharmacologic treatment of lower urinary tract dysfunction in geriatric patients. *Am. J. of Med. Sci.* 1997; 314: 262-267.
[41] White WM, Pickens RB, Doggweiler R, Klein FA. Short term efficacy of botulinum toxin A for refractory overactive bladder in the elderly population. *J. Urol.* 2008; 180: 2522-2526.
[42] McAchran SE, Daneshgari F. Sacral neuromodulation in the older woman. *Clin. Obstet. Gynecol.* 2007; 50: 735-744.
[43] Amundsen SL, Webster GD. Sacral neuromodulation in an older, urge-incontinent population. *Am. J. Obstet. Gynecol.* 2002; 187: 1462- 1465.
[44] Amundsen SL, Romero AA, Jamison MG et al. Sacral neuromodulation for intractable urge incontinence are there factors associated with cure? *Urology.* 2005; 66: 746-750.
[45] Resnick NM, Yalla SV. Detrusor hyperactivity with impaired contractile function. *JAMA.* 1987; 257: 3076-3081.
[46] Lui S, Chan L, Tse V. Clinical outcome in patients with detrusor hyperactivity with impaired contractility (DHIC). *BJU Int.* 2011; 107 supp: 7.
[47] Leung FW, Schnelle JF. Urinary and fecal incontinence in nursing home residents. Gastroenterol *Clin. N Am.* 2008; 37: 697-707.

[48] Ogan J, Cody JD, Rogerson L. Minimally invasive synthetic suburethral sling operations for stress urinary incontinence in elderly. Cochrane Databases of Systematic Reviews. 2009; 4 Art No: CD006375. DOI: 10/1002/ 14651858.CD006375.pub2.
[49] Rehman H, Bezerra CCB, Bruschini H, Cody JD. Traditional suburethral sling operations for urinary incontinence in women. Cochrane Databases of Systematic Reviews. 2011; Issue 1. Art No; CD001754.D0I: 10.1002//14651858.CD001754.pub3.
[50] Sevestres S, Ciofu C, Deval B, Troxier O, Amarenco G, Haab F. Results of tension-free vaginal tape technique in the elderly. *Eur. Urol.* 2003; 44: 128-131.
[51] Lo TS, Huang HJ, Chan CL, Wong SY, Horng SG, Liang CC. Use of intravenous anesthesia for tension-free vaginal tape in elderly women with genuine stress urinary incontinence. *Urology* 2008; 59: 349-353.
[52] Kim J, Lucioni A, Govier F, Kobashi K. Worse long term surgical outcomes in elderly patients undergoing SPARC TM retropubic midurethral sling placement. *BJU Int.* 2010; 108: 708-712.
[53] Karantasis E, Fynnes MM, Stanton S. The tension-free vaginal tape in older women. *BJOG.* 2004; 111: 837-841.
[54] Groutz A, Cohen A, Gold R, Pauzner D, Lessing JP, Gordon D. The safety and efficacy of the “inside-out” transobturator TVT in elderly versus younger stress incontinent women. A prospective study of 353 consecutive patients. *Neurourol. Urodyn.* 2011; 30: 380-383.
[55] Liap A, Bakas P, Christopoulos P, Giner M, Creatsas G. Tension-free vaginal tape for elderly women with stress urinary incontinence. *Int. J. Gynecol. Obstet.* 2006; 92: 48-51.
[56] Touloupidis S, Papatsoris, Thanopoulos, Charalambous S, Giannakopoulos S, Rombis V. Tension-free vaginal tape for the treatment of stress urinary incontinence in geriatric patients. *Gerontology.* 2007; 53: 125-127.
[57] Campeau L, Tu LM, Lemieux MC, Naud A, Karsenty G, Schick E, Corcos J. A multicentre, prospective randomized clinical trial comparing tension-free vaginal tape and no treatment for the stress urinary incontinence in elderly women. *Neurourol. Urodyn.* 2007; 26: 990-4.
[58] Haidinger G, Temml C, Schatzel G, Brossner C, Roehlich M, Schmidbauer CP, Maderbacher S. Risk factors for lower urinary tract symptoms in elderly men. For the Prostate Study Group of the Austrian Society of Urology. *Eur. Urol.* 2000; 37: 413-20.
[59] Roehrborn CG. BPH progression: concept and key learning from MTOPS, ALTESS, COMBAT, and ALF-ONE. *BJU Int.* 2008; 101: 17-21.
[60] Roehrborn CG, Siami P, Barkin J, Damiao R, Major-Walker K, Nandy I, Morrill BB, Gagnier RP, Montorsi F on behalf of the CombAT study group. The effects of combination therapy with dutasteride and tamsulosin on clinical outcomes in men with symptomatic benign prostatic hyperplasia: 4 year results from the COMBAT study. *Eur. Urol.* 2010; 57: 123-131.
[61] McConnell JD, Roehrborn CG, Bautista OM, Andriole GC, Dixon CM, Kusek JW, Lepor H, McVary KT, Nyberg LM, Clarke HS, Crawford ED, Diokno A, Foley JP, Foster HE, Jacobs SC, Kaplan SA, Kreder KJ, Lieber MM, Lucia MS, Miller GJ, Menon M, Milam DF, Ramsdell JW, Schenkman NS, Slawin KM, Smith JA. The long term effect of doxazosin, finasteride and combination therapy on the clinical progression of benign prostatic hyperplasia. *NEJM.* 2003; 349: 2387-98.

[62] Madersbacher S, Pycha A, Schatzl G, Mian C, Klinger CH, Marberger M. The aging lower urinary tract: A comparative urodynamic study of men and women. *Urology*. 1998; 51: 206-212.
[63] Montorsi F, Moncada I. Safety and Tolerability of Treatment for BPH. *Eur. Urol. Supp.* 2006; 5: 1004-1012.
[64] Blouin MC, Blouin J, Lapointe A, Perreault S, Dragomir A. Intraoperative floppy-iris syndrome associated with alpha-1 adrenoreceptors: comparison of tamsulosin and alfuzosin. *J. Cataract*. Refract. Surg. 2007; 33: 1227-1234.
[65] Davis BR, ALLHAT officers and coordinators for the ALLHAT collaboration research group. Major cardiovascular events in hypertensive patients randomized to doxazosin vs chlorthalidone. The Antihypertensive and Lipid-Lowering treatment to prevent Heart Attack Trial (ALLHAT). *JAMA*. 2000; 283: 1967-78.
[66] Chung DE, Wysock JS, Lee RK, Melamed SR, Kaplan SA, Te AE. Outcomes and complications after 532nm laser prostatectomy in anticoagulated patients with benign prostatic hyperplasia. *J. Urol.* 2011; 186: 977-981.
[67] Miano RM, De Nunzio C, Tubaro A, Asimakopoulos A. Treatment of benign prostatic hyperplasia in the geriatric patient. *Eur. Urol. Rev*. 2009; 4: 15-19.
[68] Krogh J, Jensen JS, Iverson H-G, Andersen JT. Age as a prognostic variable in patients undergoing transurethral prostatectomy. *Scand. J. Urol. Nephrol.* 1993; 27: 225-229.
[69] Bruschini H, Simonetti R, Anatunes AA, Srougi M. Urinary incontinence following surgery for Bph: the role of aging on the incidence of bladder dysfunction. *Int. Braz. J. Urol.* 2011; 37: 380-387.
[70] Cucchi A, Quaglini S, Roverto B. Development of idiopathic detrusor underactivity in women: From isolated decrease in contraction velocity to obvious impairment of voiding function. *Urology*. 2008; 71: 844-848.
[71] Nordling J. The aging bladder: a significant but underestimated role in the development of lower urinary tract symptoms. *Exp. Geronto*l. 2002; 37: 991-999.
[72] Marcus E-L, Ababanel J. Impaired detrusor contractility in community-dwelling elderly presenting with lower urinary tract symptoms. *Urology*. 2007; 69: 436-440
[73] Taylor JA, Kuchel GA. Detrusor underactivity: Clinical features and pathogenesis of an underdiagnosed geriatric condition. *JAGS*. 2006; 54: 1920-1932.
[74] Cucchi A, Quaglini S, Rovereto B. Proposal for a urodynamic redefinition of detrusor underactivity. *J. Urol*. 2009; 181: 225-229.
[75] Ou R, Pan C, Chen H, Wu S, Wei X, Deng X, Tang P, Xie K. Urodynamically diagnosed detrusor hypocontractility: should transurethral resection of the prostate be contraindicated. *Int. Urol. Nephrol.* 2011 June 10. DOI 10.1007/s11255-011-2.
[76] Abrams P. Bladder outlet obstruction index, bladder contractility index and bladder voiding efficiency: three simple indices to define bladder voiding function. *BJU Int.* 1999; 84: 14-15.
[77] Krishnamoorthy S, Kekre NS. Detrusor underactivity: To tone or not to tone the bladder? *Indian J. Urol*. 2009; 25: 407-408.
[78] Barendrecht MM< Oelke M, Laguna MP, Michel MC. Is the use of parasympathomimetics for treating underactive urinary bladder evidence-based? *BJU Int.* 2007; 99: 749-52.
[79] Han DH, Jeong YS, Choo MS, Lee KS The efficacy of transurethral resection of the prostate in patients with weak bladder contractility index. *Urology*. 2008; 71: 657-661.

[80] Anderssen K-E. Detrusor underactivity/ underactive bladder: New research initiatives needed. *J. Urol.* 2010; 184: 1829-1830.

Index

#

A

H

I

J

K

L

M

N

O

P

Q

R

S

T

U

V

W

X